INTEGRATING EA
ASIAN MEDICINE
CONTEMPORARY
HEALTHCARE

Commissioning Editor: Claire Wilson
Development Editor: Helen Leng
Project Manager: Vinod Kumar
Design Direction: Kirsteen Wright
Illustration Manager: Bruce Hogarth

INTEGRATING EAST ASIAN MEDICINE INTO CONTEMPORARY HEALTHCARE

Edited by

Volker Scheid PhD
Reader and Director EAST*medicine* Research Centre,
School of Life Sciences, University of Westminster,
London, UK

Hugh MacPherson PhD
Senior Research Fellow, Department of Health Sciences,
University of York,
York, UK

Foreword

Ted J Kaptchuk
Associate Professor of Medicine
Harvard Medical School
Boston, USA

CHURCHILL
LIVINGSTONE

ELSEVIER

Edinburgh London New York Oxford Philadelphia St Louis Sydney Toronto 2012

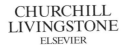

CHURCHILL LIVINGSTONE
ELSEVIER

ISBN 9780702030215

British Library Cataloguing in Publication Data
A catalogue record for this book is available from the British Library

Library of Congress Cataloging in Publication Data
A catalog record for this book is available from the Library of Congress

Notices

Knowledge and best practice in this field are constantly changing. As new research and experience broaden our understanding, changes in research methods, professional practices, or medical treatment may become necessary.

Practitioners and researchers must always rely on their own experience and knowledge in evaluating and using any information, methods, compounds, or experiments described herein. In using such information or methods they should be mindful of their own safety and the safety of others, including parties for whom they have a professional responsibility.

With respect to any drug or pharmaceutical products identified, readers are advised to check the most current information provided (i) on procedures featured or (ii) by the manufacturer of each product to be administered, to verify the recommended dose or formula, the method and duration of administration, and contraindications. It is the responsibility of practitioners, relying on their own experience and knowledge of their patients, to make diagnoses, to determine dosages and the best treatment for each individual patient, and to take all appropriate safety precautions.

To the fullest extent of the law, neither the publisher nor the authors, contributors, or editors, assume any liability for any injury and/or damage to persons or property as a matter of products liability, negligence or otherwise, or from any use or operation of any methods, products, instructions, or ideas contained in the material herein.

Printed in China

CONTENTS

Contents

FOREWORD

Historical exchanges between East Asian medical practices and other healing systems, and the dilemma of transplanting East Asian medical practices to the West

Ted J. Kaptchuk
Harvard Medical School
Boston, Massachusetts

Illness is surrounded by irreducible uncertainty. Medical doctors and physicians in the East Asian medical traditions commonly try to navigate this uncomfortable dilemma with appeals to canonical texts and/or thousands of years of experience. Western biomedicine hides behind laboratory science and stochastic inferences from randomized controlled trials (RCTs). Healers can provide perfect treatments, good plans and the best intentions, but outcomes are often less than optimal. Practitioners continue to strive to do better.

One repercussion of this uncertainty is a constant search, explicitly or implicitly, for new knowledge, treatments and theoretical constructs. Standardized textbooks, established pharmacopeias, precise acupuncture point locations and the details of immunology and genetics maintain a solid appearance, but there is always a need to find new and better treatments. This book is one of the first attempts to directly engage the uncertainty and complexity inherent in Western attempts to integrate East Asian medicine into contemporary healthcare systems. The questions are raised primarily in the present tense.

Historical exchanges

There is a long history of medical interaction between East and West – exchange has been a constant. Great cultures only develop through contact with other cultures and no major medical system has existed in isolation for any length of time. Certainly this is true for the relationship between East Asian medical practices and other cultures. A well-studied example is the materia medica. From the earliest times, China, and probably to a greater extent Korea, Japan and Vietnam, was constantly borrowing from other cultures. The *Pharmacopoeia Classic of the Divine Husbandman* (*Shen nong ben cao* 神農本草 *c.* 1st century CE) included many herbs that originally came from outside China, such as *Saussaura lappa*, and *Kochia scoparia* (Hu 1990). During the Tang dynasty, Chinese physicians borrowed many herbs from Central Asia and the Near East. For example, thriving Arab-owned pharmacies located in Guangzhou (then known as Nanhai) provided Euro-Asian herbs to pharmacies throughout China (Hu 1990). Sun Si-Miao, in his *Supplemental Wings to the Thousand Ducat Prescription* (*Qian jin yifang* 千金翼方 682 CE) (1982), wrote an entire chapter on Ayurvedic healing methods and freely discussed what he learned from Tibetans, Hindus and Sogdians (members of a Persian-language Central Asian culture practicing Galenic medicine). Many herbs, such as *Piper nigrum* and *Terminalia chebula*, were transformed into 'Chinese' herbs during this period. During the

Song dynasty's expansion of Chinese territory, the number of herbs that crossed cultural barriers escalated exponentially. For example, *Carthamus tincorium* and *Psoralea corylifoia* became common ingredients in Chinese herbal formulas. By the time of the Yuan dynasty, in 1292 CE, the information highway of the Silk Route allowed for the creation of a Muslim Medical Office within the China Imperial Academy of Medicine. In both Beijing (Dadu) and Chabar (Shangdu), Muslim pharmacies dispensed herbs based on Euro-Asian pharmacopeias (Hinrichs 2003). The subsequent compilation of the Chinese-language *Islamic Formulary* (*Hui hui yao fang* 回回藥方, early 1300s CE) was a momentous achievement and clearly influenced subsequent Chinese materia medicas (Kong & Chen 1996). Modern reminders of these Islamic interactions can been seen in contemporary Xinjiang, where Uighur schools of medicine teach a system based on Greek and Ayurvedic sources (Rudelson 1997), and in the continued Han Chinese interest in 'Uighur' medicine (Song et al. 2007). As part of the search for better medicine in the Yuan period, in 1285, 1288 and 1290 Khubilai Khan sent envoys to South India to investigate Ayurvedic and Siddha medicine (Russabi 2009).

The Qing dynasty saw another expansion of interest in Western herbals. Well-known examples are the Kangxi emperor's interests in 'alternative' healing, including his famous experimentation with Jesuit's Bark or quinine (*Chincona succirubra*) in 1693 (Hanson 2007) and the incorporation of American ginseng (*Panax quinquefolium*) into the Chinese materia medica.

An analogous interest in Eastern medicine occurred in the West. Two relatively well-studied examples concern Chinese pulse diagnosis and acupuncture. A Persian text by the title *Chinese Pulse Lore* was written by Radhid ad-Din Fadlallah (c.1247–1318 CE). Many scholars believe that Avicenna (Ibn Sina) had an intimate knowledge of a translated version of the Chinese *Classic of the Pulse* (*Mai jing* 脈經 280 CE), sections of which appear verbatim in his *Canon of Medicine* (1025 CE) (Hsu 2000). Avicenna's text was widely used in medieval and early modern Europe, and by the 17th century explicit Latin and French discussions of Chinese pulse diagnostics were beginning (Hsu 2000). Likewise, Linda Barnes (2005) has extensively described the remarkable European interest in and study of acupuncture that began at least in the 16th century, if not earlier. This interest went through periods of expansion and contraction, culminating in the present widespread societal acceptance of acupuncture.

Historically, the information highway of the Silk Route and the later Ocean Route facilitated medical exchanges between East and West. The recent explosion of the Internet and Asia's rise to global prominence has exponentially increased interest in the East and accelerated the movement of knowledge to the West. Practitioners of East Asian medicine have access to many translated classical texts, visits from leading Asian physicians and many opportunities to study in the East. East Asian medicine has developed solid professional infrastructures, legal recognition and thriving academic training institutions in the West. This easy access has made knowledge more available than in the past. Unlike earlier periods of cultural exchange, the discussion now is how to transplant wholesale the entire system of East Asian medicine. But more information has not necessarily transformed into greater certainty. This book addresses major issues where certainty and uncertainty still collide. Specifically, it raises the contested issues of authenticity, best practice and the evidence mosaic.

Authenticity

Authenticity is concerned with attempts to adopt Eastern practices and theories that are genuine and congruent with their points of departure. If the West is going to integrate East Asian practices, we need an accurate understanding of what is being imported. As this book shows, authenticity is not obvious. For me, the immediate questions are: What is genuine East Asian medicine? Which of the various Chinese, Korean, Japanese or Vietnamese versions has the best interpretation of this literate historical tradition? How can one possibly decide such a question?

The problem does not disappear once one has somehow selected a particular cultural tradition. If, for example, one decides to work within the Chinese tradition, new problems immediately arise. Take acupuncture, for example. Is authentic acupuncture based on the *Classic of Difficulties* (*Nan jing* 難經, 2nd century CE), the *Great Compendium of Acupuncture* (*Zhen jiu da cheng* 針灸大成, 1601 CE) or the modern version of traditional Chinese medicine (TCM) that was shaped to conform to the needs of a developing communist state (Taylor 2007)? At the very least, these are not entirely congruent interpretations.

Take a more specific problem: Sun Si-Miao's 13 ghost points are commonly interpreted in modern Chinese medicine as specific for treating mental illness. But is it authentic to disregard Sun Si-Miao's original extensive discussions modifying treatments according to the color of the eyes of the various ghosts? Can we afford not to grapple with Sun Si-Miao directly, and depend only on what certain later commentators felt should be discarded? In the search for authenticity, who decides which part of a discussion was delusional and which part was accurate? What would it mean if we decided that some of Sun Si-Miao's teachings were delusional and some not? Where to draw the line? What a can of worms this would open up!

Or take the issue in acupuncture of '*de qi*' (得氣, obtaining the qi). Should we adopt the most common modern Chinese interpretation of the *Inner Canon of Huangdi* (*Huang di Nei jing c.* 100 BCE) that the patient feels the *qi,* or the most common current Japanese interpretation that the practitioner feels the *qi* in their hand (Kong et al. 2007)? Which is the more authentic reading of the original text?

Or with respect to herbs, does authenticity prohibit the use of the category of herb formulas based on *Drive Out Stasis from the Mansion of the Blood Decoction* (*xue fu zhu yu tang* 血府逐瘀湯) developed in *Correction of Error Among Physicians* (*Yi lin gai cuo* 醫林改錯, 1830 CE) just because they are based on the author's, Wang-Qing-ren's, poor understanding of Western notions of physiology?

What makes something 'genuine' in a world replete with multiple interpretations of the same thing and where cultures are always borrowing from one another? Should we believe the official TCM line that the author of the *Discussion on Cold Damage* (*Shang han lun* 傷寒論 *c.* 220 CE) really would have felt that Ye Tianshi's *Discussion of Warmth and Heat* (*Wen re lun* 溫熱論 1746 CE) was a benign complementary interpretation? To some historians, at least, it would seem that Ye Tianshi's new ideas represent a bold reformulation of herbal medicine based on cultural, ethnic and regional geographic issues (Hanson 1997). It seems that authenticity is not stable and a taken-for-granted objective fact, but rather represents an ongoing collective discussion and debate that allows for growth and new discoveries.

Best practices

I think 'best practice' represents a desire to perform East Asian medicine in an optimal manner. If one is not a 'fundamentalist', perhaps best practice also includes the need for a creative and sensitive adaptation that balances new options with the routines, requirements and expectations of existing healthcare systems. How then does one adopt best practices from China, Korea or Japan? Obviously, the practice and regulation of Asian medicine is different in each of these countries and, from what I can tell, there is no reliable way of knowing which is optimal for the West.

Even within a single culture, best practices are difficult to determine. Take cancer as an example. The first problem is that in pre-modern China cancer was recognized only in terms of visible lesions of the skin, jaw, neck, tongue or breast, and maybe discharges due to uterine cancer (and such visible lesions were not necessarily clearly distinguished from carbuncles, polyps, tubercles, pustules, etc.). Historical discussions of cancer were limited to these categories. Today, any discussion of cancer is necessarily based on Western nosological categories. In general, TCM has expanded the older Chinese notions of cancer to include all cancers recognized by biomedicine. So how does one treat cancer in modern China? Rather than a single answer, one finds a spectrum of practices. At one extreme is a complete reliance on a traditional diagnosis and disregard for the Western diagnosis of cancer. At the other extreme, practitioners use large doses of herbs that have been found to inhibit the growth of cancer cells in laboratories. The majority of practitioners seem to work at various points along a continuum between these two poles. Compounding the confusion, the last time I visited cancer wards at different well-known Chinese medical hospitals in China, I could not find a single cancer patient who was not also taking Western drugs alongside their herbs or acupuncture.

It is not easy to figure out what is best practice in China or East Asia. Knowing what that would mean in the West is even more difficult. Do we really want to emulate the current general practices in, say, China or Japan? In China, it seems that Chinese medicine healthcare often provides, in addition to Chinese medicine treatments, versions of substandard Western medicine (Jin 2010). In Japan, licensed acupuncturists are isolated from Western medical practitioners and cannot prescribe traditional Kampo herbal treatments. Neither system appears to be a candidate for best practice in the West.

And even if we understand what is best practice in any single East Asian nation, there is still the question of how best to adapt Asian medicine for a Western healthcare system (this assumes that Asian medicine will not be suppressed or completely assimilated – see Chapter 11; Kaptchuk and Miller 2005). At the very least, best practice is a social category and requires conformation to licensing registration standards and safety requirements. It also requires learning new ways of communicating with other healthcare providers and patients. Current scholarship already points to the fact that Asian medicine is undergoing a profound transformation as it adapts to the West. For example, in many situations in the West, clinical discussions are much more psychological than in the East (Barnes 1998), and in Eastern clinical practice targets such as illness prevention, health promotion and healthy lifestyles are often overlooked (Zhan 2009, Napadow and Kaptchuk 2004).

Undoubtedly, best practices will evolve and diminish, and will always be contested. The ways in which Cuba (see Chapter 13) and Tanzania (Hsu 2002) have incorporated East Asian medical practices are important examples of how possibilities are discovered, interpreted and implemented.

Evidence

A key question for all stakeholders in this process, therefore, is how do we decide whether something is good for patients? An evidence mosaic asks what is the basis for making decisions about whether a treatment 'works' and provides health benefits for an individual, family, community or society. Obviously, many societal factors go into such decision-making. These include such non-medical issues as guild monopolies, power, racism, class issues, commerce, imperialism (both Western and Eastern), nationalism and post-colonialism. Both Asia (Hinrichs 2003) and the West (Kaptchuk and Eisenberg 2001) have a long history of suppressing heterodox healing to reinforce the social domination and cultural hegemony of particular medical systems.

Leaving aside these social issues and limiting the question to a simple discussion of what determines whether an intervention directly provides benefits to individual patients does not do away with complexity. To my knowledge, there are no extensive discussions on epistemology or methodology in East Asian medical writings. If this is correct and does not reflect my ignorance, I think the assumptions implicit in the East Asian medical tradition for determining 'what works' depends on a convergence of:

- critical reading of revered classical texts (evidential scholarship)
- historical interpretations of the literature tradition
- modern syntheses as portrayed in contemporary textbooks
- compiled historical and contemporary clinical cases
- close observation of teachers, mentors and colleagues.

All this input is amalgamated with the gradual accumulation of clinical experience and feedback from a practitioner's patients.

How sacred texts, historical commentaries, contemporary standardized textbooks and learning in clinic are balanced has not, to my knowledge, been adequately studied.

The bottom line, the basic unit of evidence for what an intervention does, is a careful observation of whether and to what extent a patient improves between their first visit and after a course of treatment. This kind of causality does not seem to significantly differ from traditional Western Galenic methodology. Even after the Enlightenment and until World War II, Western medicine continued to value evidence based on single patient responses. Although laboratory science could produce important knowledge, medicine remained an art that applied such new knowledge to a unique and a highly variable and non-replicable human being. Until World War II, the basic unit of evidence and confidence was observation of individual patient improvement or its absence.

Only after World War II did the concept of acceptable evidence undergo a radical shift, with the development, consolidation and adoption of the randomized controlled trial (RCT). This new methodology required that novel treatments be compared, ideally, to placebo controls (see Chapter 8; Kaptchuk 1998a,

Kaptchuk and Kerr 2004). Whether patients improved from baseline was now no longer important. Instead, what became important was whether a group of patients improved more than a cohort concurrently treated with placebos (Kaptchuk 1998b, Sullivan 1993). An individual's improvement from baseline, the old version of evidence, was thereby reduced to an anecdote. In this new world of RCTs, 'really working' (legitimate healing) means that any amelioration detected in a group of patients must be more than the improvement found in the placebo control group. Observing improvement without a comparison group (the basis of pre-World War II medicine) becomes nothing more than telling stories.

This new 'evidence-based medicine' standard reduces the accumulated experience of Asian classical texts to unverified clinical narratives. Implicit in applying evidence-based medicine to East Asian medicine is the supposition that Asian medicine, if it is to gain widespread legitimacy in the West, should start over and validate each and every one of its interventions. Research protocols insist on standardized interventions, otherwise an RCT become hopelessly heterogeneous. Protocols also require the goal of the intervention to be defined in terms of biomedical diseases and assessments. Efforts to comply with this recent biomedical model have not been especially positive for East Asian medicine and acupuncture (Madsen et al. 2009, Cummings 2009). The response from the Euro-American East Asian medicine profession has been tremendously diverse, ranging from complete rejection of 'criminal controlled trials' to 'let's try harder and modify the RCT methodology', to 'be more sensitive to the variability in Asian treatment and diagnoses' (Kaptchuk et al. 2010). Importantly, alternative Western models have been proposed, such as whole-systems research (Paterson and Dieppe 2005), anthropological investigation (see Chapter 10; Barry 2006) and mixed-method quantitative–qualitative research (Kaptchuk 2011). At present, there is no consensus on how East Asian medicine should value RCTs, and some acupuncture researchers have called for a cessation of acupuncture RCTs (Paterson 2008). What role and weight the profession of East Asian medicine will assign to the RCT is a big question facing practitioners in the West.

Contributions to this book

I do not think that the editors and most of the contributors to this book claim to have definitive answers regarding the questions of authenticity, best practice and the epistemology they address. My sense is that the aim of the book is to promote discussion and open a new space for readers to ponder important, deep and complex issues. Critical questions are asked that are essential for deliberate and careful integration of the East into the West. The book assumes that medical facts, medical practice, knowledge of 'what works' and theories of healing are embedded in complex cultural and social discourse. Instead of simple answers, it brings the reader into the heart of conundrums. This honest openness is a positive omen demonstrating that scholars and practitioners of East Asian medicine are ready to work together and grapple with hard questions. Besides being a good sign for the West, this holds promise for the East. For the first time in East Asian medical history, it will be possible to compare Chinese, Korean, Japanese and Vietnamese variants and interpretations in the context of critical input from Western scholars and practitioners.

Such a dialogue will not eliminate complexity and uncertainty, but will undoubtedly make for a revitalized and genuinely cosmopolitan version of East Asian medicine. The scholars and practitioners in this book are brave pioneers in the current East–West and North–South encounters that hold the promise of transforming East Asian medicine from a regional medicine to a world medicine. The integration of East and West depends on the kind of honesty and creativity that is shown here.

ACKNOWLEDGMENTS

Work on this foreword was partially supported by grant # K24 AT004095 from the National Center for Complementary and Alternative Medicine (NCCAM) at the National Institutes of Health. All opinions are the author's alone.

REFERENCES

Barnes, L.L., 1998. The psychologizing of Chinese healing practices in the United States. Cult.Med. Psychiatry 22, 413–443.

Barnes, L.L., 2005. Needles, Herbs, Gods, and Ghosts. Harvard University Press, Cambridge.

Barry, C.A., 2006. The role of evidence in alternative medicine: considering biomedical and anthropological approaches. Soc. Sci. Med. 62, 2646–2657.

Cummings, M., 2009. Modellvorhaben Akupunktur–a summary of the ART, ARC and GERAC trials. Acupunct. Med. 27, 26–30.

Hanson, M.E., 1997. Inventing a Tradition in Chinese Medicine: From Universal Canon to Local Medical Knowledge in South China: the Seventeenth to the Nineteenth Century. Unpublished PhD Dissertation. University of Pennsylvania, Philadelphia. ProQuest Paper AA1984853.

Hanson, M.E., 2007. Jesuits and medicine in the Kangxi Court (1662–1722). Pacific Rim Report July, 1–9.

Hinrichs, T.J., 2003. The Medical Transforming of Governance and Southern Customs in Song Dynastry China (960–1279 C.E.). Unpublished PhD Thesis. Harvard University, Cambridge, MA.

Hsu, E., 2000. Towards a science of touch, part I: Chinese pulse diagnostics in early modern Europe 7, 252–268.

Hsu, E., 2002. 'The medicine from China has rapid effects' in Tanzania. Anthropology & Medicine 9, 291–313.

Hu, S.Y., 1990. History of the introduction of exotic elements into traditional Chinese medicine. Journal of the Arnold Arboretum 71, 487–526.

Jin, L., 2010. From mainstream to marginal? Trends in the use of Chinese medicine in China from 1991 to 2004. Soc. Sci. Med. 71, 1063–1067.

Kaptchuk, T.J., 1998a. Intentional ignorance: a history of blind assessment and placebo controls in medicine. Bull. Hist. Med. 72, 389–433.

Kaptchuk, T.J., 1998b. Powerful placebo: the dark side of the randomised controlled trial. Lancet 351, 1722–1725.

Kaptchuk, T.J., 2011. Placebo studies and ritual theory: a comparative analysis of Navajo, acupuncture and biomedical healing. Transactions of the Royal Society Part B in press.

Kaptchuk, T.J., Eisenberg, D.M., 2001. Varieties of healing, 1: Medical pluralism in the United States. Ann. Intern. Med. 135, 189–195.

Kaptchuk, T.J., Kerr, C., 2004. Unbiased divination, unbiased evidence and the patulin clinical trial. Int. J. Epidemiol. 33, 247–251.

Kaptchuk, T.J., Miller, F.G., 2005. What is the best and most ethical model for the relationship between mainstream and alternative medicine; opposition, integration, or pluralism. Acad. Med. 80, 286–290.

Kaptchuk, T.J., Chen, K.J., Song, J., 2010. Recent trials of acupuncture in the west: responses from practitioners. Chin. J. Integr. Med. 16, 197–203.

Kong, J., Gollub, R., Polich, G., Napadow, V., Hui, K., Vangel, M., et al., 2007. Acupuncture deqi, from qualitative history to quantitative measurement. J. Altern. Complement. Med. 13, 1059–1070.

Kong, Y.C., Chen, D.S., 1996. Elucidation of Islamic drugs in Hui Hui Yao Fang: a linguistic and pharmaceutical approach. J. Ethnopharmacol. 54, 85–102.

Madsen, M.V., Gotzsche, P.C., Hrobjartsson, A., 2009. Acupuncture treatment for pain: systematic review of randomized clinical trials with acupuncture, placebo acupuncture and no acupuncture group. BMJ 388, a3115.

Napadow, V., Kaptchuk, T.J., 2004. Patient characteristics for outpatient acupuncture in Beijing, China. J. Altern. Complement. Med. 10, 565–572.

Paterson, C., 2008. The colonization of the lifeworld of acupuncture: the SAR conference. J. Altern. Complement. Med. 14, 105–108.

Paterson, C., Dieppe, P., 2005. Characteristic and incidental (placebo) effects in complex interventions such as acupuncture. BMJ 330, 1902–1905.

Rudelson, J.J., 1997. Oasis Identities: Uyghar Nationalism Along China's Silk Road. Columbia University Press, New York.

Russabi, M., 2009. Khubilai Khan: His Life and Times. University of California Press, Berkeley.

Song, G.H., Halmurat, U., Geng, J.C., Feng, L.C., Yilihamujiang, S., Ma, C., et al., 2007. Clinical study on the treatment of premature ejaculation by Uighur medicine Gu-jing-mai-si-ha Tablet. Chin. J. Integr. Med. 13, 185–189.

Sullivan, M.D., 1993. Placebo controls and epistemic control in orthodox medicine. J. Med. Ethics 18, 213–231.

Sun, Si-miao, 1982. Supplemental Wings to the Thousand Ducat Prescriptions (Qian-jin Yi-fang). People's Press, Beijing (682 CE).

Taylor, K., 2007. Chinese Medicine in Early Communist China, 1945–63. A Medicine of Revolution. RoutledgeCurzon, London.

Zhan, M., 2009. Other-Worldly. Making Chinese Medicine Through Transnational Frames. Duke University Press, Durham, NC.

ACKNOWLEDGMENTS

This book is a novel attempt to bring together different voices, perspectives and stakeholders in the ongoing modernization of East Asian medicines and their integration into contemporary healthcare. Anything new and different is not only exciting but also brings with it all kinds of risks. We therefore wish to acknowledge our great debt to all those who not only shared in the excitement but were also willing to take on the various risks involved in writing this book. These are, first and foremost, our fellow authors and all those who joined us in two workshops we organized at the University of Westminster in April 2007 and July 2009. All of them contributed their unique insights and were willing, in the process, to engage with ideas, perspectives, and concepts quite different to those they usually deal with. Without their willingness to travel to London, most at their own expense, and to enter into a dialogue with scholars of a multitude of different academic and research backgrounds, this project would not have taken off.

We wish to thank the sponsors of these two workshops and the individuals involved in organizing them: the University of Westminster, the Acupuncture Research Resource Centre (ARRC), the Arts and Humanities Research Council (AHRC), Elsevier, the International Association for the Study of Traditional Asian Medicines (IASTAM), the Coca-Cola Company, the Daiwa Foundation, the Foundation for Research into Traditional Chinese Medicine, the TCM Development Trust, the Wellcome Trust for the History of Medicine, Hal Andrews, Michelle Aris, Mark Bovey, Emma Cook, and Huaying Zhang.

We also wish to thank Elsevier for its editorial support, specifically Karen Morley and Mary Law who took the risk of commissioning the book, and Helen Leng, who has been midwife in bringing the book to fruition.

Volker Scheid specifically wishes to thank three colleagues at the University of Westminster: Peter Davis, former Dean of the School of Integrated Medicine, and Jane Lewis, Dean of the School of Life Sciences, who granted him the space to make this project happen, and Felicity Moir, Course Leader for Chinese Medicine, for her continued support throughout its entire duration.

Hugh MacPherson would like to thank the many colleagues who have supported him at the University of York, especially Professor Trevor Sheldon who has provided encouragement as a mentor throughout the period of this book's gestation. He also thanks the Trustees at the Foundation for Research into Traditional Chinese Medicine who have been enthusiastic in their support for this project throughout. Throughout the period of preparing this book, Hugh was supported by a Career Scientist Award funded by the National Institute for Health Research.

Last but not least, we would like to acknowledge the role of our managing editor, Karen Overend. Karen contributed far more than she was contracted to do, gently but persistently coaxing contributors into meeting their deadlines and facilitating communication between editors, authors and publishers. She has also contributed her copyediting skills, providing suggestions to authors which have helped their chapters become more accessible to a wider audience. The compiling and editing of this volume would not have been possible, nor proceeded as smoothly or quickly as it did, without her hard work and dedication.

CONTRIBUTORS

Hen-hong Chang MD PhD
Vice Superintendent of the Center for Traditional Chinese Medicine, Chang Gung Memorial Hospital; Professor in the Graduate Institute of Traditional Chinese Medicine, Chang Gung University, Taoyuan, Taiwan, Republic of China

Judith Farquhar PhD
Professor of Anthropology, University of Chicago, Chicago, USA

Andrew Flower PhD MBAcC MRCHM
Practitioner and Researcher, Complementary and Integrated Medicine Research Unit, Department of Primary Medical Care, University of Southampton, Southampton, UK

Elizabeth Hsu PhD
Reader in Social Anthropology, School of Anthropology, University of Oxford, Oxford, UK

Paul Kadetz APRN-BC, LAc, MSc, MSOM, MSN, MPH
DPhil Candidate, Department of International Development, University of Oxford, Oxford, UK

Ted J. Kaptchuk
Associate Professor of Medicine, Harvard Medical School, Boston, USA

Myeong Soo Lee PhD
Principal Researcher, Brain Disease Research Centre, Korea Institute of Oriental Medicine, Daejeon, South Korea

Sean Hsiang-lin Lei MSc PhD
Associate Research Fellow, Institute of Modern History, Academia Sinica; Associate Professor, Institute of Science, Technology and Society, Yangming University, Taiwan, Republic of China

George Lewith MA DM FRCP MRCGP
Professor of Health Research, Complementary and Integrated Medicine Research Unit, Department of Primary Medical Care, University of Southampton, Southampton, UK

Chiao-ling Lin MA
Editor, Rive Gauche Publishing House, Taiwan, Republic of China

Vivienne Lien-Ying Lo PhD
Senior Lecturer, University College London, London, UK

Hugh MacPherson PhD
Senior Research Fellow, Department of Health Sciences, University of York, York, UK

Kathryn Montgomery PhD
Professor of Medical Humanities & Bioethics and of Medicine, Northwestern University Feinberg School of Medicine, Chicago, USA

Laurent Pordié PhD
Research Lead, Cluster of Excellence, University of Heidelberg, Germany

Sonya Pritzker LAc, PhD
Researcher, Department of Anthropology, University of California, Los Angeles, USA

Adrian Renton BSc MB BS MSc MD FFPH
Professor of Health and Human Development, Director of the Institute for Health and Human Development, University of East London, London, UK

Volker Scheid PhD
Reader and Director EAST*medicine* Research Centre, School of Life Sciences, University of Westminster, London, UK

Ayo Wahlberg PhD
Postdoctoral Research Fellow, Department of Anthropology, University of Copenhagen, Copenhagen, Denmark

Trina Ward MPhil
PhD Candidate, University of Westminster, London, UK

Claudia M. Witt MD MBA
Professor of Medicine, Vice Director, Institute for Social Medicine, Epidemiology and Health Economics, Charité University Medical Center, Berlin, Germany

Christopher Zaslawski PhD
Associate Professor, College of Traditional Chinese Medicine, School of Medical and Molecular Biosciences, University of Technology, Sydney, Australia

BIOGRAPHIES OF LEAD AUTHORS

Judith Farquhar

Judith Farquhar is Professor of Anthropology at the University of Chicago. Her research has focused on the development and practice of traditional Chinese medicine in modern China and on cultures of health and embodiment in both rural and urban China. She is the author of *Knowing Practice: The clinical encounter of Chinese medicine* (1994) and of *Appetites: Food and Sex in Post-Socialist China* (2002). A volume co-authored with Qicheng Zhang of the Beijing University of Chinese Medicine will appear in 2011: *Ten Thousand Things: Nurturing Life in Contemporary Beijing*. Ongoing research in China is also collaborative, with Lili Lai of Beijing University; this work focuses on modernizing processes affecting the traditional medicines of China's minority nationalities. Some recent articles have also extended Farquhar's early work in the historical epistemology of Chinese medicine in China.

Andrew Flower

Andrew Flower has been practicing acupuncture and Chinese herbal medicine (CHM) since 1992. He is a past President of the UK Register of CHM. He recently completed a PhD exploring the role of CHM in the treatment of endometriosis that included an innovative double blind, randomized, placebo-controlled trial using individualized herbal decoctions. He is currently employed at the Complementary and Integrative Medicine Research Unit at the University of Southampton and is developing a post-doctoral project relating to recurrent urinary tract infections. He has a special interest in developing research methodologies that are appropriate for CHM.

Elisabeth Hsu

Elisabeth Hsu is Reader in Social Anthropology at the School of Anthropology, University of Oxford. Her research contributes to medical anthropology and ethnobotany; language and historical textual studies; and, more recently, explores new approaches to the study of kinship and relatedness. She authored *The Transmission of Chinese Medicine* (CUP, 1999) and *Pulse Diagnosis in Early Chinese Medicine* (CUP, 2010) and edited *Innovation in Chinese Medicine* (CUP, 2001), *Wind, Life, Health* (Blackwell, 2008; with C. Low), *Plants, Health and Healing* (Berghahn, 2010; with C. Harris) and several volumes on the globalization of Chinese medicine, initiated by her current field research in East Africa. In 2006, she founded a post-doctoral research centre, the Anthropology research group at Oxford on Eastern medicines and religions (ArgO-EMR), not least, to enhance critical medical anthropological research on Chinese and other East, Central, South and South-East Asian medical traditions.

Paul Kadetz

Paul Kadetz is completing a doctorate in the Department of International Development at The University of Oxford. He has served as a consultant for several projects for the Western Pacific Region Office of the World Health

Organization and has conducted research in medical anthropology in the Philippines, Guatemala, China, and post-disaster New Orleans. His articles on chronic malnutrition, post-disaster studies, and the political economy of heterodox healthcare have been published in *Biosocieties, Disaster Medicine and Public Health, Asian Medicine/Tradition and Modernity* and *The Yale Journal of Public Health*. He is a board certified acupuncturist and nurse practitioner in the United States and an Associate of the China Centre for Health and Humanity at University College, London.

Sean Hsiang-lin Lei

Sean Hsiang-lin Lei is Associate Research Fellow in the Institute of Modern History, Academia Sinica in Taiwan and the Institute of Science, Technology and Society, Yangming University. He co-edited two Taiwan Science and Technology Studies Readers: *Techno-science Aspires for Society* and *Techno-science Aspires for Gender* (Socio, 2005). He has been working on a book manuscript, *When Chinese Medicine Encountered the State, 1910–1949*, which analyzes the historical confrontation between modern biomedicine and traditional Chinese medicine in China, with special focus on the co-emergence of public health and the state, and the radical re-making of traditional Chinese medicine.

Vivienne Lo

Dr. Vivienne Lo is Convenor of the UCL China Centre for Health and Humanity in the History department. For forty years she has been a practitioner of various martial arts and Qi gong. In 1979 she qualified as an acupuncturist and has been in practice ever since. She also specializes in the history of Chinese medical practice, translating and analyzing excavated and recovered manuscripts from the early imperial and mediaval period concerned with the development of acupuncture, moxibustion and therapeutic exercise. Current projects include a cultural history of nutrition in China and an edited volume on the history of sports, medicine and immortality. Publications also include an online annotated catalog of Chinese medical imagery.

Hugh MacPherson

Hugh MacPherson, PhD, trained as a practitioner of acupuncture and Chinese herbal medicine in the early 1980s and continues to practice in York. He subsequently founded the Northern College of Acupuncture, based in York, and steered the College towards achieving university validation for the first acupuncture degree course in the UK. As a result of his interest in research, he set up the Foundation for Research into Traditional Chinese Medicine and subsequently joined the Department of Health Sciences, University of York, as a Senior Research Fellow. He is currently supported by a Career Scientist Award and a Programme Grant for Applied Research, both from UK's National Institute for Health Research. His research includes conducting clinical trials and systematic reviews to evaluate the effectiveness and cost-effectiveness of acupuncture for a variety of conditions. He is lead editor of the books *Acupuncture in Practice: Case History Insights from the West* (Elsevier 1997) and *Acupuncture research: strategies for building an evidence base* (Elsevier 2007).

Kathryn Montgomery

Kathryn Montgomery, PhD, is Julia and David Uihlein Professor of Medical, Humanities & Bioethics and Professor of Medicine at Northwestern University's Feinberg School of Medicine, where she directs the graduate program in medical humanities and bioethics. Professor Montgomery's research interests include the epistemology of medicine and the use of literature in medical education. She is the author of *Doctors' Stories: The Narrative Structure of Medical Knowledge* (Princeton University Press 1991) and *How Doctors Think: Clinical Judgment and the Practice of Medicine* (Oxford University Press, 2006). A past president of the American Society for Bioethics and Humanities, she was recently elected to the Hastings Center Fellows' Council.

Laurent Pordié

Laurent Pordié, anthropologist, is a Research Lead with the Cluster of Excellence 'Asia & Europe' at the University of Heidelberg. He is currently teaching at the Ecole des Hautes Etudes en Sciences Sociales (EHESS) in Paris. His work concerns the social studies of science and medicine in South Asia, transnational healthcare, pharmaceutical innovation and drug discovery in Indian medicine. Among his recent works are *Healing at the Periphery* (in press with Duke University Press) and *Tibetan Medicine in the Contemporary World* (Routledge, 2008), winner of the International Convention of Asia Scholars (ICAS) Book Prize 2009.

Sonya Pritzker

Sonya Pritzker, PhD, is a medical anthropologist and a licensed practitioner of Chinese medicine. She is a clinician and researcher at the UCLA Center for East-West Medicine and an instructor at Pacific College of Oriental Medicine. Her research focuses on the global translation and dissemination of Chinese medical knowledge, including the linguistic choices of specific translators as well as the transfer of research findings into clinical practice, the interpretation of textbooks by teachers, and the explanation of Chinese medical concepts to patients.

Volker Scheid

Volker Scheid, PhD, is Reader and Director of the EAST*medicine* (East Asian Sciences and Traditions in Medicine) Research Centre in the School of Life Sciences at the University of Westminster, London. His research and publications focus on the development of traditional medicine in China, Japan and Korea in the late imperial and modern periods and its translation into contemporary healthcare systems. He is the author of two monographs, *Chinese Medicine in Contemporary China* (Duke UP 2002) and *Currents of Tradition: Chinese Medicine 1626–2006* (Eastland Press 2007), as well as numerous articles across a wide range of disciplines including medicine, history, and science studies. He is president of the International Association for the Study of Traditional Asian Medicines (IASTAM), and a visiting professor at the Zhejiang University of Chinese Medicine in Hangzhou, China. Besides his academic work he maintains a practice of Chinese medicine. He is editor with Dan Bensky, Andy Ellis and Randal Barolet of *Chinese Herbal Medicine: Formulas & Strategies* 2nd Edition (Eastland Press 2007).

Trina Ward

Trina Ward is a practitioner-researcher of Chinese medicine, currently writing up a PhD funded by the United Kingdom Department of Health. Following a degree in anthropology and extensive travels to Asia she trained as a Chinese medicine practitioner in Australia and China, finishing with an internship at the Shuguang Hospital in Shanghai. She completed an MPhil on the safety of Chinese medicine, funded by the Register of Chinese Medicine in 2002, as a response to government concerns over the potential hepatotoxicity of Chinese medicine. She has run an acupuncture service in both primary and secondary National Health Service clinics for over ten years, and provided treatments through various charities and prison services, as well as running a private practice in London for sixteen years.

Claudia Witt

Dr. Claudia M. Witt, MD, MBA is Professor for complementary medicine at the University Medical Center Charité in Berlin, Germany. She is a trained medical doctor and epidemiologist. Since May 2008 she has held the first chair for research in complementary medicine in Germany. Additionally, she serves as Vice Director of the Institute for Social Medicine, Epidemiology and Health Economics at the Charité and is the head of the CAM research group. Although she is most well known for some recently published large acupuncture trials, she has also conducted basic and clinical research on other CAM methods. She is the president of the International Society for Complementary Medicine Research (ISCMR), has more than 90 publications in peer reviewed journals and developed the first international summer school on complementary medicine research methods which is offered annually.

Chris Zaslawski

Associate Professor Chris Zaslawski is currently Director of the College of Traditional Chinese Medicine and Associate Head of School, (Medical and Molecular Biosciences) at the University of Technology, Sydney. He has been practicing acupuncture for 31 years and is also a physiotherapist. He has been a short term consultant for the World Health Organization for a number of acupuncture related projects in the areas of education, research and clinical practice guidelines. Chris is an active researcher in the areas of acupuncture and pain, acupuncture clinical research design and human research ethics. He has been involved in several acupuncture clinical trials on stress, male sub-fertility, hepatitis C, lateral elbow pain and has just had published a Delphi study on a the development of a rating scale for assessing the adequacy of acupuncture in clinical trials. Chris has also been English editor for three acupuncture texts, which were published in conjunction with Chinese medicine colleagues from the Guangzhou University of Traditional Medicine and has published 25 papers of which 19 were in peer reviewed journals. He is also deputy editor of the *Australian Journal of Acupuncture and Chinese Medicine,* Australia's only peer reviewed journal on acupuncture and Chinese herbal medicine. In addition he is also on several journal international editorial boards including *Acupuncture Research and Journal of Acupuncture and Tuina Science.* More recently he has also been involved in the development of international standards for TCM within the International Organization for Standardization (ISO) and is on the national Australian mirror committee for Chinese medicine for Standards Australia.

VIGNETTE WRITERS

Sang Young Ahn PhD
Senior Researcher, Korean Institute of Oriental Medicine, Daejeon, South Korea

Gerard Bodeker EdD EdM(Harvard) MPsych
Adjunct Professor, Epidemiology, Columbia University, New York; Senior
Clinical Lecturer, Public Health, Division of Medical Sciences, University of
Oxford; Chair Global Initiative for Traditional Systems of Health, Oxford, UK

Gretchen De Soriano MSc (Oxon)
Complementary Medicine Team, Cavendish Health Centre; President,
International Society for Japanese Kampo Medicine, London, UK

Mary Garvey MLitt MHS
PhD Candidate, Lecturer, College of Traditional Chinese Medicine,
University of Technology, Sydney, Australia

Nicholas Harkness PhD
Korea Foundation Postdoctoral Fellow, University of Illinois,
Urbana-Champaign, Chicago, USA

Marian Katz PhD
Assistant Research Sociologist, Division of General Internal Medicine
and Health Services Research, University of California, Los Angeles, USA

Jongyoung Kim PhD
Assistant Professor, Department of Sociology, Kyung Hee University, Seoul,
Korea

Seonsam Na KMD MA MSc
DPhil Candidate in Anthropology, University of Oxford, Oxford, UK

Arielle Rittersmith BA
DPhil Candidate, Department of Social Anthropology, University of Oxford,
Oxford, UK

Paulo Wangoola PhD
Founder and President, Mpambo Afrikan Multiversity, Kampala, Uganda

Jon Wardle ND MPH
National Health and Medical Research Council Public Health Scholar, School
of Population Health, University of Queensland, Herston, Australia

Mei Zhan PhD
Associate Professor, Department of Anthropology, University of California,
Irvine, USA

Introduction

Volker Scheid • Hugh MacPherson

This book is designed to break new ground in debates over how traditional East Asian medicines might best be integrated into contemporary healthcare systems that are invariably dominated by biomedicine. Such debates have been ongoing in East Asia for over a century since newly emergent nation states decided to modernize healthcare along models imported from the West. As a consequence, the relationship between traditional medicine and biomedicine in countries such as Japan, China, Korea and Vietnam is inevitably bound up with the history of various imperialisms (that of the Western colonial powers but also of Japan), with the development of the modern nation state, and with the integration of science and technology into these processes. Different Asian countries resolved the attendant tensions between tradition and modernity, between a desire to safeguard national culture and compete with Western powers economically as well as politically in different ways and usually only after prolonged and often bitter struggles (Lock 1980; Zhao Hongjun 趙洪俊 1989).

In China biomedicine and Chinese medicine are now officially accorded equal rights within the boundaries of a single, albeit plural, healthcare system. In Japan biomedical physicians within the state healthcare system may elect to practice traditional herbal medicine, whereas acupuncture practiced by non-physicians remains outside. Korea and Taiwan opted for dual systems with traditional medicine and biomedicine existing side by side. Although traditional medicine has survived in all of these countries, its status continues to be precarious and clearly constrained by what Margaret Lock (1990) refers to as 'orchestrated pluralism' – the domination of ostensibly plural healthcare systems by one of its constituent parties, namely biomedicine.

In the West, the practice of East Asian medicines dates back centuries (Barnes 2005). Debates regarding the desirability of integration into official healthcare, however, only began in earnest in the final decades of the 20th century. Until then, the selective assimilation of techniques such as needling by individual physicians, or of *taiqiquan* into personal health regimes was seen as a personal choice, while East Asian medicines as alternative medical traditions were assumed to exist only at the fringes of acceptable healthcare or in the various East Asian diasporas. Since then traditional East Asian medicines have rapidly moved from these fringes towards the mainstream. In the UK, for instance, Chinese pharmacies can today be found in every high street offering cures for anything from impotence and weight loss to migraines; *qi gong* and *taiqiquan* classes are available at local gyms or village halls; and acupuncture for the treatment of chronic backache has recently become a standard option in the UK's National Health Service (NHS) on the recommendation of the National Institute for Health and Clinical Excellence (NICE 2009).

Yet, unlike in China, Korea or Japan, no official consensus has yet been reached regarding the value and use of East Asian medicine in Western healthcare systems. Furthermore, in spite of their very different cultural and historical provenances they are generally lumped together in both official and public discourse with all kinds of other practices – with which they share nothing whatsoever apart from not being taught in conventional medical schools – under the single label 'complementary and alternative medicines' (CAM). Conversely, Western practitioners of acupuncture, a treatment method that historically as well as conceptually is tied to the wider domain of traditional East Asian medicine, often downplay or even deny the importance of these roots. Instead, they describe themselves as 'medical acupuncturists' or simply as 'acupuncturists' and seek to create professional identities independent from and sometimes in outright opposition to those who would see acupuncture as part of more comprehensive traditions such as Chinese medicine.

Furthermore, just as biomedicine did not enter a vacuum when it moved East and South during the period of empire and imperialism, East Asian medicines spreading around the world as part of contemporary processes of globalization encounter existing cultures of healing, perceptions of self and the body, and different economic and legal contexts of practice that impact in various ways on what they are and how they are practiced (Zhan 2009). Acupuncture in California became psychologized, used no longer to treat disease but to help patients realize themselves (Barnes 1998). In this it shares a common path of development with other forms of complementary and alternative medicine in both the US and Europe, where earlier attachments to 1960s' counterculture have increasingly given way to forms of practice that reinforce dominant ideologies of individualism and consumption (Baer 2002). Moving in the opposite direction but only superficially contradictory to the above, other commentators have noted that acupuncture today is simultaneously becoming physiologized as educators, practitioners and researchers seek to divest it of all pseudoscientific attachments to traditional knowledge in order to discover its 'real' mode of action and measure its 'true' effectiveness (Tao 2008).

In Cuba, where healthcare is still directed primarily at the public, acupuncture is integrated into primary care and used, free of charge, in hospital emergency rooms (see Chapter 13). In Tanzania Chinese medicine is perceived to have rapid effects, distinguishing it from much slower-acting local medical traditions (Hsu 2002). In China, where most Chinese physicians in the 1930s still made their living from treating acute disorders, Chinese medicine is today perceived as particularly useful for chronic conditions (Scheid 2002). In the West, Korea and Japan, where acupuncture is largely practiced outside the official healthcare system and thus in competition with biomedicine, much research effort has been spent on demonstrating its effectiveness. In China itself, where Chinese medicine is supported by the state and practiced in an officially plural healthcare system, researchers are increasingly uninterested in such comparative questions, directing their efforts instead to measuring what therapies such as acupuncture might add to conventional care.

Clearly, therefore, what a medicine is, what its practitioners do, and how they and others perceive what they do depends on how physicians and their patients are connected to each other and the rest of society through mutually constitutive webs of knowledge, technology, and governance. Scholars in the humanities have learned this lesson. Anthropologists initially sought to understand traditional medical systems as reflecting in terms of their structure and conceptual makeup the broader social and cultural systems in which they were embedded. This effort failed, largely because medical practices proved too complex, diverse and changeable to be pressed into static analytic frameworks like health beliefs, explanatory models of illness, and medical systems. Humanities scholars now largely accept that these frameworks were largely figments of their own imaginations – attempts to detect behind the diversity of their informants' statements more stable structures that fulfilled their own need for certain types of explanation (Littlewood 2007). Historians of medicine, likewise, have moved on from the study of the canonical texts that were once seen as repositories of tradition to more sophisticated analyses of how a medicine was really practiced at any given time and place. What emerges as a result of these shifts of perspective is an understanding of East Asian medicines as diverse and constructed by local currents and transnational flows of knowledge, technology, and people that makes it difficult to define what it is about something like 'Chinese medicine' that is enduringly 'Chinese,' or even where the boundaries of medicine should be drawn (Hinrichs 1998). Historically, traditional East Asian medical practices blur distinctions between what we in the West would designate as medicine and religion; and even now, in the tonic soups taken daily by millions of southern Chinese, it is difficult to make out where medicine ends and cooking begins. Hence, rather than taking notions of stable traditions or cultural difference as starting points for inquiries into traditional East Asian medicines, contemporary research in anthropology and medical history is concerned with understanding how the very notions that create difference – 'medicine', 'Korean', 'science', 'tradition' – are constructed, negotiated, and deployed.

By and large, practitioners, clinicians and regulators in the West have not yet engaged with these changed understandings. They continue to think of what they do, examine or regulate in terms of stable entities that can be clearly described in textbooks; that can be compared with each other along dimensions such as holism/reductionism or science/belief; that are assumed to have universal validity; and that can be evaluated *in toto* in terms of their effectiveness. On closer inspection, however, such research and regulatory practices are riven by the same internal contradictions and unexamined assumptions that caused the shifts in humanities' research outlined above.

For instance, if medical traditions are indeed stable and systematic, why then do East Asian nation states expend quite so much effort on standardization and regulation? Are these not rather tools of domestication that allow for easier regulation and governance? Or are perhaps regulation and standardization an intrinsic aspect of the process of fashioning 'invented traditions' that can then be inserted into the global economy in the same way as one would market any other commodity? Are researchers investigating the therapeutic effectiveness of traditional medicines perhaps failing to see that the real effectiveness of 'traditional Chinese medicine' (TCM) lies not in its ability to treat disease but in its capacity to compete as a recognizable brand in a global healthcare market, created with much forethought precisely to meet the needs

3

of a modern Western audience (Taylor 2000)? Consequently, is what should be of interest to us not the authenticity or not of any given practice, but who controls systematization, regulation, standardization or branding, and who benefits from its success?

Similar tensions are replicated within the domains of clinical practice and research. Westerners, for instance, rarely study Asian languages and therefore lack access to most of the ancient and contemporary literatures in their field. Yet, they present themselves to their patients and the public as representatives of authentic Asian medicines. Likewise, although the examination of an intervention's effectiveness should be entirely disinterested in its historical provenance or modes of explanation – and hence of what is culturally familiar and what is not – notions of plausibility significantly influence research agendas. Proponents of traditional East Asian medicines insist, somewhat inconsistently, that the theories underpinning their practices are universally valid yet also culturally specific insofar as they embody uniquely Chinese/ Japanese/Korean/Vietnamese understandings of health, disease, and the body. Clinical researchers who are meticulous in their discussions of research methodology fail to extend the same diligence and evidence-based attitude to the claims they make regarding the objects of their study. Hence, when researchers claim to examine the effectiveness of acupuncture or Chinese medicine they choose to ignore an entire research literature documenting the enormous diversity of these practices.

Perhaps the general lack of interest by clinicians and clinical researchers in humanities and social science research on East Asian medicine is simply reflective of power relations within the field and in society at large. Perhaps it is indicative of the stubborn persistence in modern society of what CP Snow (1964) famously referred to as a breakdown in communication between the 'two cultures.' Certainly, when leading figures in the field of complementary and alternative medicine research describe the social sciences as 'generally unintelligible' and as essentially useless (White 2000), this does not bode well for dialogue of any kind. Likewise, labeling a study of the transformation of traditional medicine by evidence-based medicine as 'randomized controlled crime' (Adams 2002) is easily interpreted as a lack of desire to open channels of communication on the other side of the culture wars. The entrenched divisions between the humanities and the natural sciences that Snow identified as a major hindrance to solving the world's problems thus continue to exist in the domain of East Asian medical research, disabling the search for meaningful solutions to the problem of their managed integration into modern healthcare.

This book is a conscious effort to overcome these divides. It is the result of more than three years of cooperation between the editors, the authors of the various chapters and vignettes, a number of other academics and clinical researchers around the world, and the publishers. These efforts have included the organization of two innovative workshops under the same title as the book, initiated by the editors at the University of Westminster in April 2007 (Scheid 2008) and again in July 2009. We received the generous support of Elsevier, the International Association for the Study of Traditional Asian Medicines (IASTAM), the Acupuncture Research and Resource Centre (ARRC), the Wellcome Trust for the History of Medicine, the Daiwa Foundation, and the

Coca-Cola Company. These workshops brought together over 40 different researchers from fields as disparate as medical anthropology, science studies, the history of medicine, epidemiology, clinically applied research, public health, clinical governance, teaching and clinical practice. They created opportunities for discussing in a collegiate atmosphere the many questions that attend the ongoing modernization and transformation of East Asian medicines and their integration into contemporary healthcare. The workshops also served as platforms for launching the collaborative writing project between a smaller number of individuals that has resulted in this book.

For many reasons, we believe our book constitutes a unique achievement that will hopefully guide a new generation of researchers towards developing approaches, methods and projects that transcend the many limitations of the current state of the field. First, the very writing of the book demonstrates that Snow's 'two cultures' – like much else in the domain of traditional East Asian medicine – can be bridged. Second, although much of the book is a survey of the field rather than an attempt to proscribe research methods or programs, it also begins the process of offering concrete suggestions for how things might be done differently, and why. Third, in consistently breaking the three taboos (outlined below) that have for some time beset research in the domain of East Asian medicine, the various contributors are ushering in what we hope will be a new era of interdisciplinary studies in the field.

The first of these taboos is what Nathan Sivin has called the 'Awesome Taboo' – the reluctance by writers in the humanities to make use of primary texts in science, technology and medicine, or to engage directly with the practice of these disciplines (Elman 2005). The second encompasses what Benjamin Elman (2005) refers to as the 'Science Taboo' – the unwillingness of natural scientists to engage with scholars and research in the humanities and social sciences. The third taboo is what we label the 'Effectiveness Taboo.' This prescribes that clinical researchers must think about the effectiveness of medical practices only in naturalist terms, whereas scholars in the humanities and social sciences are allowed to think of effectiveness only in symbolic terms. The notion of a taboo implies that breaking it invariably results in terrible consequences such as producing meaningless or even false knowledge. We believe this book demonstrates the opposite.

Critically minded readers might object that breaking taboos for their own sake is meaningless unless it is accompanied by constructive suggestions for what to put in their place. We believe this is precisely where this book goes beyond other writings in the field. We agree with the proponents of evidence-based medicine that all effectiveness claims made should be subjected to comprehensive factual evaluation. However, we go beyond current research in that we would extend such critical evaluation to all knowledge claims. We agree equally with cutting edge scholarship in the humanities and social sciences that refuses to accept any of the terms or practices that would seem to provide a stable foundation for our inquiries – 'tradition', 'Asia', 'acupuncture', 'tongue diagnosis', 'the placebo effect' – as other than created, negotiated and stabilized within specific and constantly changing syntheses (Scheid 2002). We advocate the integration of such scholarship into clinical research itself, which may be difficult and often inconvenient, but to us it is the only way to make the term 'evidence-based' live up to its claims.

The issues and challenges associated with the integration of East Asian medicine into contemporary healthcare are addressed within this book in four themes. In Chapters 2, 3 and 4, the focus of the first theme is primarily on the practices and practitioners of East Asian medicine. In the first of these chapters, Volker Scheid sets out two contrasting views: on the one hand, the conventional biomedical approach seeks to objectively define disease and standardize procedures in order to develop what might be called 'best practice.' The evidence-based medicine movement, with its emphasis on population health and equality of access to those healthcare interventions that have been shown to be safe and effective, has further reinforced this approach. On the other hand, the more traditionally minded physicians and practitioners of East Asian medicine assert the importance of the uniqueness of each case and the need to address the underlying patterns that provide coherence to the case. Based on this, Scheid emphasizes the central role of the practitioner's judgment and skill in providing the best treatment outcome for the individual patient. Having highlighted this tension between best practice and best practitioner, Scheid goes on to provide a broader context within which both positions and their apparently competing knowledge bases can be understood. Then, in the key section of the chapter, he sets out an agenda that moves beyond this dichotomy of either generating best practice or cultivating best practitioners. In six innovative theses, he opens up the possibilities of a fruitful integration through interdisciplinary dialogue and research. He argues that only by bringing together insights and expertise from the arts, humanities, social sciences and natural sciences can there be a successful movement towards the modernization and integration of Chinese medicine into contemporary healthcare.

In Chapter 3, Judith Farquhar continues the theme of best practice versus best practitioner. She identifies the context in which there are global pressures to modernize East Asian medicines, with an emphasis on developing standards of 'best practice.' As an aspect of this, she describes the electronic pulsometer, a mechanical way to evaluate the qualities of the pulse. This was developed several decades ago with the intention of standardizing the qualities of the pulse so as to help develop best practice in the clinic, and potentially to play a role in randomized controlled trials. To its proponents, the pulsometer was deemed to be more 'objective' and therefore more authoritative. Despite these early good intentions, the pulsometer is no longer widely used in clinical practice. Practitioners of Chinese medicine perceive their practice as involving so much more than that which can be guided by the readings of a machine. Judith introduces the 28 pulse qualities and describes the way a practitioner of Chinese medicine configures from these qualities the patient's overall pulse picture. In turn, the pulse picture is integrated into the complex process of diagnosis and treatment, a process that requires the art of a human practitioner. In her research, Judith has found that pulse taking can be seen as an embodied experience, one that taps into a sensitivity to qualities that exceed mechanical quantity. Judith presents two case histories as illustrations of the complexity of such practice, which highlight both the limitations of mechanical quantification and the way the task of the best practitioners is to give coherence to the treatment process for each individual. For Judith this links to the inherent social value in medicine, which is to address the complexity of the individual with the aim of achieving better health.

In Chapter 4, Trina Ward examines a variety of different ways in which the practice of Chinese medicine is enacted by practitioners in China and the UK. Based on empirical research she carried out as part of her doctorate, Trina challenges the assumption that there exists one single definable Chinese medicine, an assumption reinforced by terms such as traditional Chinese medicine (TCM) and by the institutions that create and, in turn, depend on such narrow definitions. In her study, Trina first examined the different ways that practitioners think and talk about the relationship between biomedicine and Chinese medicine, both in their own practices and in the world at large. Using a mixed qualitative and quantitative methodology, she was able to identify six distinct groupings of practitioners in terms of the way these positioned themselves with regard to biomedicine. Innovatively she describes each of these styles as 'enactments', as this captures in our minds the sense that the practitioners themselves are actively producing and reproducing Chinese medicine. These coexisting styles of practice, or enactments, draw on a mixture of competing and overlapping knowledge bases. We gain a clear sense from Trina's research that Chinese medicine is not only diverse but also constantly evolving. Her research, and the conclusions that she explores in her chapter, have important implications for our understanding of all East Asian medical traditions, and especially the challenge of trying to define what exactly such traditions are.

The second theme of the book, in Chapters 5, 6 and 7, is focussed on the standardization of East Asian medicines from a number of different perspectives. Worldwide, many initiatives to standardize East Asian medicine have been instigated at both national and international levels over recent decades, driven by a number of diverse agendas linked to the overall project of modernizing and globalizing traditional medical practices. These chapters draw out the issues and challenges associated with such areas as the standardization of terminology, of acupuncture point locations, of needle design and of clinical practice (best practice) guidelines. In Chapter 5, Sonya Pritzker focuses on the terminology and language that have been central to the standardization agenda. She sets out for us an understanding that language is a living entity, something that comes to life in the interactions between people, in the dialogue between students and teachers, and in the debates between East and West. In her chapter, Sonya presents four case studies, or 'snapshots', that illustrate her perspective on the role of language, and which highlight the pros and cons of standardization. Throughout she emphasizes the role of interactions and the way these can involve not just interpersonal processes, but also economic, political and moral influences. She gives us a clear sense that the language of Chinese medicine is evolving, with implications for what its practice is becoming in our globalized world.

Chapter 6 continues with the theme of standardization. Chris Zaslawski and Myeong Soo Lee, writing from an international perspective, document the growing trend, especially among East Asian countries, to actively pursue standardization across many aspects of traditional medical practice. This trend is fuelled by the desire to promote national medical practices on a global stage. Standardization is seen as a positive force in the technological developments in needle manufacture, in the commercialization of herbal medicine, in the integration of traditional medical practices with biomedicine, in the support for regulation of non-physician practitioners and in the promotion of research agendas to demonstrate therapeutic benefits. The authors explore the developments in standardization that have been taking place in the Western Pacific region as exemplars of this wider process, specifically with respect to the forces that drive it both nationally and internationally. Chris and Myeong Soo outline some of the limitations within the methods used to agree standards. Many decisions have been made based on expert opinion rather than high-quality evidence; national and cultural differences are not easily resolved; the complexity of practice may be lost in standardized clinical practice guidelines; and fundamental differences in perspective may be glossed over when there is pressure to reach a consensus. Although the proponents of standardization are convinced of the benefits, there are others who are questioning the longer-term effects. For example, will standardization have a limiting effect on diversity and innovation? Will it lead inadvertently to a biomedicalization of traditional medical concepts, such that therapeutically important aspects are lost? Chris and Myeong Soo avoid taking sides in these debates in order to set out the advantages and disadvantages of standardization in a way that helps the reader to understand current issues and the challenges that lie ahead.

In Chapter 7, Sean Lei and his colleagues approach standardization from a different angle. Original ethnographic research was used to understand the methods and processes used by a research team in Taiwan to standardize tongue images using photography. Tongue diagnosis has long been an established part of the diagnostic process in many East Asian medicines. Using image processing technology, the Taiwanese research team captured photographic images of the tongue, intending to use them to improve the precision of tongue diagnosis compared to the traditional methods based on practitioners' subjective views. Interestingly, the research team was also aware of the importance of the subjective view of the practitioner and did not want to lose the human judgment that has traditionally been integral to tongue diagnosis. Sean and his colleagues describe how, as a result, they aimed to integrate the objectivity of the photographic images with the subjectivity of the practitioner. This integration moves beyond the apparent opposition between innovation and authenticity, and between those who would have traditional medicine leave behind its traditional roots and those who would preserve all aspects of traditional medicine irrespective of modern developments. In this chapter the authors suggest a spectrum of possibilities for integration that might bridge these apparently irreconcilable positions.

In Chapters 8, 9 and 10, the focus of the third theme of the book is on clinical research in East Asian medicine, exploring the methods used to build an evidence base for East Asian medicines and identifying their strengths as well as their limitations. In Chapter 8, Claudia Witt and her colleagues present definitions of efficacy, effectiveness and efficiency through a focus on the role of the randomized controlled trial (RCT), seen by many as the 'gold standard' in evaluative research. Although randomized controlled trials can generate considerable controversy in the field of East Asian medicine, Claudia and her colleagues argue that they have a role when used appropriately, and when they are properly designed to answer specific questions. What is not always well understood is that different research questions should lead to different designs of RCT, namely explanatory and pragmatic. The authors illustrate these two designs by comparing the methods used in trials of acupuncture for low back pain conducted in Germany and the UK. They also describe how evidence from RCTs can affect decision-making in different ways. In the context of acupuncture as a treatment for low back pain, they contrast the policies resulting from a German explanatory trial with that from a pragmatic trial in the UK. In the concluding section of the chapter the authors explore some of the broader aspects of such decision-making processes, concluding that the way new evidence is used can be influenced by both the science and the politics.

In Chapter 9, Andrew Flower and his colleagues pick up on the previous chapter's concerns regarding the political dimensions of implementing research evidence. Their starting point is an analysis of the evidence-based medicine movement, including its origins and development over recent years. The good intentions of its founders are clearly set out, with the aim of using best evidence combined with clinical judgment to deliver rational and effective healthcare. However, Andrew and colleagues also contend that a positivist philosophy permeates the practice of evidence-based medicine, allowing its proponents to consider themselves the arbiters of truth, even as they themselves conveniently ignore evidence of the socioeconomic forces that influence evidence-based medical practice. Based on this analysis, the authors raise concerns about the use of the standard tools of evidence-based medicine in the evaluation of East Asian medical practices. These concerns relate to the differences between the Eastern and Western philosophical approaches that impact directly on practice, the difficulty of incorporating the individualized nature of the consultation process, and the need to capture the appropriate expertise and judgment of the practitioner. The authors do not accept the existence of incommensurable paradigms, for example that evidence-based medicine should not be used to evaluate East Asian medicine. Rather, they raise specific questions about what sort of methodologies might be appropriate with regard to research in this field. To this end, they critically appraise a broad range of research methods and set out a convincing research strategy that calls for a less hierarchical approach to the generation of evidence.

Chapter 10 continues the theme of treatment evaluation with an anthropological perspective by Elisabeth Hsu. She interweaves her own findings as ethnographer with examples from the literature. She reinforces the view that conventional randomized controlled trials can evaluate only a limited range of treatment effects and shows what might be gained by widening the perspective. Medical anthropological approaches have included a reinterpretation of the placebo effect as a 'meaning response' to color and other symbolisms, and insight into 'social efficacy', which shows the benefit of medical treatment in supporting and reinforcing social and family bonds. Elisabeth's own contribution draws on literature that frames medical treatment as a ritual process, which depends on the subjectivities of the patient and practitioner as well as on the interpersonal processes between them. However, where anthropologists of religion have emphasized the psychological and symbolic persuasiveness of ritual efficacy, Elisabeth suggests that this ritually induced efficacy may depend on sophisticated body techniques that medical traditions have developed, which are grounded in an entirely different treatment rationale from biomedicine. Medical efficacy may well depend on culturally induced synchronicity in patient–practitioner interactions, effected through these body techniques, which thereupon trigger vitality-enhancing processes in the patient. Examples include the deqi needle sensation during acupuncture, and the purging and vomiting in the initial period of a panchakarma treatment. Elisabeth ends with a call to health researchers to stop focusing just on patient outcomes and to broaden the focus of evaluation to include the context of treatment. An effective medical treatment from this perspective triggers processes that can lead to an all-encompassing transformation of not only the patient but also the practitioner, and their social and material environment.

The final theme of the book, in Chapters 11, 12 and 13, has a focus on issues related to the globalization of traditional medicines and their integration into official healthcare systems that are invariably dominated by biomedicine. These chapters explore these issues in the context of relatively recent developments in the Philippines, India and Cuba. In Chapter 11, Paul Kadetz describes the political and economic forces that have shaped the healthcare system in the Philippines, which includes a range of local, informal and unsystematized healthcare practices. In this context, Paul presents a number of interpretations and misinterpretations of concepts such as 'traditional medicine', 'integration' and 'standardization.' For example, he describes how the use of the term 'traditional' has often been used inconsistently, inappropriately and pejoratively, yet that there is also a logic to such usage that places these traditions in an implicitly inferior position with regard to biomedicine. He also argues that many 'traditional' medical practices are actually invented, that is, they have been reshaped to serve a particular political and/or economic agenda. Finally, the approach to the integration of traditional medicines promoted by the World Health Organization and many nation states, including the Philippines, is modeled on that of the People's Republic of China of the 1950s and 1960s. This model not only embodies all of the above biases, but its emergence within the specific historical context of the modernization of healthcare in China raises practical questions about its appropriateness to other places and times. Paul presents specific examples drawn from his research in the Philippines, highlighting some of the potential challenges of integration and their unintended consequences. He concludes by speculating whether integration is something that needs to be 'done to' a population, 'done with' a population, or something that a population might organically arrive at 'from within.' What this chapter clearly illustrates is that the specific context within which integration is being implemented will have a profound effect on the outcome.

In Chapter 12, Laurent Pordié presents an innovative approach to discussing the globalization of East Asian medicines. Based on an ethnographic case study examining how a successful chain of spas in India has succeeded in establishing a presence within what is a transnational healthcare space, Laurent argues that a focus on branding overcomes the analytical deficiencies associated with the more common view that examines the globalization of tradition through a focus on the preservation or loss of authenticity. The chain of spas provides a standardized set of 'Indian' therapies, including massage and yoga. Despite claims for the authenticity of the therapies provided, for example stating that they are drawn from 'ancient Indian healing wisdom', Laurent shows that the therapeutic practices within the spas are to some extent invented traditions. Innovation has been determined by a number of factors, both internal and external to the chain. Within the chain, the entrepreneurial approach of the managing director has been instrumental in reshaping the services in response to client feedback. However, the creative processes involved in making and sustaining the brand are equally strongly influenced by the global wellness industry, supported by international trends that include increasing levels of tourism with a focus on wellness. Also of relevance are the transnational linkages and networks that support contacts and interactions between individuals within and across nation states. The combined impact of these local and transnational influences have helped reshape the developments within the spa chain and facilitated the development of a recognizable brand of 'Indian aromatherapy' through a process of innovation that stands in its own right as one of the ways in which medical traditions integrate into the contemporary world.

In Chapter 13, Vivienne Lo and Adrian Renton continue to explore the different ways in which traditional medical practices are blended into new and different contexts of practice, this time in Cuba. They survey the historical development of Chinese medicine in Cuba, from the time of the indentured Chinese laborers on the sugar plantations in the eighteenth century, to the first acupuncture seminars in Havana in the 1960s, and through to the socialist military networks that existed for the transfer of knowledge between China, Vietnam and North Korea. With Cuba's commitment to the patient as a biopsychosocial being, issues of efficacy have to be understood against the broader historical background. After the withdrawal of Soviet aid, the Cuban government encouraged the practice of traditional and natural medicine in the 1990s because of economic necessity and national pride. This produced a 'Chinese' medicine all of its own, one that is tied to the Cuban revolution as much as it is to the Yellow Emperor, that integrates Cuban herbs into Chinese medicine, just as it fits acupuncture treatment to the specific needs of the Cuban people. Hence, unlike in the West, Chinese medicine in Cuba is not only used for chronic ailments but is also used in emergency rooms to treat cardiovascular accidents, heart attacks and acute asthma. By 2008, between 20 and 30 million patients a year in Cuba were treated with traditional and natural medicine, and one hospital visited by the authors recorded that 10% of patients passing through the accident and emergency service and 50% of inpatients received some form of traditional and natural medicine. Drawing on such evidence, the authors show that Chinese medicine in Cuba is a 'living tradition', a blend of aspects of an authentic tradition with appropriate innovation to meet local needs. This form of authenticity may be far more important in evaluating how well a medicine fulfills its role in society than attempts to embody or evaluate 'authentic traditions' existing outside history.

And finally, Chapter 14 by Kathryn Montgomery concludes the book by tying together the perspectives advanced in the previous chapters into one single argument: that medicine, of whatever kind, is at core a practice, and will remain so no matter what resources it draws on. In the last instance, medicine is about making decisions in contexts of uncertainty, taking risks, shouldering responsibility, and extending help to others even if that effort might often fail. It is this shared perception that allows physicians practicing any kind of medicine to speak to each other if they wish, and which provides us with the best hope for managing the integration of East Asian medicines into contemporary healthcare in a reasoned and reasonable manner.

Adams, V., 2002. Randomized controlled crime: postcolonial sciences in alternative medicine research. Soc. Stud. Sci. 32 (5/6), 659–690.

Baer, H.A., 2002. The growing interest of biomedicine in complementary and alternative medicine: a critical perspective. Med. Anthropol. Q. 16 (4), 403–405.

Barnes, L.L., 1998. The psychologizing of Chinese healing practices in the United States. Cult. Med. Psychiatry 22, 413–443.

Barnes, L.L., 2005. Needles, herbs, gods, and ghosts: China, Healing, and the West to 1848. Harvard University Press, Cambridge, MA.

Elman, B.A., 2005. On Their Own Terms: Science in China, 1550–1900. Harvard University Press, Cambridge, MA.

Hinrichs, T.J., 1998. New geographies of Chinese medicine. In: Low, M.F. (Ed.), Beyond Joseph Needham: Science, Technology, and Medicine in East and Southeast Asia, Osiris (2nd Series), vol. 13. University of Chicago Press Journals, Chicago, IL, pp. 287–325.

Hsu, E., 2002. 'The medicine from China has rapid effects': Chinese medicine patients in Tanzania. Anthropol. Med. 9 (3), 291–313.

Littlewood, R. (Ed.), 2007. On Knowing and Not Knowing in the Anthropology of Medicine. Left Coast Press, Walnut Creek.

Lock, M.M., 1980. East Asian Medicine in Urban Japan: Varieties of Medical Experience, Comparative Studies of Health Systems and Medical Care. University of California Press, Berkeley.

Lock, M., 1990. Rationalization of Japanese herbal medicine: the hegemony of orchestrated pluralism. Hum. Organ. 49 (1), 41–47.

NICE, 2009. Low Back Pain: Early Management of Persistent Non-Specific Low Back Pain. National Institute for Health and Clinical Excellence, London, UK.

Scheid, V., 2002. Chinese Medicine in Contemporary China: Plurality and Synthesis. Duke University Press, Durham.

Scheid, V., 2008. Authenticity, best practice, and the evidence mosaic. The challenge of integrating traditional East Asian medicines into Western Healthcare. Complement. Ther. Med. 16 (2), 107–108.

Snow, C.P., 1964. The Two Cultures: and a Second Look, second ed. University Press, Cambridge.

Tao, I., 2008. A critical evaluation of acupuncture research. East Asian Sci. Technol. Soc. 2 (4), 507–524.

Taylor, K., 2000. Medicine of Revolution: Chinese Medicine in Early Communist China 1945–1963. Ph.D. Department of History and Philosophy of Science, University of Cambridge, Cambridge.

White, A., 2000. Review of P Tovey [eds.]. Contemporary primary care. Buckingham: Open University Press. Complement. Ther. Med. 9, 52–53.

Zhan, M., 2009. Other-Worldly: Making Chinese Medicine Through Transnational Frames. Duke University Press, Durham.

Zhao Hongjun, 趙洪俊, 1989. History of the Polemics Between Chinese and Western Medicine in Modern Times 近代中西醫論爭史. Anhui kexue jishu chubanshe, Hefei.

Defining best practice or cultivating best practitioners

Volker Scheid

2

> **"**It's always good to know what went down before you, because if you know the past, you can control the future.**"**
> Bob Dylan

In 1999, when writing my ethnography of Chinese medicine in late 20th century China, I searched for an image that would convey to the reader from the very outset the diversity of practice I was dealing with. In the end, I wrote that if someone were to seek out ten famous Chinese medicine physicians for the treatment of the same illness, they would most likely walk away with ten different prescriptions all of which might potentially be effective (Scheid 2002a). I did not realize at the time that the very same example had been used by the early 20th century philosopher and cultural critic Liang Shuming 梁漱溟 in his juxtaposition of Western and Chinese medicine.

> *"What is referred to as medicine in China is in fact [nothing but] art. Prescribing in Western medicine proceeds on the basis of matching specific diseases with specific prescriptions [so that there is] little variation [between individual physicians' treatment]. The highest calibre Chinese physicians however rely on context and individual ability in writing out their formulas. Ten different physicians will thus write out ten different formulas that can, moreover, be extremely different [from each other]."*

> Liang Shuming 梁漱溟 1921 (2002)

Western medical science in the eyes of its early 20th century Chinese admirers embodied an empiricist objectivism that had many advantages when compared to the subjective diversity of indigenous medicine. Above all, it offered the promise that the same disease would always be responded to in the same manner, and that once an effective treatment had been found everyone could be cured. It would have come as a surprise to Liang Shuming to learn that when put to the test by John Wennberg in 1973 clinical decision-making in biomedicine was shown to be influenced by a wide range of contingent and subjective factors (Wennberg & Gittelsohn 1973). These findings were so surprising, in fact, that they ushered in a fundamental re-evaluation of biomedical practices. This eventually led to the rise of evidence-based medicine (EBM) as the dominant medical paradigm of our time.

Before EBM biomedical practice was seen as rooted in scientific knowledge that physicians applied to clinical practice guided by the professional skills they acquired during their training. After Wennberg the notion of professional expertise became increasingly suspect. Perceived as open to all kinds

13

of cognitive biases what had hitherto been celebrated as the 'art of medicine' was now seen in need of replacement by best-practice guidelines and protocols (Berg 1995). Sackett and Rosenberg, two leading exponents of EBM, explain:

> "Equally powerful methods [to those adopted in clinical research] have been developed and applied to validate the clinical history and physical examination, diagnostic tests, and prognostic markers. When performed in collaboration with seasoned clinicians these methods often have made explicit the expert's implicit, non-verbal diagnostic, prognostic and therapeutic reasoning, making it possible for their trainees to replace mere mimicry with understanding, and avoiding the necessity for decades of experience as the only pathway to sound clinical judgement."

Sackett & Rosenberg 1995

But let us return, for a moment, to early 20th century China and Liang Shuming's assumptions regarding the essential difference between objective Western and subjective Chinese medicine:

> "[Chinese medicine is so diverse] because neither with regard to diseases nor the medicinals by which these are treated do there exist objective standards. Actually, what diseases are [Chinese physicians] treating? Where is the site of the lesion? In the absence of any standard method of investigation, the examination of disease states must necessarily be subjective! ... Treating illness [under such conditions], how could ten different people not arrive at ten different treatments."

Liang Shuming 梁漱溟 1921 (2002)

The distinction between objectively defined disease and the subjective practices of traditional physicians is not unique to Liang. As a recurring theme around which the modernization of Chinese medicine in the course of the last century has been enacted, it provided structure to argument and debate and thereby shaped the very constitution of China's modern healthcare system (Andrews 1996; Scheid 2002a; Lei 1998; Karchmer 2004). Within this system biomedical diseases now constitute the top-level diagnostic category. In the Chinese medical domain disease is subsequently broken down into the manifestation patterns (zhenghou 證候) that are said to reflect the uniqueness of Chinese medical practice (Farquhar 1994a). Such patterns have been extensively discussed both in modern textbooks and in classic canons and their precise definition and application to a given case explicitly evokes the personal experience and craftsmanship of each individual physician (Farquhar 1994b; Qin Bowei 秦伯未 1957 [1983]; Scheid 2002b).

Institutionally supported by the full power of the Chinese state the present compromise is nevertheless intrinsically unstable. For it does not resolve the tension between disease (standing for medicine as an objective science grounded in universal biology) and manifestation patterns (standing for the ultimate uniqueness of each illness episode that can be understood and reacted to but never exhaustively mapped in all its details). Attempts to further integrate Chinese and Western medicines at the level of the official healthcare system resulted in the increasing objectification of patterns now called types (xing 型). Compared to patterns, which are determined by the physician at the bedside, types are subcategories of disease standardized at both national and international level (Scheid 2002a). In opposition to this process, more traditionally minded physicians – increasingly disillusioned by the results of Chinese medicine's modernization and generally able to create for themselves spaces outside official healthcare – are advocating a return to a practice that self-consciously avows all reference to biomedical disease (Liu Lihong 劉力紅 2006).

These different enactments of Chinese medicine, to use a term employed by Trina Ward in Chapter 4, reflect not merely two different positions in the struggle for Chinese medical modernization. They embody two opposing interpretations of cultural history and of the limits and possibilities of the encounter between China and the West. The first of these implies a belief that at their heart, and in spite of whatever differences may exist at the surface, Chinese and Western medicine are essentially similar in nature. Facing the same problems they are amenable to the same solutions and, by extension, will eventually be merged into one integrated medicine. The second enactment assumes that an essential difference exists between China and the West and, by implication, between authentic Chinese and Western biomedicine. From this position, if a tendency towards objectivity, transparency, and standardized practice is inherent in biomedicine, then that cannot also be the case for Chinese medicine wedded as it is to entirely different cultural values. It follows that Chinese medicine as "Chinese" medicine must either be accepted as intrinsically different or abandoned as a throwback to a more primitive local understanding of illness that universal (Western) biomedical science has already overcome.

The goal of this chapter is to examine these opposing enactments specifically in relation to the notion of best practice and the integration of Chinese medicine into contemporary healthcare systems. To this end, I will first briefly analyze the relationship of EBM to Chinese medicine from the perspectives of political economy and the history of ideas. This will help us to understand more clearly what is at stake in this encounter, and to define more precisely the nature of the tensions between East and West, tradition and modernity enacted within these apparently irreconcilable positions. From there I will move on to an investigation of how Chinese physicians engaged with the issue of best practice prior to their encounter with Western medicine. I will tease out some of the key concepts that oriented this discourse to ask how they can be made to fit into a medical system embodying the values and objectives of EBM. Finally, I will introduce a model of knowledge management that can account for the apparently irreconcilable differences between the two approaches while also offering novel strategies for their resolution.

TWO PERSPECTIVES ON EBM, BEST PRACTICE, AND THEIR ENCOUNTER WITH CHINESE MEDICINE

To avoid a conflation of the terms biomedicine and EBM we need to remind ourselves that although the EBM movement has emerged organically out of the biomedical tradition, it functions simultaneously as an instrument aimed at its systematic reorganization (Armstrong 2007; Rodwin 2001; Runo 1998; Wahlberg & McGoey 2007). This transformation is multidimensional and tied at its core to the accelerated industrialization of medical practices that define official healthcare systems in contemporary neoliberal economies (Rees 2008). Oriented towards maximizing efficiencies at all levels of scale, these economies institutionalize, wherever possible, a division of labor based on routinization and task specification. In an increasingly global economy national healthcare systems are linked to each other by means of transnational technoscientific networks that require streamlined processes of production, distribution and consumption of goods, services, information and knowledge. This is achieved via the imposition of standards (terminological, practical, ethical, educational) and the formulation of best-practice guidelines centered on explicit evidence through agencies as diverse as the nation state, the World Health Organization (WHO), the International Standards Organization (ISO), national and transnational professional bodies and educational institutions as described in detail by Chris Zaslawski in Chapter 6.

Many of the motivations behind this reorganization are progressive. They address inequalities in healthcare that arise from subjective biases; they aim to reduce costs and increase efficiency in order to improve healthcare delivery; and they seek to improve the quality of care for all by guaranteeing access to effective medical practice. Yet, because they are aimed largely at populations rather than individuals, they also stand in a certain agonistic relationship to person-centered medical practices, be they East Asian or that of a traditional family physician (Armstrong 2002; Buetow 2002; Feinstein 1994).

All of these transformations have long since infiltrated the domain of Chinese medicine. In China, national standards on almost any aspect of traditional medical practice, from diagnostic categories to the definition of treatment outcomes, have been implemented since the late 1980s (Zhonghua renmin gongheguo biaozhun 中華人民共和國標準 1994, 1995; Discussion Group for Standards for Disease Names and Diagnostic Categories in Chinese Medicine 中醫病名診斷規範課題組 1987). At present, the Chinese state is pushing hard for similar standards to be accepted internationally (Niu 2005). In Germany, acupuncture treatment protocols aimed at assisting delivery are regularly administered by midwives who do not need to possess any understanding of Chinese medicine beyond a basic knowledge of point localization and needle techniques. In clinical research consensus techniques such as the Delphi process (Flower et al 2007; Schnyer et al 2005), the use of focus groups (Xu et al 2006), and the development of questionnaire-based assessments (Chen et al 2009; Ryu et al 2010; Su et al 2008) – all of which are directly borrowed from the world of commerce and industry – have become important tools in attempts at reducing the subjectivity that still defines mainstream Chinese medical practice.

The perception of EBM as but one tool in the progressive industrialization of medical practice is useful because it challenges assumptions regarding the existence of essential differences between Chinese and Western medicine posited by generations of writers. Put simply, whatever obstructs the realization of these goals must be removed, irrespective of whether this is the clinical judgment of a Western family physician or the *jingyan* 經驗 (experience) that guides the knowing practice of a Chinese *laozhongyi* 老中醫 (senior clinician). Such locally specific forms of knowing simply do not fit the large-scale technoscientific networks that sustain the globalized economies of the 21st century. Nor, as Vincanne Adams convincingly demonstrates for the case of Tibet, do all types of evidence (Adams 2002a). What counts as evidence to EBM researchers is not simply what works, but evidence that can be connected to other types of knowledge already circulating within EBM-based networks of production and consumption (Adams 2002b).

If Adams' research challenges the neutrality of the EBM project with regard to different kinds of medical practice, many proponents of EBM are not shy about admitting as much. They specifically tie EBM to 'the continuing […] rivalry between empiricist and rationalistic traditions in Western culture' and see it as a tool for overcoming anything non-empirical that may still exist within biomedicine (Parker 2005). This makes it impossible for proponents of EBM's neopositivist ideology to accept Chinese medicine if it is guided by personal insight that cannot be put into words.

Critics as well as proponents of the EBM-driven modernization of Chinese medicine generally fail to acknowledge the different nature of these two interrelated yet different positions (Shea 2006). Critics of modernization, on the whole, tend to conflate them (Fan 2003). They highlight EBM's unwillingness to understand Chinese medicine on its own terms, yet believe that some kind of formula can nevertheless be found to integrate authentic Chinese medicine into contemporary healthcare. EBM proponents tend to downplay the attachment of their program to historically and culturally distinctive epistemologies and metaphysics preferring instead to see them as the only rational way to optimize clinical outcomes (Sackett & Rosenberg 1995). As a result, they fail to understand that alternative ways of constructing evidence are always possible and often more appropriate (Barry 2006). In fact, the hegemony of the population-based methods that dominate EBM is already being challenged by an increasing number of researchers in biomedicine who are pushing to consider more fully issues of complexity and systems interaction in implementing the personalized medicine of the future (Li et al 2010).

China Mountain Zhang, a science-fiction novel by Maureen McHugh set in a 22nd century where China has become the new global superpower, explores such a future-albeit in the domain of engineering rather than medicine (McHugh 1992). In McHugh's world the best universities, now located in China, still teach sciences to their engineering students albeit, at a significantly advanced technological level. The most promising graduates are then offered a chance to apprentice with master practitioners in their chosen fields. To become true experts it is expected that they need to go beyond what can be taught in school by means of words. Through disciplined study, meditation and ongoing practice disciples learn to comprehend the uniqueness of each specific project and to discover the single optimal solution to any brief. In this alternative universe objective science and subjective insight combine, and do so to stunning effect. But because (in the novel) global power relationships have changed, the resultant synthesis now privileges Confucian and Buddhist rather than Platonic and Hegelian values and orientations. In the following section I want to explore how these orientations guided the pursuit of effective action in Chinese medicine prior to its encounter with the modern West.

As the medical historian Paul Unschuld notes in one of his essays, "The Chinese physician as a definable entity does not exist" (Unschuld 1979). Therefore, what I am discussing here is not intended as an exhaustive survey of how doctors and healers in China prior to the 19th century reflected on what they did. Rather, I limit myself to a narrow stratum of elite physicians who through their writings and commentaries on earlier classics defined Chinese medicine as a scholarly tradition. This focus seems justified in as much as it is this elite medicine to which contemporary 'traditional Chinese medicine' (TCM) explicitly relates itself; and because it is TCM, in turn, that is the main object of EBM evaluations. This scholarly tradition emerged roughly between the 12th and 15th centuries and dominated Chinese medicine until the modernizations of the Republican and Maoist periods (Karchmer 2004; Scheid 2002a; Taylor 2005). In their writings, their practice and the living of their lives these scholar physicians drew on various (Neo)confucian, Daoist and Buddhist doctrines about nature, the body and human agency, the roots of which stretch back to the Han and pre-Han eras, yet were continually revitalized in response to changing social, economical, technological and political contexts of practice (Scheid 2007).

Effectiveness – of different techniques, styles of practice and types of physician – was a recurring and important topic of debate. Scholar physicians emphasized the foundation of their practice in learning (*xue* 學) rather than mere technique (*shu* 術), even if they contested among themselves the precise content of such learning and how this was to be related to the domain of clinical practice. Following the modern scholar physician and historian Xie Guan 謝觀, these debates – and thereby scholarly medicine as an identifiable tradition – can be thought of as structured around the four key terms: *li* 理 (coherence/pattern/principle), *fa* 法 (strategies/methods), *fang* 方 (formulas/methods) and *yao* 藥 (medicinals/herbs/treatments). To these it is useful to add a fifth, namely *yi* 意 (conceptions/significations).

In this nexus of interrelated and difficult-to-translate concepts, *li* 理 refers to the coherence of a system, the pattern of relationships that holds the parts of a whole together, to our understanding of the way things should work, and also to the way they really are. Physicians employ various notational systems – yin/yang 陰陽, the five phases (*wu xing* 五行), the six pathogenic qi (*liu yin* 六淫), or the visceral systems (*zangfu* 臟腑) – in an attempt to describe and thereby capture the nature of such coherence (Volkmar 2006). Today, these notational systems have been reconceptualized as constituting the 'basic theories' (*qichu li lun* 其處理論) of Chinese medicine (Taylor 2005). This distorts the meaning of the original term for at least two reasons. First, if the identity of scholar physicians was closely tied to their familiarity with such systems, their use in actual clinical practice lacked the close integration suggested by the term theory (Sivin 1987). Rather, physicians would draw on these systems in different ways depending on the characteristics of the illness and person they were dealing with, but also on personal preference and on their affiliation to specific currents of learning (Scheid 2007). Second, even if all scholar physicians agreed that such notational systems were essential in order to understand the body/person in health and illness, they were not expected to actually describe this reality in every single detail (Volkmar 2006).

One way to explain this lack of interest in stringent theory is to ascribe to scholarly Chinese medicine, and to Chinese conceptions of effectiveness, a predominantly pragmatic orientation. If a body or person is imagined as a system of emergent relationships then, in order to act effectively, it is less important to know precisely the nature of individual constituent parts than to grasp their dynamic interactions. In the analysis of the French historian Françoise Jullien, in this view,

> *"[R]eality – every kind of reality – is perceived as a particular deployment or arrangement of things to be relied on and worked to one's advantage. Art, or wisdom, as conceived by the Chinese, consequently lies in strategically exploiting the propensity emanating from that particular configuration of reality, to the maximum effect possible."*

Jullien 1995

Or again, in the words of the 12th century Neoconfucian philosopher Zhu Xi 朱熹 (1130–1200),

> *"Reality is not something transcending affairs and things. Rather it is like making a ship travel on water or a cart travel on land."*

Tillman 1978

In this view, action does not follow from abstract ideas about how the world is, but rather validates one's understanding of reality in the process of achieving effects. That is, there can be no theory about the world independent of both actions and effects. Note that although similar in some ways, this conception of effective action is quite different from the pragmatic uses of theory that characterized general medical practice before the advent of EBM. Biomedical physicians at that time accepted that medical science provided a correct view of health and disease by means of its theories, and that it was not their task to add to or subtract from them. Instead, their art consisted in making this science work in clinical practice (Berg 1995).

Hence, in late imperial China the model for physicians in their struggle against disease was not as in the various instantiations of Platonism an all-knowing God or Nature mirrored in our minds, nor the professional doctor embodying the effective synthesis of art and science. Their model was the successful general who conquers his enemies through the flexible application of military strategies. These strategies are embodied in the formulas transmitted in the medical literature, which are realized anew in everyday medical practice through the concrete use of medicinals. The modern physician Shi Jinmo 施今墨 (1881–1969) explains the relationship of these terms and practices through a military metaphor that constitutes a recurrent trope in Chinese medical literature:

> *"Approach clinical manifestation patterns as you would approach a battle. Use medicinals as you would use soldiers. One must clearly differentiate symptoms, carefully organize one's formulas and flexibly employ one's medicinals. If one does not understand coherence it becomes difficult to differentiate patterns. If pattern differentiation is unclear, one has no way to establish a strategy and merely piles up individual medicinals in a disorganized fashion."*

Zhu Chenyu 祝諶予 1982

A key problem for any military strategist, even if he clearly understands the constellation of forces at play, is that one can never know precisely what the opponent will do in any given situation. Among these possibilities some are theoretically more likely than others. Yet, as the battle unfolds it can take sudden and entirely unexpected turns. Scholar physicians perceived illnesses in the same way: as processes constrained by the coherence of a system that was knowable in principle, but because of the potential uniqueness of each manifestation of the system in real time also extremely elusive. Textbook descriptions of disease processes and their treatment could therefore only ever function as approximations of how an illness manifested and how it needed to be responded to in the here and now. The 19th century scholar physician Fei Boxiong 費伯雄 provides a clear outline of this view, the difficulties this sets up for clinical practice, and how it might be resolved:

> *"Medicine is built on [understanding] coherence. Treatment proceeds from [received] methods. Adjusting to the changing realities [at the bedside] in a flexible manner, however, must follow conceptions [if one wants to be effective in a way that goes] beyond [what is possible by the use of] methods [alone]."*

Fei Boxiong 費伯雄 1863

The meaning of *yi* 意, which I have translated as conceptions, is notoriously difficult to capture by means of a single English word. It refers to cognitive processes such as intention, attention, reflection, thinking and imagination, but equally to the ability to grasp what lies hidden behind surface manifestations and respond accordingly. The present best guess as to the original meaning of this word is that it referred to what goes on in one's mind before speaking. According to Graham (1989), it is the image rather than the concept of a thing, and the movement to action with which one responds to it – hence my translation of conceptions. The nature of *yi* and its relation to knowledge and effective action is discussed by all major schools of Chinese philosophy. It became, over time, a central theme in physicians' attempts to define the nature of medical practice, as reflected in the adage, 'Medicine is *about conceptions*' (*yi zhe yi ye* 醫者意也). This discourse is too complex and multifaceted to trace here in all of its ramifications. Suffice to say that it is equated at times with the notion of *li* 理 or coherence, implying that by way of one's conceptions a person is able to conceive of the coherence or order of a system as system, and thereby know how to guide its development in a desired direction (Liao Yuqun 療育群 2006; Volkmar 2006).

Not surprisingly, the term came to be closely associated with definitions of effective medical practice. As early as the 7th century, the famous Tang dynasty physician Sun Simiao stated that "Those who are proficient at using conceptions are good doctors" (Sun Simiao 孫思邈 compl. 650/659). By the Ming dynasty this had become a common trope in the medical literature. The well-known scholar physician Zhao Xuemin is merely one of many who unequivocally links *yi* with clinical effectiveness:

> *"Medicine is about conceptions. It is not as good to use medicinals as it is to use one's conceptions. Whether or not a treatment works is based on one's conceptions. If one's conceptions can enter the fundamental subtleties [of the illness], one can achieve a penetrating understanding. After this, when one uses medicinals, none will not work as expected."*

Zhao Xuemin 趙學敏 18th century

As defined by Fei Boxiong, Zhao Xuemin and others, the term conceptions refers to a physician's capacity to grasp meanings and constellations that are too complex, subtle or fleeting to be captured in their entirety by words. But precisely because such conceptions are beyond words, they free themselves from the limitations of language and its irredeemable attachment to the past, including the constraint of tradition itself.

> *"Adjusting to the changing realities [at the bedside] in a flexible manner [means] to arrive at a definitive point of view without being in any way prejudiced [by established norms or conventions]. This is the most important principle [of effective clinical practice]."*

Fei Boxiong 費伯雄 1863

There was a clear awareness of the possibility that individual physicians would appeal to the non-transparent subjectivity of conceptions in order to avoid critique by patients or peers. There was a consequent concern for developing strategies that, on the one hand, fostered the development of conceptions as insight into the uniqueness of each illness episode, while on the other, detaching it from romantic notions of genius disabling reflection and critique.

Although the debates by which scholar physicians in late imperial China mapped out the development of their tradition need not concern us here in all their detail, their shared focus on conceptions does allow us to re-evaluate Liang Shuming's assessment regarding Chinese medicine's apparent lack of interest in disease. Contrary to what Liang implies this did not reflect an intellectual inability to grasp diseases objectively and understand them for what they really are but, rather, a conscious choice: to focus on the manifestation patterns (*zheng* 證, or *zheng* 症) through which illness is embodied in the present moment; to grasp how this unique and ultimately singular presentation embodies both the coherence of the body/person and its integration into the world around it; and to develop strategies for effectively acting on this relationship – in the sense of knowing by knowing what to do – through gaining a clear conception of it.

Any such conception is by definition a singular event in time/space, relevant only in the here and now. Nevertheless, it can simultaneously assume the status of a model capable of orienting similar conceptions in the future, just as it is itself informed by a shared archive of previous records of effective medical practice. Vignette 2.1 is an example of such a case record by the late Qing physician Fei Shengfu (1851–1914). In this record Fei presents a case from his practice that did not fit into received patterns of diagnosis. Thinking 'outside the box' he was able to gain a clear conception of the underlying pathophysiology and to develop an effective treatment strategy. The published case contributes to the Chinese medical tradition a new example of how coherence can manifest itself in clinical practice. Simultaneously, it serves as a model of effective scholarly medical practice for later generations of physicians to emulate.

The tools and strategies that scholar physicians employed to foster the development of clinical insight and effective medical practice included the study of texts that contained others' understanding of coherence, mindfulness and meditation practices, clinical apprenticeships that provided the

Fei Shengfu was a famous physician practicing in Shanghai at the turn of the 20th century. This is the translation of one of his case records. Its style combines elements of the medical essay (*yihua* 醫話), a genre used by Chinese physicians to communicate their opinion as well as discourse on general points of practice, and the case record (*yi'an* 醫案), which often were quite short and elucidated diagnosis and treatment of a given case. The case is of a patient whose presentation does not accord with textbook knowledge. Fei Shengfu responds to this unusual situation by using the manifestations of the case to guide him in formulating a successful treatment strategy. His short essay lucidly demonstrates the style of medical practice aspired to by elite physicians in late imperial China described in the main text.

"In cold damage [disorders] when heat enters into the Stomach [in the] middle [burner] and knots together with the stools this will [manifest] with thirst for fluids, raving, and inappropriate behavior. When heat enters into the blood chamber there will be lucidity during the day but raving at night and [the patient will appear] as if they had seen ghosts. In warm heat or damp heat [disorders] heat dispersing and flooding from the yang brightness and steaming the Pericardium [will manifest] with thirst for fluids, raving, inappropriate behavior, and consciousness that will sometimes be clear and sometimes muddled. In all these manifestation patterns outlined above there is none that is not due to heat. In warm heat and damp heat disorders this is of course due to a heat pathogen, whereas in the context of cold damage this will occur after the cold has transformed into heat as shown in writings from ancient times to the present. The condition of the son of Guo Yingtang from Guangdong was, however, entirely different. Mr Guo had come to the Yang family in the southern city [of Shanghai]. On 15 July 1907, his thirteen year old son Jinyi got a fever, headaches and diarrhea, which after eight or nine days had not diminished. When he became thirsty for fluids, was sometimes conscious and sometimes not, raved and behaved inappropriately worse at night, I began to treat him. I examined his pulse, which was floating and wiry rather than flooding and rapid [as one would have expected]. The tongue coating was slippery and moist thickly covering the entire tongue including the tip. The tongue body was not crimson either. Although the disorder had by now progressed for some days, [the boy] had not sweated a single drop. [This indicated to me] that there was still externally contracted wind cold due to insufficient warming and dispersing. [Usually] in patients suffering from wind cold the warming yang qi within the body has the inherent capacity to transform the pathogen into heat. Presently, after eight or nine days of fever there were clear manifestations of heat on the outside even though in reality no such transformation had yet taken place in the interior. This had to be due to the physicians that previously treated [the boy] inappropriately using [bitter cooling formulas] …, which trapped the pathogen and prevented it from passing [through the normal heat transformation]. Places where cold pathogens are present are [by definition] places not reached by the [body's] yang qi. If the yang qi is unable to travel throughout the protective and constructive [aspects] it will instead retract to move throughout the organs. This is a condition where the yang is inversely in the interior and the yin inversely in the exterior. A person's yang qi is like the sun. Yang overcomes the yin like the sun that disperses the clouds. If [the yang qi] does not shine brightly, [the patient] will sometimes be conscious and sometimes not. As for raving and inappropriate behavior that are worse at night, these are due to protective and constructive retreating into yin [aspects of the body] at night. When yin is exuberant yang is being shackled. Instead of being harmonized with the yin, the two contend with each other. Thirst and desire for fluids are due to the cooling herbs aiding [in the production of] dampness and phlegm, which obstruct the movement [of the qi and fluids]. If turbid fluids are not being eliminated, [physiological] body fluids cannot be generated. The disorder was originally caused by cold and the pathogen was not located in the interior. Therefore, I employed an acrid warming prescription that [helped to] push the trapped wind cold to the exterior and eliminated the phlegm dampness in the interior whereupon all the various [symptoms] of false heat disappeared by themselves.

After two doses the diarrhea stopped, and the headaches, thirst and clouding of consciousness decreased. As there was still no sweating the fever did not yet clear. Therefore, I added to the previous prescription [herbs that promoted sweating] …. Two further prescriptions produced a sweat that [caused] the fever to decrease, consciousness to become clear, the white tongue coating to transform, and wind, cold, dampness and phlegm to be entirely clarified and descended. [At this point I changed the strategy] to one of generating the fluids and augmenting qi the beneficial [effects of which] entirely cured [the disorder]. In terms of what how I treated this disorder, the use of [acrid warming herbs to promote sweating] was entirely appropriate in order to facilitate the resolving the cold pathogen trapped by the cooling herbs.

Regarding [the symptoms of] muddled consciousness and raving combined with thirst there is not one earlier author who would not define this as being due to heat. [In such a case it is essential] that even if the person prescribing the herbs is alone in holding an insight they know to be true they have complete confidence in what they do so as to ensure the patient's cooperation in spite of whatever doubts they may have. As I initially employed light and bland herbs but obtained a result and only then [proceeded] to adding stronger ones, the patient's mind remained calm because I was able to comply with their own ideals. The crude physician [who had earlier treated this patient] did not pay attention [to the actual symptoms] mistaking them for a heat pattern. By using cold and cooling [herbs] they progressively trapped the pathogen deeper [inside the body]. This, in turn, created constraint that transformed into heat, which was then mistakenly identified as true heat forcing its way into the Pericardium. A warming [strategy] will assist the yang, while cooling will trap [pathogens] making it ever more difficult to thrust them out. That is why I say, in order to treat disorders one must first differentiate patterns, but in differentiating patterns one must differentiate the [specific] hanging together of manifestations. This is why Xu Huixi said, "when one manifestation [does not accord] with the entire [pattern] one must be [especially] circumspect." This is the wisdom [contained] in the statement that it is difficult "to treat by identifying a disorder [based merely] on a knowledge of its normal presentation but not its [actual] changes."

Fei Shengfu 費繩甫, 2009. 1926? Fei Shengfu's Case Notes and Medical Essays 費繩甫醫案醫話 edited by Xu Xiangren徐相任. In: Zhou Guangrong 周光榮 (Ed.), Collection of Case Notes and Medical Essays from the Four Menghe Medical Families 孟河四家醫案醫話. Shanxi kexue jishu chubanshe, Taiyuan, p. 93.

opportunity for guided participatory learning, as well as the accumulation of a vast archive of case histories.

In fact, 'thinking in cases' is not a unique feature of Chinese medicine. As the historian of science John Forrester has shown, we can find in the Aristotelian tradition of thought a similar ideal of grasping the singular life through practical wisdom. Over time, this ideal has become deeply embedded in the expert disciplines ranging from law to medicine and, in Forrester's view, should therefore be considered as important a method for producing valid scientific knowledge as logic or experimental reasoning (Forrester 1996).

The prominent historian and philosopher of science Isabelle Stengers likewise emphasizes a broad conception of science that focuses on its openness towards the new and different, rather than on a concern for what we know with certainty:

"The true grandeur of science is not power but the enduring quest for relevance. ... How to learn? How to pay attention? How to acquire new habits of thinking? How to concentrate or explore other kinds of experiences? Those are questions that matter."

Stengers 2004

Such a broad definition of science is useful because it undercuts from yet another perspective the idea that the encounter between scholarly Chinese medicine and EBM is simply about the quest for truth and has nothing to do at all with politics or the exercise of power. We saw that EBM is aimed at transforming all medicine, biomedicine and Chinese medicine alike. It does so in the name of science, equality and accountability, but its pursuit of best practice cannot be dissociated from the biopolitics of global healthcare and its focus on populations amenable to standardized care. Scholar physicians perceived clinical effectiveness to be a function of singular clinical insights and were openly dismissive of anyone who did not possess the resources necessary for becoming an elite physician. Any hierarchy of knowledge, after all, is embedded in networks that tie the domains of epistemology and clinical practice to economy and society. As long as the encounter between Chinese medicine and EBM is filtered through these hierarchies, distortions like those apparent in Liang Shuming's uncharitable portrayal of his country's traditional medicine or, those shown in Vignette 2.2 on researchers' efforts to evaluate the Chinese medicine treatment of menopause, become inevitable. As Isabel Stengers might ask, what – apart from the exercise of power – is the sense in examining something that in order to fit into specific research paradigms has been distorted to such an extent that it is no longer really what it is claimed to be?

In order to chart a way out of this impasse, in the final section of this chapter I draw on a model of conceptualizing the world and acting within it that has its roots in the sociology of knowledge but is now widely employed in organizational management. That is, I seek a way of thinking about tradition and modernity, East and West, the singular life and universal knowledge that avoids to make *a priori* judgements as to which side of these oppositions is more desirable and should therefore be accorded more rights and more resources. Nor shall I be content with the relativist solution of passively acknowledging the existence of irreconcilable difference between incommensurable paradigms of practice.

Modern Chinese medicine textbooks claim that physicians in China have successfully treated symptoms associated with menopause for at least 2000 years. These claims are repeated by individual practitioners in their promotional materials, as well as in the reasons clinical researchers give for seeking to evaluate the effectiveness of these treatments. The same textbooks provide model diagnoses and treatments that define menopausal symptoms as being caused by what Chinese medicine calls 'Kidney deficiency' (*shen xu* 腎虛). There is evidence that these textbook models consistently inform clinical practice and also clinical research.

There are several problems with these claims. There is no evidence that physicians in China or other East Asian countries considered the menopausal transition to be a medical problem much before the second half of the 20th century. It can also be shown that the Kidney deficiency model of menopausal syndrome in Chinese medicine emerged in the early 1960s, and that it constitutes a translation of the estrogen deficiency model in biomedicine into Chinese medicine. This was then reconnected to older ideas about aging as well as to treatment strategies for Kidney deficiency that had originally been used to treat disorders as varied as slow development in infants, tuberculosis and infertility. However, this creative process of *bricolage* has been completely edited out of modern textbook discussions and it is simply accepted today that menopausal syndrome in biomedicine equals Kidney deficiency in Chinese medicine.

Interestingly, during the same period that Chinese physicians succeeded in globalizing a newly invented traditional understanding of menopause, Western anthropologists began to show that the experience of menopause significantly varies across cultures. They coined the term 'local biologies' in order to draw our attention to the fact that the manifestations of a process such as the menopause are not determined by biology alone. Rather, they constitute the surface of a web of interactions between factors as varied as diet, individual constitutions, climates, life stresses and beliefs. In other words, anthropologists critiquing disease arrived at an understanding of individualized patterns, whereas Chinese physicians were doing their best to make Chinese medicine match the biomedical understanding of disease.

Not surprisingly, perhaps, East Asian medical traditions less influenced by biomedical modernity, such as Japanese Kampo or Korean medicine but also Chinese medicine in Taiwan, do not generally equate menopausal symptoms with Kidney deficiency. A survey of the mainland Chinese case record literature shows that how individual physicians treat menopausal symptoms in actual clinical practice, including physicians listed as authors of modern textbooks, is far more varied than textbook models and national standards would make us believe.

Similar stories could be told about a whole range of conditions that Chinese medicine claims to have treated successfully for thousands of years: hypertension, for instance, which can only be detected by means of technologies not widely available in China prior to the 20th century; depression, which only very recently has been accepted as an illness in China, and whose clear and precise definition continues to elude the compilers of the International Classification of Disease (ICD); or irritable bowel syndrome, another ill-defined disorder with its roots in the 19th century, for which Chinese medicine textbooks, by and large, recommend a herbal formula that treats painful diarrhea even though the biomedical syndrome is specifically defined as being characterized by alternating constipation and diarrhea.

This raises the question of what clinical researchers interested in the effectiveness of Chinese medicine should examine. Should they ignore the history of inventions as well as the diversity of medical practice on the ground and examine textbook treatments because there they can find clear diagnostic categories matched to model treatments? Should they consult experts in order to produce a consensus regarding best diagnosis/treatment, knowing that the experts will generally tend to reproduce textbook models? Should they simply select one of the many treatment models available on the ground? And if so, which one? These questions defy easy answers. They demand, above all, that we accept and engage with the issue of Chinese medicine's historical diversity rather than seeking to control it, even if such diversity can appear to get in the way of clinical research.

One of the possibilities we are currently exploring at the University of Westminster is action research. This provides opportunities for a group of practitioners to treat menopausal women, to systematically pool individual experiences, to adjust treatment on the basis of group discussions, and to seek to develop a systematic understanding of how to effectively treat menopausal women in London with Chinese medicine. The outcome of this action research project might later become the basis of a more systematic clinical trial. In this manner, we aim to facilitate the development of individual skill and experience as well as collectively shared knowledge and best practice.

Notes

This vignette draws on a long-term research project on Chinese medicine and menopause carried out at the EAST*medicine* Research Centre at the University of Westminster funded by a Department of Health Research Capacity Development Grant to Dr. Volker Scheid. Initial findings have been published in a series of papers listed below.

Scheid, V., 2007. Traditional Chinese Medicine – What are we investigating? The case of menopause. Complement. Ther. Med. 15 (1), 54–68.

Scheid, V., 2007. Acupuncture for hypertension: a tale of two trials. From the perspective of the anthropologist. Forschende Komplementär Medizin 14 (6), 371, 374–375.

Scheid, V., 2009. Globalising Chinese medical understandings of menopause. East Asia Science, Technology and Society: An International Journal 2 (4), 485–496.

Scheid, V., Tuffrey, V., Ward, T., 2010. Comparing TCM textbook descriptions of menopausal syndrome with the lived experience of London women at midlife and the implications for Chinese medicine research. Maturitas 66, 408–416.

Scheid, V., Ward, T., Cha, W.S., Watanabe, K., Liao, X., 2010. The treatment of menopausal symptoms by traditional East Asian medicines: review and perspectives. Maturitas 66, 111–130.

Ward, T., Scheid, V., Tuffrey, V., 2010. Women's mid-life health experiences in urban UK: an international comparison. Climacteric 13 (3), 278–288.

FRAMING PROBLEMS: FROM THE SIMPLE TO THE COMPLEX

Hierarchies of knowledge like those that underpin Chinese medicine and EBM assume that there is a best way of knowing the world; that this way applies to all situations and contexts; and that applying such knowledge to the solution of practical problems guarantees maximum effectiveness. As argued above, such epistemic hierarchies are embedded in matching social and cultural hierarchies and thus resistant to change. Problems arise when different epistemological and social systems meet, or when the solutions they offer no longer match the problems they were designed to solve. Chinese medicine's focus on the individual and the subjectivity of knowing practice is unsuitable, for instance, for solving problems of social medicine that necessarily require a focus on populations. Conversely, EBM's focus on populations creates a bias towards framing medical problems in a manner amenable to population statistics that downplays the uniqueness of individual illness experience.

A non-hierarchical approach to knowledge management undercuts these assumptions by placing different approaches to problem solving on an equal footing. The Cynefin (pronounced /kʌnɨvɪn/) framework of sense-making, developed by Dave Snowden and Cynthia Kurtz on the basis of earlier work by the British anthropologist Mary Douglas, is a useful starting point for developing such an approach (Snowden & Boone 2007). It examines different potential operative contexts that exist within large complex organizations and our ability to make sense of them. To this end it posits five ideal typical domains, labeled Simple, Complicated, Complex, Chaotic, and Central (Fig. 2.1).

The domain of the Simple is characterized by the existence of well-known linear cause-and-effect relationships between agents in a system. As long as

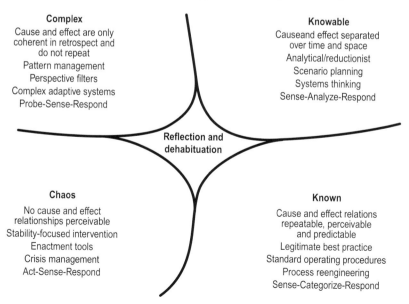

FIG. 2.1 Five ideal typical domains (Based on Kurtz, C. & Snowden, D. 2003, The New Dynamics of Strategy: Sense-making in a Complex-Complicated World, IBM Systems Journal, vol. 42, no. 3, pp. 462–83).

the system operates under given conditions, the same cause will invariably produce the same effect. Actions are therefore predictable, routine, highly transparent and can be organized by way of best-practice guidelines and standardized interventions. Such contexts of practice tend to be managed by way of hierarchical chains of command and the social status of most people in these systems is low given that they simply do what they are told to do.

The domain of the Complicated is equally characterized by the presence of linear cause-and-effect relationships, though here they are not immediately apparent and need to be identified first. Put another way, for any given problem a number of different solutions appear to be available and it requires expert knowledge to identify those that are applicable. Chinese medicine textbook practice, on which much current EBM research is based, would be a typical example of this domain. It is assumed that for each biomedically defined disease a limited number of manifestation types and associated treatments exist that can be matched to a given case by the expert knowledge of the Chinese medicine practitioner.

The domain of the Complex is defined by the presence of non-linear connections between agents within the system. How specific actions change the system is knowable but not as easily predictable as in the previous two domains. In fact, they often make sense only after events have occurred. Detailed knowledge about specific cause-and-effect chains here is less advantageous than understanding patterns that reflect how the system behaves and can be influenced as a whole. This is the domain explored by contemporary systems science, or by the pragmatic trials discussed by Claudia Witt and her co-authors in Chapter 8, and by Chinese physicians who attempt to relate surface manifestations to the coherence of the body/person as a whole.

The fourth domain is the Chaotic. Here, no cause-and-effect relationships of any kind can be discerned. In such contexts people tend to become fatalistic, relinquishing control of their actions to unknown and unknowable forces; or they proceed by way of trial and error, often at high risk, requiring courage and strong leadership. The Chaotic is therefore the domain of radical invention as well of sectarianism and irrational beliefs, where people frequently disengage actions from consequences.

The fifth domain, finally, is conceived of as a central space that connects to all the others but belongs to none. It allows for critique and reflection from where habituated patterns may be understood and changed.

It is assumed that all social organizations, systems and cultures contain within them all of these domains; if not actually, then at least potentially. For instance, although I have focused on scholarly Chinese medicine as being concerned with finding solutions to complex problems, there is also ample evidence for the use of specific herbs to treat specific symptoms (so called 'simples' or, in Chinese, *danyao* 單藥), and for physicians seeking to understand disease in reductionist terms as being due to specific causes (Unschuld 1987). Likewise, many biomedical physicians emphasize the art of medicine and the understanding of complex problems that cannot be expressed in simple algorithms as essential to what they do (Battista et al 1995). Yet, whatever specific similarities may exist across domains, situations and cultures, individual physicians as well as social systems also exhibit a bias to favor some solutions over others. It is such bias that allows us to demarcate Chinese medicine in late imperial China from modern TCM, or TCM from 21st century biomedicine practiced in a large modern hospital setting.

The tendency of systems towards such bias is reflected in the name of the Cynefin model, a Welsh word that can be roughly translated as "habitat," but also as "an adjective used to convey the meaning of 'acquainted' or 'familiar'." The notion of habitat implies that people have an innate tendency to revert to the domain of sense-making where they feel most comfortable. Taking a less individualistic stance we might say that the social systems have an inbuilt bias towards framing problems in ways that reflect the epistemological, economic and social biases that constitute that system. For instance, as an instrument of the industrialization of medicine EBM actively seeks to constitute medical practice as governed by best practice. Epistemologically, it is influenced by Platonic idealism and scientific reductionism. It is used by those who believe that complex problems can be reduced to simple ones because the world is made up of simple cause-and-effect chains between discrete agents or forms. Physicians in the scholarly Chinese medical tradition, on the other hand, but also biomedical physicians emphasizing the art of medicine or researchers working in the emerging field of systems biology, will tend to focus on medical problems as complexities requiring tailor-made responses. From a neutral perspective, each of these perspectives has advantages and is best at solving particular types of problem. They are also, however, exclusive of each other, and misidentification of problems of a particular type can lead to a waste of resources and to multiple negative consequences that may not be immediately apparent.

For instance, treating bacterial infections with antibiotics is based on the assumption that such infections constitute a simple problem that is amenable to simple solutions. A more complex assessment might include factors such as the environment in which bacteria live and the ability of bacteria as complex beings to adapt to changes in that environment. From this perspective simply killing bacteria might appear to be a misguided short-term solution to a larger and more complex problem that will inevitably lead to the emergence of antibiotic-resistant bacteria. Configuring complex problems such as criminal behavior, depression or obesity as simple problems amenable to solutions by genetic determinism is another example. Vice versa, viewing epidemic disorders as resulting from the relationship between complex individuals and complex weather patterns prevented elite physicians in late imperial China from adapting more simple models of contagion available in popular culture.

The Cynefin model therefore places a fifth domain at the centre of the grid on which the other domains are mapped. This central domain describes a space where, rather than habitually or systemically reverting to established ways of sense-making, it becomes possible to reflect on the pay-offs that result from viewing concrete problems in different ways. This is the domain of critique and debate: a somewhat idealized space given the power relationships that arise in any social system, but a space that can be occupied nevertheless. It is from the perspective of this space that we can reflect on the encounter between Chinese medicine and EBM and ask what are the real differences between generating best practices and cultivating best practitioners; whether realizing one must necessarily exclude the other; and how we might envisage the integration of scholarly Chinese medicine into contemporary healthcare as a dialogue between equals instead of enforcing apparently natural hierarchies of knowledge?

CHINESE MEDICAL MODERNIZATION REVISITED: SIX THESES

Rather than providing yet another set of prescriptive solutions to the problem of modernizing Chinese medicine the Cynefin model of sense-making, especially when it is accepted that sense-making always occurs in specific economic and cultural contexts, leads us to a conceptual reframing of objectives and processes. Throughout the last century it was widely assumed that modernization must lead to an inevitable curtailment of diversity and that the simplification of Chinese medicine's diagnostic and therapeutic instrumentarium is a precondition for improving its effectiveness. In other words, only when anything specifically 'Chinese' has been removed from Chinese medicine will it become truly effective medicine.

From the perspective of the Cynefin model this reductionist bias towards the simple is just that: bias, preference, habit. Biases, habits and preferences, however, can always be changed. For the world is not 'either/or' but contains both the simple and the complex and even more besides. Defining clinical problems is not an objective mapping of the world but a way of making sense in order to orient what we believe to be effective agency. Such definitions may be more or less suitable to the problem at hand. Treating problems in one way rather than another will have some advantages but also comes with both intended and unintended consequences. The Cynefin model of knowledge management does not treat the existence of different options as a problem but as a resource. Instead of following habitual pathways of problem solving it asks us to occupy the central space of potentiality whenever something does not work, no longer works as intended, or when we are faced with an entirely new problem. Treating the modernization of Chinese medicine as such a problem allows me to propose six theses intended to function as starting points for a possible re-evaluation of this process in light of the wider aims outlined above.

First, seeking to optimize healthcare by focusing on the development of best practices rather than cultivating best practitioners, or vice versa, reflects choices: about how we perceive the world and about how we want to live in it. It does not reflect a better understanding of the world per se. In general such choices are not made on a case-by-case basis. More often they gather together into self-authenticating styles of reasoning and problem solving. These in turn, are embedded in institutions that over time become traditions defining but also limiting horizons of inquiry. Changing course with regard to the modernization of Chinese medicine is therefore not an easy undertaking for it involves transforming more than just ideas. Many interests are invested in the establishment and maintenance of traditions and these are likely to resist change. Nevertheless, especially because the term 'science' is consistently mobilized in order to steer Chinese medical modernization into specific directions, those doing so need to be reminded equally persistently that science is an open-ended process of inquiry that is not tied to any one method of viewing and solving problems.

Second, in making the choices outlined above it will be useful to view this process as one of knowledge and healthcare management rather than one geared to distinguishing between what is true and false. Such a shift in orientation creates a space in which we can reflect on how different problem-solving strategies may best be matched to the nature of different problems at hand. Taking Chinese medicine itself as an example, physicians have long distinguished between the need to deal differently with the root (*ben* 本) and manifestations (*biao* 標) of a disorder. Although both are of necessity linked to each other, physicians need to decide whether to first attend to the manifestations or to the root, or perhaps to both at the same time. Attending to the manifestations may require symptomatic treatment aimed at simple cause-and-effect chains that pays scarce attention to complex individual difference. Treating the root effectively, on the other hand, may be impossible unless the complexities of such difference are taken fully into account. Similar distinctions apply when making choices between treatment aimed at the individual person and clinical decision-making based on aggregate populations, be that the allocation of societal resources or deciding on how to combine these in actual clinical practice.

Third, honesty and transparency constitute essential aspects of effective knowledge management. For instance, Chinese medicine may offer a range of simple solutions to simple problems that have not yet been realized within the development of the Chinese medical tradition. These might include the use of specific acupuncture points for specific symptoms, or the use of single herbs or the chemical constituents of herbal medicines for the treatment of biomedically defined diseases. However, the methods currently used for extracting these need to be acknowledged as a form of bioprospecting that is likely to have no regard for the integrity or survival of the Chinese medical tradition. Likewise, simplifying Chinese medical interventions for the purposes of EBM evaluation while simultaneously selling these approaches to consumers, funding bodies and fellow researchers as embodying authentic Chinese medicine validated by 2000 years of clinical experience is simply not true and disables critical debate and reflection. This means that assumptions and claims by researchers or practitioners regarding the objects of their research or the practices they claim to represent need to be subjected to the same critical scrutiny we would routinely apply to the methods or results section of a clinical study. Given that the professional expertise to do so will be found not among clinicians or clinical researchers but among historians, anthropologists and other science study experts, it is crucial to redesign current research efforts along broader and more comprehensive interdisciplinary lines.

Fourth, viewed from a knowledge management perspective the real potential of scholarly Chinese medicine may lie not in its medicines and formulae but in the capacity of its practitioners to understand complex and even chaotic problems and to formulate possible pathways to resolve them. This claim resonates with that of Chinese physicians themselves who repeatedly remind us that the ultimate source of clinical effectiveness is located not in herbs or acupuncture needles but in the insights and skills of the individual practitioner. Not surprisingly given this bias the Chinese medical tradition developed specific technologies to foster the development of such skills. These include practiced-based learning and thinking in cases; the reliance on polysemic concepts such as *qi* that, precisely because they are exceedingly difficult to capture in a single English word, allow flexibility in practice; of an approach to diagnosis and treatment that consistently demands to switch between different perspectives without the expectation that these perspectives will ultimately come together in a single picture or 'theory'; and of an acceptance that explicit verbal knowledge may limit our ability to grasp the coherence of complex phenomena. Because such insights apply to all kinds of complex situations, the dividing lines between medicine, statecraft and art in traditional Chinese culture were not rigidly drawn. There exists no reason, therefore, to limit them to specific medical disciplines. It could be imagined, for instance, that the ability of Chinese medicine physicians to detect patterns might also guide the prescribing practices of pattern-based treatment using biomedical drugs, especially as biomedical practice itself is moving in the direction of polypharmacy and multiple combined interventions. At the same time, emergent technologies in the biosciences and statistics may facilitate the definition of patterns in a more objective manner than Chinese medicine – relying solely on the ability of humans to detect complex relationship patterns through a combination of cognition and feelings – has so far been able to do.

Fifth, Chinese medicine and the wider East Asian medical tradition constitute complex practices that contain within themselves different approaches and biases with respect to managing knowledge and solving clinical problems. For instance, Japanese physicians during the Edo period rebelled against the many subjective biases inherent in the Chinese medical tradition. They replaced these biases with an evidence-based approach that focused on direct observation, yet one that perceived such observation not as a recording of objective facts but of making fine discriminations in the process of a body-centred differential diagnosis. Greater attention to such difference and their relation to specific historical contexts of emergence will contribute to our ability to develop strategies for effectively adopting East Asian medicines to current contexts of practice.

Sixth, modernizing Chinese and East Asian medicine viewed from the knowledge management perspective I have outlined here is intrinsically ecological in orientation. Effective knowledge management demands the preservation and cultivation of the foundations of such practice in the same way as the preservation of biodiversity increases our own chances of survival. It is thus intrinsically opposed to viewing such traditions as nothing but resources of raw materials – be they knowledge, techniques or medicinals – to be mined without regard for their own integrity. As Laurent Pordié's vignette on best practitioners of Tibetan medicine in rural Ladakh vividly demonstrates, traditional medical practices already constitute attempts to combine within them the various problem-solving strategies that the Cynefin model of sense-making separates (see Vignette 2.3). Similar claims could be made for elite Chinese medicine or Korean medicine in the late imperial eras. In that sense, any attempts to break apart such forms of practice, whether by means of bureaucratically driven efforts at standardization or by seeking to reduce traditions analytically to stable types, carry within them seeds of destruction as well as of development.

VIGNETTE 2.3   IDEAL QUALITIES AND THEIR RELIGIOUS MATRIX: BEST PRACTITIONERS OF TIBETAN MEDICINE IN RURAL LADAKH
LAURENT PORDIÉ

2

In the Himalayan region of Ladakh, the rural practitioners of Tibetan medicine, or *amchi*, divide their time between agricultural or pastoral works and the practice of medicine. Most of their activity in this domain includes learning the traditional medical theory, supplying themselves with medicinal materials, making medicines and treating patients. The *amchi* emphasize that a good practitioner should be equally knowledgeable in the practice of pharmacy and that of medicine. He or she should show perfect mastery of medical and pharmacological theory, and of clinical and pharmaceutical practice. This underlies most claims of therapeutic efficacy. This is why the specialization found today in urban, institutional settings is said to undermine the practice of Tibetan medicine as a whole, for it alters or reduces the knowledge of the ideal therapist.

Like most Tibetan erudite forms of knowledge and practices, however, medicine (the 'science of healing,' *gso ba rig pa*) unfolds on different registers, which include Buddhism (the 'interior science,' *nang gi rig gnas*). The practitioners call our attention to these overlapping registers when they evoke the moral dimension in the act of healing, a dimension that is expressly a matter of Buddhism. Besides theoretical, clinical and pharmaceutical considerations, what essentially makes a good *amchi*, they assert, is his or her adherence to the religious doctrine and the practice of Buddhist ritual. This is meant to improve their medical practice and more broadly the fate of each of them.

The *amchi* reveal an entire series of behavioral and moral codes that, ideally, they should follow. The 'qualities' most often mentioned, based on a sample of more than 90 *amchi*, are compassion, respect for living beings, honesty and generosity. They also hold that assistance, generosity, an open smile and candid words are very important. The development of altruistic qualities also occupies a central place and enhances, perhaps more than the rest, the healing power of the therapist. In Mahayana Buddhism, altruism is a notion that involves oneself and others and has a twofold function of creation of social relations and of universal solidarity, leading to the salvation of sentient beings. The practice of medicine enables the practitioner to develop compassion. A limited number of practitioners mention the obligation to follow the ideal of the bodhisattva (being oriented toward Enlightenment), which many found rather presumptuous.

The practitioners in rural Ladakh often cite the rare passages alluding to the strictly Buddhist domain that are to be found in the canonical medical text the *Rgyud bzhi*, above all in the introduction and in the section concerned with the ideal qualities of the therapist in Chapter 31 of the explanatory treatise (*Bshad-pa'i rgyud*). In this text, the ideal physician 'must fulfill the 'six basic requirements' [*rgyu*]: to possess vast knowledge, to present a spirit of bodhisattva and devotion to the good of all creatures, to be sustained by bonds of consecration, to possess a certain adroitness of body, speech and mind, to be assiduous in one's task and to conform to the customs of this world (*mi chos*) while practising the Noble Religious Law.' The *Gyiconshi* also recommends endeavoring to abstain oneself from the ten negative actions: killing, stealing, sexual misconduct, speaking lies, involvement in idle gossip, speaking harsh words, speaking with the risk of sowing discord, covetousness, malicious thinking and wrong views. The *amchi* know this part of the text and recite it almost identically when they wish to mention the *ideal qualities* of the therapist. This centuries-old text has considerable repercussions on today's therapists. It marks out their medical practice, shapes their ideal type and, to a lesser extent, their daily religious practice.

OUTLOOK AND CONCLUSION

How to integrate East Asian medical traditions into modern healthcare systems is a complex problem that defies simple 'one size fits all' solutions. The knowledge management perspective advocated in this chapter establishes one possible framework for handling such complexity by creating a space where different options can be discussed and evaluated. Showing up intrinsic biases not only guides critical reflection regarding existing solutions but actively encourages us to explore different ones.

Vignette 2.2 on 'Researching East Asian Medicine in the Treatment of Menopausal Symptoms' demonstrates the practical utility of applying this perspective to a specific research problem. Many other research projects already pursue similar paths. The 'whole systems research' movement emanating from the United States, which is now actively integrated into research in the domain of East Asian medicines, is one example. The emerging interface between systems biology, which itself aims at a fundamental transformation of biomedicine, and East Asian medicines owing to a mutual interest in personalized medicine and complex interventions is another. It should be clear, however, that none of these solutions is ideal, and – as also highlighted by Sean Lei in the conclusion to Chapter 7 – that every effort at change will by definition destroy something else. As shown especially by the authors of Chapters 11, 12 and 13, this means that seeking to preserve the authenticity of traditional practices fails to understand the fluid nature of living traditions. We should therefore subject all claims made by those participating in the ongoing transformation of East Asian medical practice to scrutiny and not accept anything as necessarily and invariably given.

I therefore suggest that only interdisciplinary research drawing on the humanities as well as on the social and natural sciences is able to ensure that complex problems are treated as such without in any way hindering the search for effective and sometimes simple solutions. For reasons that emerge from all of the various chapters of this book, bringing critical historical and cultural scholarship to bear on such issues does not merely add another inconvenience to an already difficult process. It is essential in order to disentangle the intermingling of nature, culture and politics in medicine that any knowledge management perspective takes for granted.

Adams, V., 2002a. Randomized controlled crime: postcolonial sciences in alternative medicine research. Soc. Stud. Sci. 32 (5/6), 659–690.

Adams, V., 2002b. Establishing proof: translating science and the state in Tibetan medicine. In: Nichter, M., Lock, M. (Eds.), New Horizons in Medical Anthropology: Essays in Honour of Charles Leslie. Routledge, New York.

Andrews, B.J., 1996. The Making of Modern Chinese Medicine. 1895–1937. Ph.D., History of Medicine, Cambridge.

Armstrong, D., 2002. Clinical autonomy, individual and collective: the problem of changing doctors' behaviour. Soc. Sci. Med. 55 (10), 1771–1777.

Armstrong, D., 2007. Professionalism, indeterminacy, and the EBM project. Biosocieties 2, 73–84.

Barry, C., 2006. The role of evidence in alternative medicine: contrasting biomedical and anthropological approaches. Soc. Sci. Med. 62 (11), 2646–2657.

Battista, R.N., Hodge, M.J., Vineis, P., 1995. Medicine, practice and guidelines: the uneasy juncture of science and art. J. Clin. Epidemiol. 48 (7), 875–880.

Berg, M., 1995. Turning a practice into a science: reconceptualizing postwar medical practice. Soc. Stud. Sci. 25 (3), 437–476.

Buetow, S., 2002. Beyond evidence-based medicine: bridge-building a medicine of meaning. J. Eval. Clin. Pract. 8 (2), 103–108.

Chen, L.L., Lin, J.S., Lin, J.D., et al., 2009. BCQ+: a body constitution questionnaire to assess Yang-Xu. Part II: Evaluation of reliability and validity. Forsch. Komplementmed. 16 (1), 20–27.

Discussion Group for Standards for Disease Names and Diagnostic Categories in Chinese Medicine 中醫病名診斷規範課題組, 1987. Standards for Disease Names and Diagnostic Categories in Chinese Medicine: A First Draft 中醫病名診斷規範初稿. Hubeisheng zhongyiyao yanjiusuo 湖北省中醫藥研究所, Zhengzhuang.

Fan, R.P., 2003. Modern Western science as a standard for traditional Chinese medicine: a critical appraisal. J. Law Med. Ethics 31, 213–221.

Farquhar, J., 1994a. Knowing Practice: The Clinical Encounter in Chinese Medicine, Studies in the Ethnographic Imagination. Westview Press, Boulder.

Farquhar, J., 1994b. Multiplicity, point of view, and responsibility in traditional Chinese healing. In: Zito, A., Barlow, T.E. (Eds.), Body, Subject and Power in China. University of Chicago Press, Chicago, IL.

Fei Boxiong 費伯雄, 1863. Refined medicine remembered 醫醇剩義. In: Zhang Yuankai 張元凱, (Ed.), The Collected Medical Texts of the Four Menghe Medical Families 孟河四家醫集.

Feinstein, A.R., 1994. 'Clinical Judgment' revisited: the distraction of quantitative models. Ann. Intern. Med. 120 (9), 799–805.

Flower, A., Lewith, G.T., Little, P., 2007. Seeking an oracle: using the Delphi process to develop practice guidelines for the treatment of endometriosis with Chinese herbal medicine. J. Altern. Complement. Med. 13 (9), 969–976.

Forrester, J., 1996. If p, then what? Thinking in cases. Hist. Human Sci. 9 (1), 1–25.

Graham, A.C., 1989. Disputers of the Tao: Philosophical Argument in Ancient China. Open Court, La Salle, Ill, p. 501.

Jullien, F., 1995. The Propensity of Things: Toward a History of Efficacy in China. Zone Books, New York.

Karchmer, E.I., 2004. Orientalizing the Body: Postcolonial Transformations in Chinese Medicine, Anthropology. University of North Carolina, Chapel Hill.

Lei, S.H., 1998. When Chinese Medicine Encountered the State: 1910–1949. Ph.D., University of Chicago, Chicago.

Li, N.Y., Abbott, K.V., Rosen, C., et al., 2010. Translational systems biology and voice pathophysiology. Laryngoscope 120 (3), 511–515.

Liang Shuming 梁漱溟, 1921 [2002]. Eastern and Western Cultures and Their Philosophies 東西文化及其哲學. Taiwan shangwu 台灣商務, Taibei.

Liao Yuqun 療育群, 2006. Medicine is yi 醫者意也. Guangxi shiyuan daxue chubanshe, Guilin.

Lihong 劉力紅, Liu, 2006. Sikao zhongyi 思考中醫, third ed. Guanxi shifan daxue chubanshi, Guilin.

McHugh, M.F., 1992. China Mountain Zhang, first ed. Tom Doherty Associates, New York.

Niu, C.Y., 2005. Program on international standardization of traditional Chinese medicine nomenclature has been started. Zhong Xi Yi Jie He Xue Bao 3 (1), 79–82.

Parker, M., 2005. False dichotomies: EBM, clinical freedom, and the art of medicine. Med. Humanit. 31 (1), 23–30.

Qin Bowei 秦伯未, 1957 [1983]. A preliminary discussion of pattern differentiation and treatment determination 淺談辨證論治. In: Wu Dazhen 吳大真, Wang, Fengqi 王鳳岐 (Eds.), A Collection of Essays on Medicine by Qin Bowei 秦伯未醫文集. Hunan kexue jishu chubanshe, Changsha.

Rees, J.L., 2008. Evidence and the industrialization of medicine. Clin. Exp. Dermatol. 33 (4), 390–393.

Rodwin, M.A., 2001. The politics of evidence-based medicine. J. Health Polit. Policy Law 26 (2), 439–446.

Runo, A., 1998. Towards an evidence based health care management. Int. J. Health Plann. Manage. 13 (4), 307–317.

Ryu, H., Lee, H., Kim, H., et al., 2010. Reliability and validity of a cold-heat pattern questionnaire for traditional Chinese medicine. J. Altern. Complement. Med. 16 (6), 663–667.

Sackett, D.L., Rosenberg, W.M., 1995. On the need for evidence-based medicine. J. Public Health Med. 17 (3), 330–334.

Scheid, V., 2002a. Chinese Medicine in Contemporary China: Plurality and Synthesis. Duke University Press, Durham.

Scheid, V., 2002b. Remodeling the arsenal of Chinese medicine: shared pasts, alternative futures. Ann. Am. Social Assoc. Global Perspect. Complement. Altern. Med. (September), 136–159.

Scheid, V., 2007. Currents of Tradition in Chinese Medicine, 1626–2006. Eastland Press, Seattle.

Schnyer, R.N., Conboy, L.A., Jacobson, E., et al., 2005. Development of a Chinese medicine assessment measure: an interdisciplinary approach using the delphi method. J. Altern. Complement. Med. 11 (6), 1005–1013.

Shea, J.L., 2006. Applying evidence-based medicine to traditional Chinese medicine: debate and strategy. J. Altern. Complement. Med. 12 (3), 255–263.

Sivin, N., 1987. Traditional medicine in contemporary China. In: Sivin, N. (Ed.), Science, Medicine and Technology in East Asia. The University of Michigan Centre for Chinese Studies, Ann Arbor.

Snowden, D.E., Boone, M.E., 2007. A leader's framework for decision making. Harv. Bus. Rev. (November).

Stengers, I., 2004. The challenge of complexity: unfolding the ethics of science. In Memoriam Ilya Prigogine. Emerg. Complexity Organ. 6 (1–2), 92–99.

Su, Y.C., Chen, L.L., Lin, J.D., et al., 2008. BCQ+: a body constitution questionnaire to assess Yang-Xu. Part I: establishment of a first final version through a Delphi process. Forsch. Komplementmed. 15 (6), 327–334.

Sun Simiao 孫思邈. compl. 650/659. Prescriptions Worth a Thousand Pieces of Gold Beiji qianjin yaofang 備急千金要方. (Critically annotated ed., Li Jingrong 李景榮, Ed.). Renmin weisheng chubanshe, Beijing.

Taylor, K., 2005. Chinese medicine in early communist China, 1945–63: a medicine of revolution. (Vol. Needham Research Institute studies). RoutledgeCurzon, London, New York.

Tillman, H.C., 1978. The idea and the reality of the 'thing' during the Sung: philosophical attitudes toward wu. Bull. Sung Yuan Stud. 14, 68–82.

Unschuld, P.U., 1979. Medical Ethics in Imperial China: A Study in Historical Anthropology. University of California Press, Berkeley.

Unschuld, P.U., 1987. Traditional Chinese medicine: some historical and epistemological reflections. Soc. Sci. Med. 24, 1023–1029.

Volkmar, B., 2006. Die Fallgeschichten des Arztes Wan Quan (1500–1585?). Medizinisches Denken und Handeln der Ming-Zeit. Urban & Fischer Bei Elsevier.

Wahlberg, A., McGoey, L., 2007. An elusive evidence base: the construction and governance of randomized controlled trials. BioSocieties 2 (01), 1.

Wennberg, J., Gittelsohn, 1973. Small area variations in health care delivery. Science 182 (117), 1102–1108.

Xu, W., Towers, A.D., Li, P., Collet, J.P., 2006. Traditional Chinese medicine in cancer care: perspectives and experiences of patients and professionals in China. Eur. J. Cancer Care (Engl.) 15 (4), 397–403.

Zhao Xuemin 趙學敏, 1998. 18th century Connecting Elegance: Core Section 串雅內編. Zhongguo zhongyiyao chubanshe 中國中醫藥出版社, Beijing.

Zhonghua renmin gongheguo biaozhun 中華人民共和國標準, 1994. Standards for Diagnosis and Therapeutic Effect of Diseases and Syndromes in Traditional Chinese Medicine 中醫病證診斷療效標準. Zhongguo bioazhun chubanshe, Beijing. Document ZY/T001–94.

Zhonghua renmin gongheguo biaozhun 中華人民共和國標準, 1995. Classification and Codes of Diseases and Pattern of Traditional Chinese Medicine 中醫病證分類與代碼. Zhongguo bioazhun chubanshe, Beijing. Document GB/T15657–1995.

Zhu Chenyu 祝諶予, (Ed.), 1982. The Collected Clinical Experience of Shi Jinmo 施今墨臨床經驗集. Renmin weisheng chubanshe 人民衛生出版社, Beijing.

Defining best practice or cultivating best practitioners

Pulse-touching: qualities and the best practitioner

3

Judith Farquhar

Picture a Chinese medical clinic. Each patient in turn sits down at a corner of the doctor's desk, hands over his case record booklet and registration number for the day, and offers his hand, inner side of wrist up, on the small pillow provided. The doctor places the tips of his first three fingers close together on the patient's wrist, just below the thumb and on the proximal side of the wrist bone. This may be done while some preliminary questions are asked, or the practitioner may remain silent for the several minutes it takes to palpate three points on the wrist at two depths (shallow and deep).[1] Before proceeding much further, he or she will have looked at the patient's tongue, focusing on its colors and the characteristics of its coating, and asked some questions about symptoms and history. Writing in the patient's case record booklet, his or her observations are expressed in a mostly conventional language.

Add to this picture another image: down the hall in the hospital a mechanical pulsometer sits, gathering dust in a storeroom. It may be occasionally brought out to play a role in a randomized controlled clinical trial that aims to 'objectively' evaluate Chinese medical diagnosis and treatment. And perhaps several decades ago it was heavily used even in the clinic, when seeing patients. This scene of technology use in scientific research is, and was, part of a Chinese effort to practice evidence-based medicine and contribute good data for the international dialogue on 'best practices' in medicine.

However, global participation in the establishment of best practices does not require 'high-tech' pulsometers. 'Traditional' pulse-taking too can claim scientific rigor and global reach. The classic technique in which doctor touches patient is part of a global complementary and alternative medicine movement whose advocates often invoke values such as 'experience', 'embodied knowledge', 'medical art' or 'clinical craft,' even – among the more traditional – 'wisdom' or 'virtuosity.'[2] In deploying these terms, and insisting on a touching diagnostics in which the bodily qualities of doctor and patient resonate together, traditionalists think of themselves not as operators of technologically proven best practice, but as embodiments of good medicine: as best practitioners.

---

[1] As will be noted throughout this discussion, the techniques of pulse examination are the subject of much debate among specialists, both in the present institutions of Chinese medicine and at many times in the long history of the field. Here I develop one very common model, that of 'the 28 *maixiang*', to make a more general anthropological point, one that should be valid no matter which pulse-examination system a practitioner subscribes to.

[2] For a discussion that illustrates these kinds of usages, see Zhan 2009: 63-88 .

In this chapter, then, I explore in greater depth the focus on 'best practitioner' as opposed to that of 'best practices' in an effort to extend the theme introduced in Chapter 2. The pulsometer is here only an entry point for the deeper problem of shared standards and judgments in medicine, traditional or otherwise. Practitioners and scholars alike know that Chinese medicine has offered considerable resistance to standardization in research or clinical protocols; there are always potential or actual disagreements over the most authentic methods, the proper diagnosis and the optimal treatment strategy. Not only do we need to ask how much room there is for variable clinical judgment in responsible medicine; not only do we seek to retain a fully human form of judgment to supplement the machine functions of diagnostic and therapeutic technologies; we also need to better understand the foundations of medical judgment and knowledge themselves. The discussion that follows, then, seeks such a foundation in the embodied perceptiveness of pulse-touching, understood as an engagement with qualities.

The traditional pulse examination in Chinese medicine is thoroughly embodied. It is a lingering, attentive, signifying *touch* of one person's fingers to the wrists of another; it is a connection made for a few minutes between two living states of qi-transformation,[3] the patient's body expressing a condition to the responsive attentiveness of the doctor's body. Do electronic pulsometers, with their sensitive pressure sensors and complex inscribed waveforms, model the perceptions of a doctor's fingers? Do all doctors respond identically to 'the same' pulsings on the wrists of patients?[4] Pulsometers report their results both as a unique waveform and as a qualisign, a pulse image or condition [*maixiang* 脉象], of which more below. Vignette 3.1, 'Qualities, Qualia, and Qualisigns: The Case of Softer Soju in South Korea,' by linguistic anthropologist Nicholas Harkness, explains the appeal of qualisigns for understanding pulse conditions. Pulsometers may even offer a more nuanced, more qualitative picture than that achieved by doctors. Ultimately, embodied and electronic–mechanical perceptions are not so different. In the case of pulse-touching diagnosis, both sort variation at the body's surface into standardized pigeonholes known (at least in modern textbooks) as the 28 pulse conditions.[5] The sensors provide information in *quantitative* form about motion in time,

---

[3] Qi transformation (*qihua* 气化) is a term that names the most general process of human physiological activity; as a concept it has proved useful in some of the philosophical and 'theoretical foundations' writing of Chinese medicine in China, especially to link natural processes of genesis and development with bodily processes such as metabolism. See, for example, Yin and Zhang 1989: 144–145; Huang et al. 1988: 42–44.

[4] In the early 1980s I studied a clinic in Guangzhou for a few days where a pulsometer was being pitted against the fingers and senses of the senior doctor who anchored this 'rheumatic diseases' (*fengshi bing* 风湿病) clinic. Several evaluations were being conducted at once. The findings of the machine were being calibrated to match more closely the judgments of the doctor. And the pulsometer, after collecting these comparisons at this station, was soon to move on to another clinic and another senior doctor to check how well the two doctors matched up, with the machine as a kind of arbiter (but one that was always in need of more subtle calibration). After this research project was over the senior clinicians did not return to working alongside a pulsometer. According to my interviews at the time, no-one expected the doctors to fully agree, and they wondered how the pulsometer could achieve reliable consistency in the long term.

[5] As practitioners will recognize, all 28 standard modern pulse conditions are seldom if ever all used by any one practitioner, and in each case only a few non-normal pulse conditions are noted for the case record. Moreover, though in theory any of the available pulse conditions could be discerned at any of the positions palpated (see below), usually only one or two wrist positions (or all at once) show a pulse condition of clinical interest.

For the past decade or so, people in South Korea have become increasingly concerned with the softness of their soju. Advertisements for, and reported experiences of, this clear spirit focus on the various qualitative dimensions through which this valued softness can be felt. The lowered alcohol content (currently 19.8%, down from as high as 30% in the 1980s) is understood to produce a softer taste, a softer sensation on the throat, softer sonic reactions to consumption, a softer feeling of inebriation, a softer mood among friends and colleagues, and softer embodiments of both masculine and feminine personhood. But how can the quality of softness be present in all of these different dimensions? Can the quality of a single substance really be experienced through all of these different modalities? Is the softness of one really the same as the softness of another? To clarify this seeming transitivity of quality across different sensory and embodied dimensions, I turn to the semiotician Charles S. Peirce's distinction among *qualities*, *qualia*, and *qualisigns* (1998 [1903]).

Part of Peirce's project was, as John Dewey (1935) put it, to consider 'the matter of experience as experienced' and to give 'a logical analysis of experience.' To develop a semiotic theory that would account for the richness of experience, Peirce (1997[1897], 2.228) defined the sign simply as 'something which stands to somebody for something in some respect or capacity.' Since, within this definition, all experience potentially stands for something, Peirce outlined three basic categories to structure his analytic framework. *Firstness* refers to the category of feeling and indeterminacy, 'not referring to anything nor lying behind anything' (i.e., a monadic state, a *ground*; Peirce 1997[1890], 1.356–357). *Secondness* refers to the category of response, resistance, instantiation, or event (i.e., a dyadic *relation* where something stands for something else by means of a ground). And *Thirdness* refers to the category of convention, mediation, and habit (i.e., a third position, an *interpretant*, which interprets and regiments the ground of dyadic standing-for relations). In the flow of experience, different dimensions of this trichotomy are accentuated and combined in different ways and at various levels of complexity (see Parmentier 1994, Keane 2003, Kockelman 2005, 2006).

According to Peirce (1997[1896], 1:422), quality belongs to the category of firstness; it is 'a mere abstract potentiality', not dependent on the mind, on some material entity, or on the senses. Qualitative experience, however, is made up of what Peirce termed *qualia*, the instantiations of quality that are inflected by and related to thought, materiality, sensory channels, etc. Whereas quality itself belongs to the realm of firstness, qualia as 'facts of firstness' (Peirce 1998[1903]) are more complex. They are instances, i.e., secondnesses, that stand for quality in two ways: *iconically* (by seeming to exhibit some quality), and *indexically* (by suggesting a contiguity with some quality). In this way, the abstraction of qualities is experienced and known through particular qualia (e.g., abstract redness versus the redness of a particular apple).

If, however, as Peirce wrote, 'the pure indescribable *quale* [singular of qualia]…is gone in the twinkling of an eye and…bears no resemblance to any memory of it' Peirce 1998[1903], how can a person perceive two qualia as instances of the same quality? How can contemporary soju drinkers associate a reduced burning feeling in the throat and a lighter feeling of drunkenness with the same quality of softness? How is this qualitative 'sameness' achieved? This manner of inference obtains through the regimentation of qualic relations, i.e., through habituation and representation as forms of thirdness in different contexts and at various scales. Insofar as a sign points to both an object and an interpretant, then qualia which 'stand to somebody for something in some respect or capacity' are termed 'qualisigns.' Qualisigns are not symbols representing qualities (e.g., the word 'red'), but rather are qualia serving as signs.

My interpretation of the qualisign is more complex than the well-known example of a paint chip, where the particular combination of hue, saturation, brightness, and gloss as qualia of color serve to signify a more general quality of a color. In this example, 'color' serves as a category of explicitly coded quality. Although the qualisign is necessarily an icon (Peirce 1997[1897], 2.254), the nature of qualitative iconicity in the realm of 'feeling' is not always so straightforward. For one person, a dull feeling of pain in the elbow might signal the first stages of arthritis. For another person, such a pain might signal nefarious witchcraft. For a third, such pain might reinforce an overall experience of painfulness. Or it could signal all three. The issue is whether some aspect of the signifying quale is also projected onto its object, e.g., whether painfulness and witchcraft (or even the redness of an apple and its ripeness) are understood to have a qualitative similarity or some shared essence within a cultural system, or merely to have an indexical relation of causality or contiguity.

In general, cultural convention and institutionalized practice turn elements of qualitative experience into meaningful signs which people rely on to interpret and engage with their world. Thus, we can begin to see how the different qualia of soju consumption in contemporary Korea can serve as culturally meaningful qualisigns of value (Munn 1986), which signal the valorized quality of softness that has emerged in recent decades as an abstract point of cultural orientation. Then the larger cultural question becomes: 'Why softness?'

distributed across the small space of the wrist: split seconds, pulses per minute, mapped, averaged and classified at three points and two depths on each of the two wrists. This is a great deal of information; its very richness demands a quantitative metrics that can limit the available qualities, find signal in noise. Such a metric is provided by the 28 official pulse conditions, which, in theory at least, offer a system of discrete categories by means of which pulses can be distinguished, named, and correlated with illness patterns in a diagnostic process. And the scientized version of Chinese Medicine adopted for medical schools has produced agreement, among textbook authors at least, that the pulsometer 'senses' the conditions in an authoritative way.

Despite this, the pulsometer has not become a common labor-saving device in Chinese medical clinics. Most Chinese doctors feel that they are better at pulse-touching than the pulsometer is, precisely because they know a significant quality when they feel one; perhaps they also feel that medical significance is both simpler and more complicated than the pulsometer can 'know.' As I will show with analysis of a published case, below, even the many diagnostic distinctions offered by the 28 pulse conditions are not nuanced enough for doctors. They insist on the role of *qualitative* insight in clinical work. They demonstrate, with their case-by-case action, that only a practitioner can know and show what practices are best in each circumstance. Part of what makes a best practitioner, in their view, is a sensitivity to qualities (and a way of using qualisigns) that exceeds and trivializes all mechanical quantity. It is this movement between quantitative or classificatory knowledge and qualitative or evaluative judgment that I will explore.

Anthropologists have long realized that evaluation is not a simple process. Contemporary working Chinese doctors have many tools for clinical evaluation. They are experienced in recognizing meaningful signs from unbroken continua of experience and expression. Their perceptions in pulse-touching may seem ineffable, but they are nevertheless conveyed somehow to apprentices, interns, and even college students – year after year, generation after generation. Standard modes of classifying perceptions help greatly in making it possible to share clinical understanding, and to make respectable judgments about the meaning of illness expressions. But the final diagnostic and therapeutic *value* of qualitative perceptions cannot be comprehended by classifications. The relative value of the 28 pulse condition qualisigns – each significant in contrast to (say) 27 others in the system – is not immediately or automatically linked to questions of social, moral, or even therapeutic value. The pulse conditions do not divide 'naturally' into indices of the normal and pathological, the well and the sick. In effect, clinicians read *from* their skilled perception of pulse qualities *to* a wise judgment about pathophysiological states of play in whole bodies. This reading toward an evaluation is done one 'case' at a time, and it also draws on observations beyond those of pulses. Classification with systems of diagnostic terms helps practitioners reach an evaluation, but it cannot guarantee the whole journey. A system of qualisigns in medicine does not sort out the normal from the pathological, the wholesome from the malignant in itself. Rather, the healing ethic that knows and seeks the good for every patient is always crafted by the practitioner from a continuous flow of qualities.

PULSE CONDITIONS AS QUALISIGNS

To show how therapeutic value is made from semiotic value, that is, from the reading and interpretation of surface signs, as well as to demonstrate the dependence of semiotic value on qualities beyond all classification, we need first to understand at least one system of pulse terms: what are the 28 pulse conditions now commonly taught in Chinese medicine? Increasingly, medical school textbooks express pulse conditions in either a very neutral language of abstract space and time (shallow/deep, fast/slow) or with reference to wave amplitudes reported in earlier pulsometer research. But students do not learn to take pulses from machines, they learn at the side of their clinical mentors, more senior doctors. The ability to discern and name 28 different pulse conditions is gained first as students practice pulse-touching on each other, and then, more effectively, as teaching doctors make interning students follow their lead in touching patients, day after day, week after week, in crowded clinics.

Perhaps the easiest discrimination to make in pulse-touching is like the familiar pulse rate of biomedical tradition. To determine whether pulse is 'rapid' (*shu* 数) or 'slow' (*chi* 迟) – two of the 28 pulse conditions – doctors count the pulses of patients against their own breathing. This is the classic method, although textbooks now express this rate in terms of pulses per second of abstract clock time. But it is still rare to see a Chinese medical clinician consult his watch while touching a patient's wrist.[6] Since it is qi and its forceful flow that is being perceived, and qi is inseparable from breath (or wind) and blood (or water), in both physiology and cosmology, the comparing of the doctor's respiratory inhaling and exhaling to the patient's circulatory diastole and systole is easy to see as a kind of shared bodiliness across a difference. Five or more leaps of (a certain configuration of) qi to the surface (of the touched) per ten breaths (of the toucher) is a rapid pulse, three or less is a slow pulse. But it is the word rapid or slow that is written down in the case record, not the pulse count: a qualisign, not a number or a rate. Interesting, too – and quite difficult to grasp for most who have never studied pulse diagnosis – is that a pulse may be rapid at one of the six pulse positions of the wrist described in more detail below but not on any of the others

However, counting breaths and pulses is only the beginning; discerning the qualities, shapes, or complex tempos of pulsing is a skill. There are, however, two main system conveniences that make pulse-touching possible to learn and practice: one is a partial set of contrasts between pulse conditions, and the other is a small collection of mnemonics. The system of contrasts, first, organizes some of the 28 pulses relative to each other (Box 3.1).

Thus, a floating pulse – detectable on light pressure but disappearing when pressed more strongly – is easily distinguished from a sunken pulse, which only presents itself to greater finger pressure. Surging – described as 'like the onrush of a flood' – offers a direct contrast to fine pulse, described as 'fine as a thread, onset not replete.' Contrastive pairs like these make sense of ten pulse conditions (i.e., there are five conventional sets). The rest, less distinct by virtue of being less directly contrasted with one other term, are pulse conditions such as 'string-like' (*xian* 弦), 'weak' (*ruo* 弱), 'scallion-stalk' (*kou* 芤) and 'skipping' (*cu* 促). Practitioners, in talking about what they feel when they

---

BOX 3.1: Ten contrastive pulse conditions

Floating (*fu* 浮) contrasts with sunken (*chen* 沉)
Slow (*chi* 迟) contrasts with rapid (*shu* 数)
Vacuous (*xu* 虚) contrasts with replete (*shi* 实)
Slippery (*hua* 滑) contrasts with rough (*se* 涩)
Surging (*hong* 洪) contrasts with fine (*xi* 细)

---

[6] Sivin (1987: 318) argues that the earliest textbooks of modern TCM, which resulted from the systematizing collective labor of newly institutionalized experts in China after the mid-1950s, converted pulse-counting to clock time (1987). He also argues that in the early classics pulse types and rates were 'on the whole independent.' When I was studying Chinese medicine in Guangzhou in the 1980s, however, students were told that counting against the doctor's breathing was the correct method to determine whether a pulse was rapid, slow, or moderate. Such expressions of 'traditionalism' in TCM pedagogy have only grown more marked since that time.

touch pulses, often turn to the second convenience, then: that of conventional mnemonics. Some of these mnemonics, such as the description of the slippery pulse as 'like a pearl rolling in a plate,' or the scallion-stalk pulse as 'like pressing a scallion' come from classic sources; others are more recent inventions coined for teaching purposes.

With pulse conditions, then, a system of classifications allows continua – an infinity of spatial and temporal patterns – to be broken up and expressed by means of a limited set of contrastive signifying units. But this is not a conventional classification system, in which we might expect a series of entities to be discretely and exhaustively sorted into tidy pigeonholes.[7] Even a quick look at the list of pulse conditions/qualisigns demonstrates that this is not a classification of entities, and pulses can never be *things* tidied away in boxes. This is clear partly because the perceptual system can only work with considerable overlap or doubling up. A floating or sunken pulse, for example, would be very likely to also display another pulse quality, such as slippery or weak. A pulse described as both floating and slippery would suggest a condition of moist-repletion in the body's superficial parts. A pulse both sunken and weak would lead the doctor to suspect an inner, and hence chronic, depletion of both qi and blood.

Further, the spatial relations discriminated in pulse-touching are classically not confined to shallow and deep. On each wrist there are three positions to touch, each correlated with a visceral system and/or a channel system (Box 3.2).

As will be seen in the case I discuss below, the quality of the pulse at the inch, bar, or cubit position makes a difference; as Shigehisa Kuriyama (1999, 17–60) has argued, the spatial relations of the whole body can be made legible in the small but highly differentiated space of the two wrists.

The system appears to work like a kind of componential analysis. Qualisigns are applied together to describe and configure – perhaps to triangulate – a more or less unique condition, the full clinical pulse picture, the *maixiang* of the individual. The possibility of discerning one of 28 qualities at any of six points already yields a large number of possible readings,[8] but when combinations are allowed, the possibilities surely approach infinity. And the usefulness of simple quantification – mere beat counting – is diminished to near irrelevancy.

BOX 3.2: Correlations of pulse-touching positions in wrist

Left *cun* inch position: Heart visceral system, arm shaoyin & taiyang tracts
Left *guan* bar position: Liver visceral system, leg jueyin & shaoyang tracts
Left *chi* cubit position: Kidney visceral system, leg shaoyin & taiyang tracts

Right *cun* inch position: Lung visceral system, arm taiyin & yangming tracts
Right *guan* bar position: Spleen visceral system, leg taiyin & yangming tracts
Right *chi* cubit position: *Mingmen* Life Gate (associated with kidney system)

---

[7] Bowker and Star (1999:10-11) make the point that few real classification systems meet the definitional criteria of classic classification: real sorting systems are rarely principled, mutually exclusive, and comprehensive.

[8] Although in such a calculation you would have to correct for 'shallow' and 'deep' – two of the 28 – already being spatial, like the six points touched.

Thoroughly qualitative continua, or infinities of pattern, are impractical. A field with no discontinuities, no classificatory pigeonholes, is difficult to navigate and offers little or no foothold for the collective production of value – and hence of course no guide to value, no clinical judgment, even no ethics. Chinese medical practitioners, then, must *reduce* the possibilities of perception, they *focus* their clinical insights to set up a meaningful relation to a history of effective practice, or, if you will, in relation to an 'evidence base.'[9] This is a form of value creation. Phenomena are prioritized and attended to in order; the similarity of a small grouping of pulse qualities to patterns that have been often perceived in the past, the 'fit' of a combination of reported symptoms with the results of a tongue and pulse examination, and with cases memorized or managed in the past – these are coherencies that make it possible to act with confidence in a field that is known. Infinite perception could only undermine this confidence.

To make this point, then, let me turn to several instances of practice. First, a field recollection. For a while in the early 1980s, when I was studying medicine at a college of TCM, I followed the work of a well-known senior physician, Dr Xu (a pseudonym), in his hepatitis clinic. Watching him work for several weeks' worth of morning clinics, I felt at the time that he had a remarkably consistent, or unvarying, approach to the conditions presented by his patients. He almost always diagnosed a liver system dysfunction, he almost always found a string-like (*xian* 弦) pulse, and he almost always prescribed a decoction that was conveniently recorded on a slip of paper under the glass on his desktop. In one sense, this style of work is not surprising or alarming. Almost all his patients had been diagnosed in a Western medical clinic as having hepatitis, so his attention to the liver system might have been quite correct in every case;[10] and his prescription was probably a good way of managing and treating the most common forms of hepatitis. But I was a judgmental graduate student, and as I compared his work with that of other doctors I had already followed, I found his clinic work unimaginative, apparently not engaged in any discovery process.

One day I met him on the street, and in our chat I told him I was trying to study pulse-touching in a class. He lit up, seeing an opportunity to educate an ignorant foreigner who no doubt had very positivist, scientistic leanings. "Ah, pulses," he said. "Pulses are the best example of the scientific objectivity (*keguanxing* 客观性) of Chinese medicine. After all, they're right here!" – putting three fingers on the other wrist. "I can feel it, you can feel it. It's not a secret, and it's not idiosyncratic." Given my doubts about both my inability to discern pulses and about his own apparently wooden hands, his point was perhaps ill judged. But this was also clearly not his view alone: it was a certain party line

---

[9] I use quotes in referring to the notion of evidence base because it could be easily demonstrated that neither clinicians nor scientists always, or even often, act on the basis of evidence. Medical action might be increasingly disciplined by the regulatory demand that a legitimate body of evidence be invoked as clinicians intervene in illness; but if doctors waited for reliable evidence to point the way, they would seldom make a decision about diagnosis or therapy.

[10] Eric Karchmer (2005) has pointed out that many modern clinicians, in turning to the liver system as the culprit for biomedical diseases such as hepatitis, are abandoning the diagnostic logic of a more classic Chinese medical literature.

about scientific Chinese medicine at the time. Moreover, his point that pulses are 'right here' where they can be felt has deep roots in a Chinese metaphysics that places value on the manifest, the 'myriad' surfaces presented to us as the flow of the Way generates a reality without depth.

On one of my last days in Dr Xu's clinic he was absent, and the morning caseload was entrusted to the apprentice doctor who had been practicing alongside him. This middle-aged resident, already an experienced clinician in his own right, took a rather different approach from Dr Xu. He named a number of different and more complex pulse conditions, he implicated other visceral systems besides the liver in his notes on pathological process, and he radically modified the prescription under the desktop glass for various patients. I asked him about this, and he freely admitted that he too found Dr Xu's practice unsubtle. But he hastened to point out that the standard prescription was a rather brilliant one that had helped many patients, and that indeed most of these patients did have a string-like pulse, though there were other fine points of pulse condition that deserved mention in the case record.

It has taken some years, and my current effort to rethink pulses, for me to reconsider Dr Xu and his seriously reductive practice in a more charitable light. Perhaps he never even considered the possibility that the life of the body is a continuous flow (qi-transformation, in the view of some Chinese medical theorists); perhaps even in his youth he had never been attracted – as I was – to those aspects of Chinese medical theory that resemble chaos theory or a Deleuzian imaginary of flows and diffuse micropowers (Deleuze & Guattari 1987). But the problem faced by Dr Xu, by his middle-aged apprentice, and by all pulse-touchers in Chinese medicine, is not how to achieve greater sensitivity, how to participate more intimately in the great flow of the Dao. Rather, the task of everyday medicine is how to reduce the possible and even intrusive proliferation of qualities, the jostle and push of the myriad perceptible conditions to a usable, known, *valuable* kind of knowledge / practice. In this task, qualisigns, however many there are, are useful, but not enough. In this task, Dr Xu was a good-enough practitioner.

CASES AND VALUES

It remains to show in more detail how semiotic value – i.e. the differential weight and signification of qualisigns in a system, conventionally established by way of contrast, quantification, and conventional mnemonics – is linked in practice to *social* value. The social values in question are those belonging to any kind of medical practice: the unquestioned ethic of therapy is to achieve an improvement in the patient's life. Illness symptoms are bad, ability to manage everyday tasks is good. Patients feel that they know what works, when it does, and doctors are relieved but seldom surprised when they see patients getting better as a result of their interventions. The *good* at which medical therapy aims is never simple, because it varies so much according to individual circumstances. But as a therapeutic goal, the health of this particular individual, here, now – a social value – is clear. Patients and doctors usually agree, without discussion, on what a treatment should achieve.

Within this framework, however, the trick is to discover the root of the bad or pathological process that is under way. Much of the logic of Chinese medicine centers on a 'roots seeking' process; the means by which a root can be chosen and characterized is, of course, highly technical, but it is not objective in the sense invoked by the unimaginative Dr Xu. Even he knew that Chinese medical clinicians differ a great deal in their diagnostic thinking on any one case.[11] And like his more philosophical colleagues, he accepted that there might be many therapeutic routes, mapped out with reference to many pathological roots, as doctor and patient aim at achieving better health in any given case.

So, let me turn to one of many cases where pulses matter as qualisigns of difference evaluated in medical practice:

SEVERE COLD WITH MORNING SICKNESS (恶阻 *EZU*)
GYNECOLOGY, DR. CHEN LIANGSHAN, JIANGXI PROVINCE MEDICAL ASSOCIATION

<u>Patient:</u> Ms Wu XX, age 19, resident of the provincial capital.

<u>Illness name:</u> severe cold with morning sickness.

<u>Reasons/sources:</u> body weak and wasted, last menstruated in the 12th month. After getting a chill and catching a cold, had coughing and a fever, and because of taking some medicinal fritillary bulb (*beimu* 贝母) steamed with pears, also developed cold phlegm congestion in her chest. Her long-time doctor treated the condition, using drugs that enrich yin and help mucus to descend. Patient's conditions worsened, with vomiting – everything she ate came right back up. With repeated changes of prescription, the vomiting only increased. The patient had tried many treatments for over three months, she was bone-thin with sallow skin, almost at her last gasp. A friend recommended that I treat her, so Ms Wu sought me out.

<u>Symptoms:</u> Constant vomiting, unable to eat, thin white-ish sputum, dry bowel movements.

<u>Diagnosis:</u> Lightly touching the pulse, it was slippery and rapid with some force (*huashu youli* 滑数有力), continuous at the two cubit points. This is the pulse condition of pregnancy. So why had there been illness for so long? Well, she hadn't known she was pregnant, and because she'd got a chill and caught cold, she thought that fritillary bulb steamed with pears would cure the cough, not knowing that it tends to cause phlegm to congeal. And her doctors had not checked the pulse condition, so they generally used gentle/weak formulas meant to move mucus to treat this disorder; but the phlegm did not go down; instead the Qi reversed and pushed against the normal downward flow, inducing vomiting. With the fetus in her belly, it was lucky that though she had been vomiting some months this condition had not yet become a major barrier [to fetal growth]; otherwise there would have been a great risk.

<u>Therapy:</u> Use Great Banxia (Pinellia rhizome) Decoction, in order to first treat the symptoms and stop the vomiting. If you don't use *banxia* you can't send the counter-flow of stomach Qi back down; if you don't use ginseng you can't supplement the depletion of middle sector Qi; and if you don't use

---

[11] In support of this point, it should be noted that there is a huge literature of cases, a genre with a long history. Many of these cases acknowledge different analyses by several practitioners, and the successful published case is often a critique of previous 'errors' in clinical judgment, diagnosis, and management.

baimi (honey) you can't moisten the dryness of the large intestine visceral system. After I wrote the prescription, Ms Wu asked, "Is there any sign of the pregnancy?" I said, "Of course there's a sign (*ande wuzheng* 安得无征)! The sign is in the pulse, and the pulse condition is quite obvious. If the signs were only of the illness, and you weren't pregnant, anyone who saw your months of vomiting and inability to eat would think, how could she not be dead?" Ms Wu knew medicine well, and seeing that I prescribed confidently, she said with a smile, "I also love Qi Bo and the Yellow Emperor, and I know a thing or two [about medicine]. Anyone could name the three drugs included in this prescription, and anyone could use Banxia Decoction, but no ordinary doctor could do it as you have." She then immediately took the medicine, and that night she stopped vomiting and slept soundly. The next morning when she saw me she said, "If it weren't for you, Master Chen, my life would still be in danger." Thereafter I set up a prescription for stabilizing the fetus and harmonizing Qi flow, in order to assure her recovery.

<u>Rx:</u> Xian Banxia, 150g. Baimi, 100g. Ginseng 75g. Boil several hours.

<u>Second Rx</u>, Fetus Quieting: [...]

<u>Efficacy:</u> One dose of the prescription immediately stopped the vomiting. It also softened the stools, and phlegm and coughing disappeared. Then, four doses of the second prescription stabilized the fetus. Eating and drinking returned to normal, and with a stronger body she delivered the baby.

<u>Comments:</u> In coughs due to Wind Cold, one must first lighten, open and disperse with pungent medicines, break up mucus to return the lung system to its downward tending function, so as to make an illness that has become impacted inside return to the body exterior and exit the body. Then lung Qi can restore itself to its normal clearing and descending function, and the cough will disappear of itself. In this case, the patient's family had wrongly given her fritillary bulb steamed with pears, and then the doctor failed to investigate the origin of the illness and wrongly used a moistening yin, clearing and bolstering approach, thus taking an excess syndrome [i.e. the pregnancy] to be a deficiency [i.e., inadequate lung system function]. Fortunately, though, the patient's Center qi was still in excess, hence the dry stools; further, yin germinal essence was not yet weakened, so there was morning sickness of pregnancy, and it was still possible to use Great Banxia Decoction to correct earlier errors, hitting on the right strategy with one try, achieving success with a responsive hand (*yiji er zhong, yingshou zougong* 一击而中，应手奏功). Using only measurement to investigate suspicious conditions is too clumsy (*tai zhong* 太重), you can still underestimate the danger (He 1959–1985: 4–5).

Ms Wu's case is a typical and classic example of a wiser clinician correcting the errors of more foolish predecessors. It is worth noting that this case from the 1940s was reprinted in 1985 as an object lesson – one of many – about finding the deeper roots of illness signs, and the sensitivity of both tactile and mental perception is highlighted in the details. Clearly there was a difference of opinion regarding the true root of the condition (mere phlegm congestion versus a very basic, inner, and stubborn physiological change called pregnancy); and, as I have argued elsewhere, the root of an illness is no more and no less than the space–time configuration, the pattern or *zhenghou* (证候) that yields best – at least in the view of the principal actors – to a correlated treatment

(Farquhar 1994). But I have cited this case here because of its implicit polemic about pulse-touching and medical evaluation.

In this text Dr Chen almost makes fun of Ms Wu's 'long-time doctor.' He had not even bothered to take the pulse – or if he did, he did not recognize the classic pulse condition of normal pregnancy! First published at a time when Chinese medicine as a regulated clinical system, employing a correlative logic, was being forged by doctors under the direction of the Ministry of Health, this most obvious point was worth making. *At least,* we learn, the subtleties to be found in classic pulse taking, and the conventions of classification long known in the field, must not only be recognized but imposed on standard clinic practice in the then-new socialist institutions of medicine. The time-honored practices of 'traditional' medicine are still and always will be needed – the argument goes – if patients are to be brought back from being 'almost at their last gasp'. It would not do to neglect pulse-touching.

Let us take a closer look at the pulses, then. 'Lightly touching the pulse', he found it was 'slippery and rapid with some force (*huashu youli* 滑数有力), but continuous at the two cubit points.' This reading gives us two of the 28 conventional qualisigns, slippery and rapid; a further qualitative along a continuum – 'with some force'; and a spatial distinction: continuous at the cubit point on each wrist. Even if this was simply, as Dr Chen argues, 'the pulse condition of pregnancy', the combination of perceptions he puts together goes rather beyond textbook medical semiotics. For one thing, his choice of two of the 28 pulse conditions is not enough. (slippery and rapid pulse could also reflect a syndrome known as 'phlegm heat collecting in the lung system'). The forcefulness of the pulsing combined with continuousness at the two cubit points – wrist positions correlated with the kidney system and the Life Gate, where pregnancies are located – strongly manifests a state of 'yang within yin', the local excess embodied by the fetus. Furthermore, 'continuous' (*buduan*) is not a standard pulse condition or qualisign.

Moreover, if this pulse is merely a classic sign of pregnancy, it cannot be thought of as a sign of pathology. The pregnancy revealed by this pulse condition is – in a 19-year-old girl with food to eat, in the 1940s or 1950s – unambiguously a good thing, not an illness. The snippets of conversation reported in the case make it clear that both the life of the mother and the health of the fetus needed to be saved. Understanding the full condition of the pulse was a first step to embarking upon positively valued actions that would achieve the obvious good of a well-nourished mother and a healthy infant.

In fact, these snippets of reported speech suggest a taken-for-granted relationship between pulse qualisigns and healing (or social) value: when she mentions Qi Bo and the Yellow Emperor, Ms Wu is not just showing off her knowledge of the Chinese medical classics, she is invoking a classical era of metaphysical speculation that we think of as Chinese protoscience, dating from the first millennium BCE. Chinese medicine in today's China owes much of its theoretical character to *The Inner Canon of the Yellow Emperor* (compiled *c.* 100 CE), and the Qi Bo who speaks as the principal expert in that text is mainly concerned with order and disorder in the Dao. Although this 'Daoism' is ethically agnostic – the Great Way is incapable of caring whether sparrows fall or people fall ill – early Chinese science founded its very social, very human ethics on a strategy of coming into accord with the Way. Ms Wu reminds us that these ancient philosophies of the relationship between natural action and human purposes can be heard echoing through this case of morning sickness. We can see that the processes under way in Ms Wu's body, both the chronic congestion and the pregnancy, are quite natural and can be easily read from superficial signs. They are not really pathological, but they are not conducive to human health, and the root of the divergence from the natural way (or the Way of the self-so, *ziran* 自然) must be properly identified.

Ms Wu's body, inside and out, was proceeding along its own little way or path. But Qi flow, especially of the lung system, was going in the wrong direction and needed to be nudged back into accord with the proper spatio-temporality of breathing, eating, and growing fetuses. These are continuous processes just like – and expressed by – those of pulse activity. Ms Wu is impressed that her new doctor has been able to capture and classify the root relationships that have been threatening her health. Dr Chen's reading of her pulses, which has classified, specified, and focused the confusion of illness signs at the same time as emphasizing the flow of continuities in pulses and the whole body, returns her to social viability through a skilled intervention into Qi-transformation. First he reads the state of flow in the whole body; then he figures out how to nudge local swirls or eddies of it toward health for his client. The semiotic values of pulse conditions as qualisigns in a system are key intermediate discriminations between a non-evaluative nature and very purposeful social ethics of medicine and healing.

Above I argued that the medical task is to reduce through classification the continuousness, the wave or flow character, of bodily manifestations. In this case Dr Chen makes a good case for knowing the pulse condition that speaks clearly and conventionally of pregnancy. But in every gesture of his argument, he also insists on the continuous qualities that underlie the traditional system of qualisigns: 'Using only measurement to investigate suspicious conditions is too clumsy (*taizhong* 太重), you can still underestimate the danger.'[12]

CONCLUSION

Both Dr Xu, with his insistence that pulses are 'objective' because 'I can feel it, you can feel it,' and Dr Chen's republished persona arguing for non-clumsy pulse-touching (both of them speaking in the 1980s context of state-systematized Chinese medicine) would argue that the only good medicine is practiced by 'best practitioners.' No wooden, clumsy, mechanical quantification could be part of standardized 'best practices.' Even if some medical workers would like to rely on a pulsometer in the clinic (and of course there are a few who would, perhaps comforting themselves with the more objective 'evidence base' they are building), the fundamental character of traditional medicine's clinical judgment is not altered by mechanical quantification. Medical perception is, however, slightly reorganized by the quantitatives and qualitatives perceived in the era of the pulsometer – the classified character of the pulse as condition-image or qualisign is broken out from 'other' kinds of

---

[12] The term I have translated as 'too clumsy' would be more literally rendered as 'too heavy.' This is in direct contrast to how Dr Chen characterized his own pulse-touching: 'lightly touching the pulse....'

information such as symptomatology reported in the process of questioning. But even this purified pulse condition must be understood and properly (re-) combined by the doctor with Chinese medicine's 'traditional' style of diagnosis, understood as a form of schooled and skilled pattern recognition. Only the human practitioner can operate this complex system. It is, after all, no mean trick to turn the qualities of the flow of the Dao into the actionable desiderata of sociable human beings. Qualisigns have value, but they do not evaluate. As Canguilhem (1978/1989) argued long ago, the medical distinction between the normal and the pathological has its roots in human desires. And as modern users of Chinese medicine insist, medical perception is only good when it is 'magical,' leaping beyond all systems.[13]

---

[13] In *Knowing Practice* (Farquhar, 1994) I have considered this notion of clinical magic at some length, noting that terms such as *linghuo* 灵活 (adept insight) or *miaoshou* 妙手 (magically effective hands) were in widespread use in the 1980s. It is not surprising that these common values are invoked in Ms Wu's praise of Dr Chen in the case discussed here.

REFERENCES

Bowker, G., Star, S.L., 1999. Sorting Things Out: Classification and Its Consequences. MIT Press, Cambridge, MA.

Canguilhem, G., 1978/1989. The Normal and the Pathological. Zone Books, New York.

Deleuze, G., Guattari, F., 1987. A Thousand Plateaus: Capitalism and Schizophrenia. University of Minnesota Press, Minneapolis.

Dewey, J., 1935. Peirce's theory of quality. J. Philos. 32 (20), 533–544.

Farquhar, J., 1994. Knowing Practice: The Clinical Encounter of Chinese Medicine. Westview Press, Boulder.

He, K. (Ed.), 1959/1985. Selected and Classified Experiential Cases of National Famous Doctors, Reprinted (Chongyin quanguo mingyi yan an lei bian 重印全国名医验案类编). Shanghai Science and Technology Press, Shanghai.

Huang, J., et al., 1988. Introduction to Chinese Medicine (Zhongyixue daolun 中医学导论). Guangdong Higher Education Press, Guangzhou.

Karchmer, E.I., 2005. Orientalizing the Body: Postcolonial Transformations in Chinese Medicine. Ph.D. Dissertation, University of North Carolina.

Keane, W., 2003. Semiotics and the social analysis of material things. Lang. Commun. 23 (3–4), 409–425.

Kockelman, P., 2005. The semiotic stance. Semiotica 157 (1), 233–304.

Kockelman, P., 2006. A semiotic ontology of the commodity. J. Ling. Anthropol. 16 (1), 76–102.

Kuriyama, S., 1999. The Expressiveness of the Body and the Divergence of Greek and Chinese Medicine. Zone Books, New York.

Munn, N., 1986. The Fame of Gawa: A Symbolic Study of Value Transformation in a Massim (Papua New Guinea) Society. Cambridge University Press, Cambridge.

Parmentier, R., 1994. Signs in Society: Studies in Semiotic Anthropology. Indiana University Press, Bloomington.

Peirce, C.S., 2000[1888]. Trichotomic. In: Fisch, M. (Ed.), The Writings of Charles S. Peirce: A Chronological Edition, vol. 6: 1886–1890. Indiana Unviversity Press, Bloomington, pp. 211–215.

Peirce, C.S., 1997[1890]. A Guess at the Riddle. In: Hartshorne, C., Weiss, P. (Eds.), The Collected Papers of Charles Sanders Peirce, vol. 1. Harvard University Press, Cambridge, MA. Electronic Edition, InteLex Past Masters, Charlottesville, VA, paragraphs 354–416.

Peirce, C.S., 1997[1896]. The logic of mathematics; An attempt to develop my categories from within. In: Hartshorne, C., Weiss, P. (Eds.), The Collected Papers of Charles Sanders Peirce, vol. 1. Harvard University Press, Cambridge, MA. Electronic Edition, InteLex Past Masters, Charlottesville, VA, paragraphs 417–520.

Peirce, C.S., 1997[1897]. Ground, object, and interpretant. In: Hartshorne, C., Weiss, P. (Eds.), The Collected Papers of Charles Sanders Peirce, vol. 2. Harvard University Press, Cambridge, MA. Electronic Edition,

InteLex Past Masters, Charlottesville, VA, paragraphs 227–229.

Peirce, C.S., 1998[1903]. Sundry logical conceptions. In: Peirce Edition Project (Ed.), The Essential Peirce, Selected Philosophical Writings, vol. 2 (1893–1913). Indiana University Press, Bloomington, pp. 267–288.

Sivin, N., 1987. Traditional Medicine in Contemporary China. Center for Chinese Studies, The University of Michigan, Ann Arbor.

Yin, H., Zhang, B., 1989. Theoretical Foundations of Chinese Medicine (Zhongyi jichu lilun 中医基础理论). People's Health Press, Beijing.

Zhan, M., 2009. Other-Worldly: Making Chinese Medicine Through Transnational Frames. Duke University Press, Durham.

Multiple enactments of Chinese medicine

4

Trina Ward

When considering how to integrate Chinese medicine into modern healthcare settings, or when seeking evidence through research to facilitate that process, it is crucial to ask what we wish to integrate, what exactly are we researching? There are clearly many different styles of practice, as every locum practitioner will have discovered. Furthermore, these differing styles rest on quite diverse and changing assumptions that underlie practice. In this chapter, I seek to understand the variety of different styles and how they connect with each other, or indeed whether they do not. In the process of examining how practitioners engage with Chinese medicine we might gain an understanding of different Chinese medicine practices.

In order to discuss the differences as well as the similarities between various styles of practice, equal weight is given to both peripheral and dominant practices. I consider how different styles arise, what forces shape this diversity and in what contexts they appear.

Chinese medicine is commonly presented as an ancient, 2000-year-old tradition, yet simultaneously as a changing practice that responds to social and cultural changes. In this chapter, I consider the diversity of practices at a single point in time, presenting snapshots of an ever-changing picture. This way, I aim to move beyond interpreting the multiplicity of Chinese medical practices in terms of gross cultural differences – for example presenting Chinese versus Western medicine, or even a 'Chinese' Chinese medicine versus a 'Western' Chinese medicine – in order to put forward a more complex evaluation of how Chinese medicine is enacted in the world.

RESEARCHING AS A PRACTITIONER

As a practitioner researcher I approach the research with questions arising directly from my own practice of Chinese medicine. For some time, I was working as an acupuncturist in a National Health Service (NHS) hospital HIV[1] outpatient clinic, surrounded by biomedical knowledge. Clinic rooms, waiting rooms and corridors were adorned with posters and leaflets explaining tests, diseases and treatments. The daily clinical routine was to collect the biomedical case notes from reception for each patient booked in. These were then carried to the clinic room, where I would read through them,

---

[1] HIV is the acronym for human immunodeficiency virus. However, as the acronym will be more familiar to most readers than the full term I have broken convention and used the acronym alone, as I also do for AIDS, below, standing for acquired immunodeficiency syndrome.

checking any entries since I last looked at them. Doctors, nurses, physio-therapists and psychiatrists as well as I all wrote in the same set of notes. Anyone within the hospital trust that treated an HIV patient used this set of notes.[2] While writing these notes I also kept independent Chinese medicine case notes. These contained information relevant to me as a Chinese medicine practitioner that other medical staff did not require, such as pulse and tongue diagnoses. The purpose of my entry in the biomedical case notes was more to do with clinical governance than any interest in that information for clinical decision making by biomedical staff. By listing the points used, my treatment of the patient was made transparent. Thus in the event of an adverse event – for example if a patient suffered a pneumothorax on the day of acupuncture treatment – the site of the points used would implicate or exclude acupuncture as a cause. In contrast, I found that the biomedical information had relevance to my practice: it was in a language in which I was conversant. However, the meaning of that information was not neces-sarily fixed, as is illustrated below.

At first glance, the situation described here appears to be the integration of Chinese medicine and biomedicine, with both being carried out at the same site and with at least a partial sharing of information. There were often discus-sions with doctors about mutual patients. From the point of view of the doc-tors, this was largely to glean any additional lifestyle information that might help them understand the course of the disease. Doctors were aware of and interested in the fact that patients chose to see an acupuncturist. They realized that patients communicated in a different way with them (as biomedical doc-tors in clinical encounters) than they did with me as their acupuncturist. In this sense I could potentially offer clinically relevant insights. For example, a patient might be more forthcoming with me than with their doctor in admit-ting that they often forgot to take their drugs at the correct time, or that they had enrolled on a drug trial to make money without revealing their HIV sta-tus. Such information could prove pivotal in understanding strange or unex-pected results for doctors. However, discussions with biomedical doctors never involved my Chinese medicine diagnosis. Thus, this apparent integra-tion was not mutual: it involved a flow of knowledge consistently couched in biomedical language, a point I return to later.

In clinic I found myself routinely asking each patient about their CD4 count.[3] This is considered a marker of disease progression in biomedicine, and at a certain level it also defines a diagnosis of AIDS. I reflected on why I, as a Chinese medicine practitioner, was asking about CD4 counts, particularly as I already had a figure on the computer screen in front of me that showed all patients' test results over time. When I asked patients what their CD4 count was, responses varied enormously. They included those not wanting to know,

---

[2] Often the patient would also have a non-HIV-associated set of notes used for any medical encounter where their HIV status was undisclosed, reflecting the enduring taboo of this diagnosis in the UK at that time (2005).

[3] CD4 is a glycoprotein receptor found on the surface of T-helper cells, which are a type of white blood cell called lymphocytes and an important part of the immune system. In HIV infection their numbers can fall, so they are used as a marker of disease progression. Viral load is a measure of the severity of viral infection. In HIV infection a high CD4 count increases the risk of suffering from opportunistic infections.

believing that ignorance is bliss. Others monitored every change, fretting if the count was a single point down. These responses occurred regardless of the fact that the accuracy of the count is often questioned by doctors. When tests revealed surprising results, doctors often presumed them to be wrong and discarded or repeated them. The unreliability of the tests was openly acknowledged, despite their carrying so much clinical weight. Other patients down to their final few CD4 cells humorously named them, stating that they had Fred, Beryl, Cuthbert and Gladys left. In light of this, a CD4 count was to me a marker of a person's identity, indicating their relationship with their HIV status and providing a window into their social world. Asking about the count therefore revealed insightful information on how a person related to their disease. The CD4 test ceased being a predictor of disease progress, but revealed instead a wealth of relevant information that contributed to a Chinese medicine diagnosis. Hence my interest in asking for a CD4 count lay in an entirely different arena from that of a doctor[4] viewing the quantitative answer as a standalone fact. It provided a means to view the wider world encompassing emotions and attitudes, as well as a person's social networks that impact on health. Although I do not deny that a CD4 count represents a materiality, its function is restricted when viewed as an objective fact, as it neglects that broader meaning. By focusing solely on the count, a range of information which may have important influences on a person's health is lost.

Clearly, medical knowledge is complex, particularly when each piece of information carries a variety of meanings depending on the function it plays in the medical encounter, as with the CD4 count. Nevertheless, looking at how practitioners negotiate such a complexity of knowledge provides an interesting starting point to explore the diversity of Chinese medicine.

A pertinent example of the creative adaptability of Chinese medicine is given below by medical anthropologist Arielle Rittersmith. Through recent ethnographic fieldwork she documents the ever-present influence of biomedicine on Chinese medicine doctors in Singapore. In Vignette 4.1 she shows how these doctors need to continually negotiate their practice relative to biomedicine, a situation I also encountered in China, England and Australia while undertaking this research and which practitioners anywhere confront daily.

One does not need to work in a biomedical hospital to be influenced by biomedical information. The dominance of biomedicine is evident in the way it pervades many aspects of modern culture. Even practitioners who actively attempt to avoid its influence will have patients who use its language: "I have high blood pressure," "my blood sugar was low this morning" and so on. There will always be a need to translate such terms into meaning relevant to us as Chinese medicine practitioners. In fact, it would be difficult to find Chinese medicine practiced anywhere today that does not bear some influence from biomedicine. In fact, Karchmer (2010) has suggested that contemporary Chinese medicine itself is defined by its relationship to hegemonic biomedicine, whose standards are held up as the scientific truth. Therefore, in my study I asked practitioners of Chinese medicine how biomedicine influenced

---

[4] I am not suggesting here that as a Chinese medicine practitioner I had privileged access to such a view, as many biomedical doctors would use such information in a similar way. It is more to do with one's approach than allegiance to a particular system of medicine.

In crafting a healthcare system the postcolonial Singaporean state (1965 to date) privileged the biomedical model set in place by their British colonial predecessors, politically marginalizing Chinese medicine on this small Southeast Asian island nation. In the last decades of the 20th century, the state's hesitancy to promote the culture of the ethnic Chinese majority over Singapore's other ethnic groups softened, in stated recognition of the economic and moral value of Chinese language and culture. Subsequently, the Traditional Chinese Medicine Practitioners Act (2002) introduced tighter controls on practitioners through mandatory registration and a code of conduct. Ongoing professionalization, standardization and 'modernization' efforts were solidified, partly through the detailed disciplining of Chinese medical institutions and bodies within. Whereas this complex, emerging process has granted Chinese medicine a degree of economic legitimacy and social status, politically speaking, biomedicine retains a monopoly on medical authority. Despite the reputed increased public trust in Chinese medicine attributed to this legislation, Chinese medical physicians must still adroitly negotiate their practice having regard to biomedicine.

With over 20 years of experience in Chinese medicine, Dr Lee, for example, holds degrees in both Chinese medicine and business. He consults for the popular Chinese food and medicine chain Hockhua, maintains a private practice, and occasionally gives public lectures or interviews on topics related to his work. These tasks require a nuanced understanding of the dynamic practice of Chinese medicine, not only in Singapore, but also in Southeast and East Asia, Europe and North America. In Singapore, Dr Lee must orient his practice within an exclusively biomedical healthcare system, against which Chinese medicine is often critically appraised. In this prevalent point of view, biomedical modes of investigation, explanation and epistemology are regarded as 'proper', frequently resulting in efforts to reframe Chinese medical practice and products within these terms.

Simultaneously emphasizing adaptability, profit and public service, Dr Lee advocates a marketing strategy that highlights aspects of Chinese medicine appropriate to transforming social values and priorities. Whereas first-generation (colonial era) Singaporean Chinese did not question Chinese medicine, under the split-stream education system second-generation (mid-20th century) Chinese-stream Singaporeans often suffered economically and socially in comparison with their English-stream counterparts. Many in this cohort therefore encouraged their third-generation (postcolonial) children to study English and 'absorb Western values.' The majority of Dr Lee's new patients thus turn to Chinese medical clinics after being dissatisfied with biomedical treatment. This leads him to the conclusion that "obviously, they [biomedical physicians] are the mainstream, we are the secondary. But in our heart[s] we told ourselves that we are the mainstream too." It is therefore the responsibility of the Chinese medical community, Dr Lee suggests, to demonstrate their capacity as a mainstream practice.

The strategies for promoting Chinese medicine in Singapore are diverse and sometimes contradictory. Competing for scarce resources, some companies and individuals engage in discourses of efficacy, consistency and modernity. Others appeal to Chinese history, collective medical experience or 'tradition', and still others promote Chinese medicine as 'complementary and alternative medicine' – a framework imported from the United States and Europe and adopted by the Singaporean government. According to Dr Lee, this last strategy particularly appeals to younger Singaporeans, who seek 'natural' remedies as an 'alternative' to biomedicine, and generates a niche market in which even the government sees potential. Although far from exhaustive, these strategies allude to the variety of dynamics within which Chinese medicine emerges, in and beyond Singapore, as practitioners vie for authority and security in an increasingly global medical market.

their daily practice. This question served as a springboard for exploring the multiplicity of practices that fall under the label of Chinese medicine today. It is a question that has relevance to every practitioner of Chinese medicine, and one on which everyone undoubtedly would hold an opinion.

METHOD

Q methodology was selected as a useful tool to carry out this research. An outline of what this method involves is woven into this text and can be explored in more detail elsewhere (McKeown & Thomas 1998). Basically, the method is a unique qualitative tool that nevertheless makes use of statistics. It is a way of exploring an individual's opinions from the perspective of that individual. First, communication on the topic is sought through interviews and literature searches. From this, a range of opinions, representing the spectrum of opinions that relate to the research question, are extracted and placed on cards. Second, practitioners are deliberately chosen to reflect a range of ages, different trainings and contexts of work. They are asked to undertake a simple ranking task, assigning a statement to a position from minus five to plus five according to their level of agreement or disagreement with the opinion stated. To reduce the complex data to simple patterns, factor analysis is then carried out on the ranked statements. Each pattern identified is a grouping of shared opinions. It is these groupings, or shared opinions, that are the theme of this chapter. The practitioners whose own opinions – as seen by their individual rankings – are most similar to those of the grouping are used to interpret that grouping. In this way it becomes possible to give each grouping a demographic profile. Important to the task of exploring diversity is the fact that this method is considered unique in its ability to allow minority voices to be heard (Watts & Stenner 2005). Hence, the method has the ability to moderate both the dominating influence of biomedicine and the influential currents of Chinese medicine, such as traditional Chinese medicine (TCM). These influences are thereby not given authority to overshadow other practices.

RESULTS

This research reveals six distinct styles of Chinese medical practice, each of which is formed by the shared opinions of the practitioners taking part and henceforth are referred to as enactments, rather than 'types,' or 'versions.' The term enactment conjures up the active influence of the practitioners in producing and reproducing Chinese medicine; it emphasizes the dynamic nature of realities, which are produced endlessly, with meaning tied to the processes of this production and reproduction (Mol 2002).[5]

The extent of variation could be conceived as reflecting a range of Chinese medicine enactments, rather than variations of a single enactment; for, as will be shown, not all these understandings have much overlap at all. Therefore, multiplicity and diversity rather than plurality are preferred terms to describe these. Albeit very similar in the subtlety of their meaning, multiplicity directly implies more than one, whereas plurality can imply a division of one into parts. These multiple perspectives have the potential to enrich us as practitioners, through reflecting on our own understandings of our daily decision making and the assumptions that these carry.

Before you read these shared opinions derived from practitioners, I invite you to leave aside your own understanding of Chinese medicine and consider the wisdom found in the following vignette by Paulo Wangoola (Vignette 4.2). His understanding and articulation of an issue as important as the nature of knowledge, as a science and as an art, is the product of an Afrikan[6] worldview and epistemology. It exposes the restriction of vision that Western knowledge

VIGNETTE 4.2   MULTIPLE KNOWLEDGES
PAULO WANGOOLA

According to the Afrikan worldview, all being and phenomena in the universe, visible and invisible, known and unknown, spiritual and material, natural and supernatural, spring from one source. This manifests itself in complementary sets of twos, female and male, the basis of differentiated being-in-becoming, balance, harmony and reciprocity, as well as longevity; in fact, perpetuity and eternity. Indeed, even the Creator, the epitome of being, has two names, one female and the other male. Yet behind the complementary sets of twos lies a picture far more complex. Hence, for example, the Creator is constituted by seven spirits, each complete in itself, with specific roles and responsibilities that bound its autonomy. Yet in order to be, in the course and by virtue of being, each of the seven spirits complement one another, none being more than or above the other, neither in rivalry or competition, but in constant mutual communion, by which together they constitute the Creator. Even then the picture is more complex, as each of the seven spirits, on the basis of complementary equality, has both a female and a male manifestation. It is this Creator whom all peoples of the world, according to Afrikan Spirituality, are called upon to worship, 'each in their respective languages', for it is in their respective languages that the Creator communicates with and sustains them, and it is in their languages that they will be judged.

---

[5] I view this term as synonymous with Foucault's use of the term discourse. However, it has the benefit of not carrying the baggage of discourse, in that this word is used to mean widely different things by different authors. It has been likened to performance, but again that word has associations with different things, such as theatre, see Law, J. 2004, After Method: Mess in Social Science Research Routledge, Abingdon.
[6] Note that this spelling makes a political point and sweeps away a colonial past of spellings imposed by a European system.

Against this background it is easy and logical to embrace the notion of multiple peoples, multiple knowledges. At creation, not as an event but as a process, each people of the world is endowed with land, language, culture and color, the ability to know, to learn, to understand, as well as creativity, as a divine heritage. In the circumstances, knowledge is what helps a people to locate and understand themselves in the universe and beyond, and their relationships with the others with whom they share time and space, the natural and the supernatural; the material, the intangible and the spiritual. The operative law that governs the nature of the universe and all being is differentiation, interconnectedness, integration, coherence and unity, both internally and externally. At its best then, knowledge is what helps a people to understand this law of being, to organize themselves in tandem with it, so as to be able to experience abundant and buoyant life in perpetuity, together and in communion with all other forms of being. The rule of thumb for such eventuality is believed to be respect, reciprocity, caring and sharing.

Land, space and time are the basic and common materials available to a people to know, learn, understand, act and observe, as the basis of extending the frontiers of knowledge. Language and culture, with all their associated baggage of value and belief system, epistemology, motivation, ways of knowing, etc., are the tools of learning and creativity. These tools and circumstances necessarily place a limit on what a people can know. This fact becomes the basis for networking and sharing between peoples and lands. The point is for each knowledge base to maintain its integrity, to self-improve through cross-fertilization, and, in the process, maintain a broad spectrum of knowledge genetic diversity, the very basis for the vibrancies of each of the knowledges, and human knowledge as a whole.

can impose on different epistemologies. It clearly shows that many enactments of Chinese medicine are possible, varying according to what is taken as authentic knowledge. Paulo describes himself as 'a community-based organic Afrikan mother-tongue intellectual, scholar and spiritualist. He is one of a people who have nothing to gain by asserting there is only one knowledge or one truth; or that the peoples of the world, their knowledge, cultures and languages are vertically ordered.'

To convey the meaning of each enactment of Chinese medical practice described I use three tools: first, labeling; second, creating a slogan for each; and third, looking for what opinions are missing from, as well as which are present, in each grouping. Labeling each enactment provides an immediate insight into the practice it describes. In the Q methodology literature it is customary to apply labels that encapsulate the meaning of each enactment (McKeown & Thomas 1998). They should not, however, be read as implying that each enactment is a discrete unchangeable entity. Furthermore, to avoid an essentialist interpretation, second-order constructs should not be added to them (Kitzinger 1984, p.130) such as, 'the authentic Chinese medicine view.' The second stage, giving a slogan to each (based on a variation of a well-known phrase) reminds us of the relatedness of each enactment while also highlighting the differences. For each enactment I have chosen to adapt Mao's famous phrase that sums up his vision for Chinese medicine:

"Chinese medicine is a great treasure house, we should strive to develop and improve it" (zhongguo yiyao shi yige weida de baoku, yingdang nuli fazhan jiayi tigao 中醫是一個偉大的寶庫，必須努力地開發提高)

This seems pertinent, as the slogan adorns the entrance to China's oldest Chinese medicine research institute, the China Academy of Chinese Medical Science, (*zhongguo zhongyi kexue yuan* 中國中醫科學院) in Beijing, which was one of the places where I carried out this research. The saying was frequently quoted to me by doctors there, to validate the value of Chinese medicine. Such a phrase can be interpreted in many ways, although Mao meant it to encapsulate his vision for Chinese medicine in the 1950s, which was to integrate it into biomedicine. Through the enactments that follow we will see whether this vision has emerged and what other visions of contemporary Chinese medicine exist. Third, when interpreting the shared opinions, the negatively ranked statements become as important in understanding each enactment of Chinese medicine as the positive ones. In this way the 'messiness' that is part of any research process is incorporated.[7] This method is interesting, as what is missing may be self-evident – a result I call 'manifestly absent.' However, what is missing from the enactment may be an opinion that needs repressing in order to maintain the integrity of what is presented as Chinese medicine in that enactment. A statement may also be so mundane as to be taken for granted. In such instances I call these statements 'othered.'[8] For example, the process of hiding the 'mess' is found in the rhetoric surrounding medical practices, where biomedicine is placed in opposition to Chinese medicine as if they were neatly bordered unities with no room for that which does not fit. The following phrase is one of many that reiterate such a view:

"Biomedicine treats organic diseases; Chinese medicine treats functional diseases" (xiyi zhiliao qizhi xingjibing, zhongyi zhiliao gongneng xingjibing 西醫治療器質性疾病，中醫治療功能性疾病)

An example of 'mess' in the above phrase would be to find that Chinese medicine can treat an organic disease. Treating organic disease would contradict the understanding from the quote, and hence would need to be hidden in such a situation.

In expressing their opinions on each statement, practitioners reveal the nature of that particular enactment of Chinese medicine. It is how each statement sits in relation to each of the others that allows them to be interpreted in a gestalt sense and to see how they all fit together. The enactment, therefore, emerges from the entire set of statements.

Each of the six enactments is a depiction, at a particular moment in time, of Chinese medical practice. The purpose here is not to reveal which of these is 'the *real* or *true* Chinese medicine.' But to move away from such a concept. None of these enactments of Chinese medical practice has privileged ownership of a correct or authentic version: each is valid in its own context, for as the

---

[7] For those interested in interpretation of research using this method see Law, J. Making a Mess with Method. http://www.comp.lancs.ac.uk/sociology/papers/Law-Making-a-Mess-with-Method.pdf. 2003. Centre for Science Studies Lancaster University. 9-6-0009, or Law, J. 2004, After Method Mess in Social Science Research, Routledge, Abingdon.
[8] Also refer to footnote seven.

ethnographic literature cited above has shown there can be no single Chinese medicine. However, each shares some similarity with all the others. When reading through these enactments, practitioners may consider which they feel most allegiance to and how and when this allegiance may vary, to reveal the flux within their own practice of Chinese medicine.

ENACTMENT ONE: MODERN, INDEPENDENT AND EQUAL

The practitioners who comprise this enactment are young to middle-aged Chinese doctors only.[9] Although all the enactments are concerned with identity, this one – strikingly – is about practitioner identity and status, reflecting the struggle that exists within China for Chinese medicine to achieve equal status with biomedicine. For example, among students wishing to study medicine, those with the highest grades are sent to study biomedicine, whereas those with lower grades are sent to study Chinese medicine. Thus, this enactment is concerned with Chinese medicine practitioners attempting to reclaim the power they believe society has afforded to biomedicine.

In this enactment, biomedicine and Chinese medicine are viewed as complementary and make up a whole. However, the ability to know this whole is placed solely within the sphere of Chinese medicine.

Enactment One is distinguished from all other enactments as it excludes the statement, 'My practice of Chinese medicine is based on what biomedicine doesn't treat well.' It thereby reduces the danger of Chinese medicine being seen as subservient to biomedicine. The implication of excluding this statement is that Chinese medicine can treat what biomedicine can treat: a further stamping of independent authority. Clearly, if the above statement had been given presence in this enactment then its domain would constantly be reduced with each new biomedical advance. In order to maintain Chinese medicine's standing as modern and equal, the statement is therefore manifestly absent.

I define the statement 'clinical decisions cannot be based on anything but knowledge from the classics' as othered, because it threatens the main message of this enactment of Chinese medicine. The importance of being seen as modern overrides any possible agreement with such a statement. Similarly, the statement 'In practice I stick to Chinese medicine principles; using herbs according to their pharmacological make-up is simply not Chinese medicine' is also othered. Pharmacology would need to be drawn on as part of the modern practice that this enactment aspires to, so naturally the statement is repressed as it contradicts that message of being modern.

Mao's phrase is adapted to sum up this enactment thus:

"Chinese medicine is a treasure house that only we (Chinese medicine practitioners) can select from and offer to biomedicine."

---

[9] It should be noted that Q methodology uses strategic sampling: the demographics of each enactment are not generalizable as with a random sample. However, they are interesting to note as they may aid in the interpretation.

ENACTMENT TWO: CLASSICAL WISDOM

Both Westerners and Chinese practitioners are active in creating this enactment. The Chinese doctors exemplifying this enactment include one who received an apprenticeship during the Cultural Revolution, and another who is a radical critic of institutionalized education of Chinese medicine in China. Both have roles within the institutionalized Chinese medicine world in China, but are known to hold critical views that challenge the government line. In this enactment, biomedicine and Chinese medicine are seen as parallel rather than complementary systems of knowledge. Although the enactment is in dialogue with biomedicine, it does not seek to mimic it.

The view of a Chinese medicine diagnosis is expanded here to include, for example, looking at X-rays. This is because modern technologies are seen as belonging to modernity, not to biomedicine. Therefore, Chinese medicine in the modern era naturally draws on these technological advances. In this enactment there is a redefining of Chinese medicine for the modern era. Unlike Enactment One, which seeks to be modern by rejecting certain aspects that are difficult to align with modernity, such as the classics and the immeasurable, this enactment does not need to be perceived as modern, or to follow a materialistic reality. The statement, 'Chinese medicine is all about *qi* 氣,'[10] it is more useful to understand *qi* than to know anything of biomedicine' is othered by Enactment One and given presence by this enactment. In Enactment One there is a pride in knowing biomedicine, whereas in Enactment Two there is more confidence in Chinese medicine knowledge as a standalone system suitable for the modern age.

The summarizing phrase used for Enactment Two is:

"Chinese medicine is a treasure house that once opened needs classical strategies for using the contents."

ENACTMENT THREE: BIOMEDICINE – THE FACTS

This enactment is formed by Chinese men, who are trained first in biomedicine. One Western participant is also associated[11] with this view; interestingly, she trained first in European herbal medicine, which also uses a biomedical understanding of the body. The main message seen in this enactment is the prioritization of biomedical knowledge as the reality, to the extent that Chinese medicine knowledge is only valid within a materialistic, mechanical, reductionist framework. Manifestly absent is the statement, 'First understand the patient's *qi*, in clinic a cure cannot be achieved without working with the patient's *qi*.' This is absent, as in such a framework *qi* cannot exist because it cannot be measured.

One participant who exemplifies this version was interviewed and asked about his views on the Chinese slogan 'inheriting and carrying forward' (*jicheng fayang* 繼承發揚). This is often part of the rhetoric of Chinese medicine

---

[10] *Qi* 氣 has been variously translated as life force, vital force and energy.
[11] In Q methodology only participants solely associated with a viewpoint are used to form the enactment. Others may be associated with this view but are not relevant to its formation, as they correlate with other viewpoints also.

doctors in China, used to idealize the bridging of modernity and tradition (Scheid 2002). The participant replied:

"the key point is try to find out something good or something better in Chinese medicine. We don't care about inheriting and carrying forward."

In this example, Chinese medicine is viewed as something to be analyzed and broken apart, in much the way that pharmaceutical companies look to indigenous medicines to 'discover' new drugs. There is no interest in the system of knowledge that came to know that a herbal formula could treat a particular condition. This approach is reductionism to the extreme, dismissing all that does not fit as useful add-ons to biomedical practice. Unsurprisingly, this enactment strongly agrees with: 'My starting point is always the biomedical diagnosis', in contrast to all other enactments that made the statement manifestly absent. Thus, the statement affirms the belief that biomedicine alone is the true reality. The same message is indicated by the presence of the words 'biomedical information provides the facts, Chinese medicine is another way of looking at them.'

Enactment Three, then, appears to be most similar to Mao's vision for Chinese medicine. As already mentioned, Mao aimed to integrate Chinese medicine into biomedicine. The result was the inevitable loss of Chinese medicine as a system in its own right. Therefore, the summarizing phrase is adapted thus:

"Chinese medicine is a treasure house to be plundered."

ENACTMENT FOUR: CHINESE MEDICINE – THE GRAND NARRATIVE

This enactment represents the discovery of qi and the importance of the immaterial in clinical medicine. A combination of Chinese and Westerners, both male and female, comprise this enactment. However, of note is that they all live in the West. The enactment views biomedicine as greatly limited by its mechanistic reductionism, whereby it inevitably misses the larger picture that is available to Chinese medicine. The belief is that biomedicine can be added on to Chinese medical practice but can never replace it.

Thus, Enactment Four carries a sense that, through discovering Chinese medicine, a new world view is opened up, one in which Chinese medicine can explain all things. The statement, 'In clinic I cannot describe an X-ray as *yin* or *yang*,'[12] is manifestly absent in this enactment, as Chinese medicine theory can be applied to all things. This example contrasts with Enactment Three in which the statement is othered for simply not being of value, since in this enactment it is believed that X-rays are real, whereas *yin* and *yang* are not considered concrete realities.

Some, including no doubt those making up the group of Enactment Three, would see Enactment Four as presenting a romanticized view of Chinese medicine. It has been suggested that such a view of Chinese medicine is found

---

[12] *Yin* and *yang* are considered (by whom?) inseparable opposing forces of a single reality; for more discussion see Wiseman, N., Ye, F., 1998. A Practical Dictionary of Chinese Medicine, second ed. Paradigm, Brookline Massachusetts.

exclusively in the West (Wiseman 2001). Similarly, Unschuld (1985) has expressed the view that Chinese medicine in the West selectively adopts concepts that fit into a solely Western cognitive aesthetic, and as a medical historian he would most likely view this enactment as a good example of such a view.

Therefore, I summarize Enactment Four as:

"Chinese medicine is a treasure house so vast that its riches will constantly amaze us."

ENACTMENT FIVE: CHINESE MEDICINE – A WAY OF BEING

This enactment is the most distinct, in that it shows the least correlation with any of the others. It is formed by a seventh-generation Chinese doctor and a Westerner who has immersed himself in Chinese culture, having lived and studied in China as apprentice to a series of elderly teachers for almost 20 years. Furthermore, practicing without a medical licence, the Westerner has escaped any government regulations regarding private medical practice. Unsurprisingly, this enactment values knowledge that is directly transmitted from master to student; it is the only one that places the following statement as presence: 'In clinic I do not rely on knowledge from books but on traditional methods of diagnosis handed down to me by my teacher.'

What is also portrayed in Enactment Five is that autonomy is important. Through such autonomy a 'pure' version of Chinese medicine can survive. From a historical perspective this attitude can be viewed as problematic, since the many influences and transformations that have constantly been part of Chinese medicine are seen as assisting in its survival rather than being responsible for its demise.

Rather than assimilate biomedical practices, more Chinese medical information is sought. By staying apart from biomedicine and its infrastructure, Chinese medicine can escape becoming engulfed by the mainstream dominant order. It is a way to reclaim or rediscover a tradition and at the same time to value difference; in interview,[13] a practitioner forming part of this enactment said, "Dr Lu at the China-Japan Friendship Hospital (*Zhongri youhao yiyuan* 中日友好醫院) is doing amazing things in gynecology, using all sorts of tests, but this for me is not Chinese medicine." The emphasis is, on the one hand, respect for biomedicine, but on the other hand it suggests the incomparability of the two systems. This position contrasts strongly with Enactment Four's grand narrative view.

Another comment from one forming this enactment was, "When a patient brings me their X-ray I like telling them that I don't know what it means and if they want to see someone who does they are in the wrong place." This attitude implies confidence in Chinese medicine knowledge as being complete without the X-ray; there is no suggestion that the two systems together make up a whole in this account. The enactment most closely echoes the view that different types of knowledge can obscure other types (Kuriyama 1999). This theory will be returned to later.

---

[13] In Q methodology interviews initially serve to generate the statements that are ranked, but they are also carried out after ranking to aid in later interpretation. After analysis the results are presented to those influential in a particular grouping, and the analysis can thus be adjusted further based on their final interview comments.

Quite unlike Mao's vision for Chinese medicine, this enactment can be summed up as:

"Chinese medicine is a treasure house that is preserved by its ability to remain hidden and re-emerge given the right conditions."

ENACTMENT SIX: PRAGMATIC COMBINERS

Enactment Six is another one formed solely by Westerners and is unusual in that it shows a similar correlation to most of the other enactments, rather than the more common pattern of greater to less affiliation. This suggests the ability to empathize with other opinions and to actually take them on as their own. Also of note is that all those exemplifying this enactment have held positions of power and leadership in the field of Chinese medicine in the West. One could thereby infer that this enactment might influence the course of the development of Chinese medicine in the West. In other words, this face of Chinese medicine is one that operates in the wider political and social sphere in which Chinese medicine is placed in the West. It repeatedly adheres to the view that the two medical systems together make up a whole picture. In this way it is similar to Enactment One. However, the emphasis is different: Enactment Six is about legitimizing Chinese medical practice, whereas Enactment One is primarily about the status and identity of Chinese medicine practitioners themselves. This mirrors the different positions of Chinese medicine as a profession in China and the West: in China it is legitimized by state sanction, even though – outside the political sphere – it is not viewed as highly, whereas in the West the profession remains largely unrecognized politically.

The use of biomedical knowledge in Chinese medical practice is accepted as a realistic part of practice. This acceptance is recognized in total agreement with the statement, 'The two systems of medicines can make reference to each other from their unique way of thinking about a particular problem the different angles reveal different things for us in clinic.' There is no sense of conflict in these two positions. Manifestly absent, then, is the statement 'I just discard Western medical information', as that would be throwing away necessary information for a complete picture. The phrase 'the creative extension of the conceptual net to fit new circumstances' (Pickering 1992) sums up this enactment well. Chinese medicine's encompassing of modern technologies and the knowledge arising from their use seeks to move the social field of practice into what is dominantly seen as 'medical' in modern society: that is, it seeks legitimacy through combining biomedical practices.

There are hints at Mao's vision of integration in Enactment Six, although the purpose is not to make a new medicine, but rather to evolve Chinese medicine suitably for the demands of a new time. This can be summarized as:

"Chinese medicine is a treasure house that is continuously added to and repackaged."

DISCUSSION

The purpose of my research has been to describe the diversity of practices that fall under the label of Chinese medicine today. This variety manifests as the six enactments described. When considering the integration of or research into Chinese medicine, it is necessary to know to which of these, exactly, we are referring. This approach moves beyond assuming that 'experts' or textbooks have privileged knowledge about the constituent parts of Chinese medicine. The method used to generate these data ensures that these six enactments represent a broad range of styles of Chinese medical practice. In part, this is achieved through generating a range of statements on how biomedicine influences Chinese medical practice, and by selecting a deliberately diverse range of practitioners for their opinions.[14]

Having mapped out these six enactments, I now examine the knowledge within each one. To achieve this, I draw on theories about knowledge production put forward by two leading historians of Chinese medicine (Kuriyama 1999; Unschuld 1987). I also consider how each enactment relates to, or mutually excludes, the other, and ask: Can practitioners actually move between these enactments, or are they bound by them? Is the knowledge within one enactment available to another? These are important questions in understanding our practices of Chinese medicine, as well as for designing research and relating the results to our own practices.

I will summarize, very briefly, the theories I refer to and illustrate them through the enactments. First, Kuriyama (1999) proposed that how we know the body alters what we can know. He specifically contrasts two medical images, Hua Shou's *Shisijing Fahui 1341*, a rotund figure with meridians, and Vesalius's *Fabrica 1543*, an athletic muscular form (Figures 4.1 and 4.2).

Such differences were first seen at the time of Galen (130–200ce) in the West and the later Han (25–220ce) in China. Looking further back to the Hippocratic corpus and Mawangdui scripts, the contrasts are not as marked as seen in these later figures. The figures therefore represent historical changes and not timeless attitudes. Kuriyama used these two figures to question how something as basic and seemingly universal as the body could be depicted in such different ways at different times and in different cultures. He suggests that conceptions of the body owe as much to ways of using the senses as to ways of thinking. With regard to feeling the pulse, Kuriyama suggests that Greek and Chinese doctors knew the body differently as they felt it differently. This divergence arose from the practice of dissecting corpses in Greece but not in China. Once Greek doctors observed that both the heart and the arteries contracted and expanded they believed this was the only thing that could be felt at the pulse. In contrast, the Chinese were not hindered by such a vision and felt many subtle tremors and other movements in the body. For example, Kuriyama (1999, p. 93) quotes from Wang Shuhe's *Mojing*, 'Floating mo: if one lifts the fingers there is abundance; if one presses down one finds insufficiency.' This belief contrasts strongly with the Greek search for the pre-existing rhythm generated by a beating heart.

Kuriyama's hypothesis opens up the potential for multiple realities, acknowledging that the world can indeed be experienced and understood in different ways. In the case given, there are differing conceptions of the human body. From such a view, rather than knowledge adding to our understanding, it could actually obscure other knowledge, as can be seen in Figure 4.1; in

---

[14] It is beyond the scope of this chapter to defend the method or describe it in detail. Q methodology holds that there is a finite range of opinions available on any topic. These are available as inter-subjectively shared accounts, with subjectivity seen to be forged in the sociocultural milieu. For further reading see Brown, S.R., 1993. A Primer on Q Methodology. Operant Subjectivity 16, 91–138; Stainton Rogers, R., 1995. Q Methodology. In: Smith, J.R., Harre, R., Van Langenhove, L. (Eds.), Rethinkiing Methods in Psychology. Sage, London, pp. 178–192; and Stephenson, W., 1953. The study of behaviour: Q-technique and its methodology. University of Chicago press, Chicago.

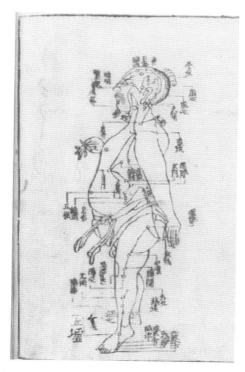

FIG. 4.1 Hua Shou, Shisijing fahui, 1341. Courtesy of the National Library of Medicine.

Hua Shou's figure the muscles are obscured by the flesh. This loss of information can be likened to the way that looking through a colored lens can obliterate the original color of an object. From such a scenario any integration project would have the effect of losing information; Chinese medicine integrated thus into mainstream healthcare would be filtered through the dominant biomedical lens and be altered. Whether this is viewed as a creative reinvention, as Sean Lei suggests in chapter 7, or whether it is viewed as a loss of vital information is clearly a matter of perspective. One could conjecture that Enactment Six – described above, with its emphasis on defining Chinese medicine in relation to external political and social powers – would view integration as a creative challenge. In contrast, Enactment Five – which values separatism in order to preserve an 'authentic' Chinese medicine – would shun such a challenge, as this approach is aware of knowledge being lost rather than gained through the process. Not only would this type of Chinese medicine actively eschew integration into a modern healthcare system, it would also be incompatible with the demands of such a system, for example standardized procedures, normative standards and clinical governance. Although this enactment does contain all these factors, they are dictated from within and not without. A further standpoint is seen in Enactment Three. This belief system would most likely view integration as a way to get rid of all that does not fit a biomedical material reality, such as *yin yang* theories, which it views as pseudoscientific and thus not real. Therefore, integration would offer Enactment Three the opportunity to eradicate large parts of Chinese medicine.

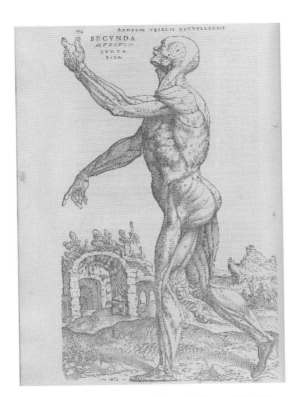

FIG. 4.2 Vesalius, Fabrica, 1543. Courtesy of the National Library of Medicine.

The question arises whether the knowledge of one enactment can be accessed by practitioners who are aligned with a different enactment. Could those making up Enactment Six, who pragmatically combine and adapt to new circumstances, for example, also make sense of knowledge in Enactment Five, which seeks to preserve an authentic Chinese medicine? This brings us to a second relevant theory about knowledge found in the Chinese medicine literature. It was observed that Chinese medicine texts frequently contradict each other, yet these texts would continue to be used in modern practice (Unschuld 1986).[15] From Unschuld's perspective, if one text was true then the other could not be, so the historian was intrigued as to how the two could coexist without conflict in contemporary Chinese medicine. Unschuld (ibid) described this phenomenon as 'patterned knowledge.' i.e., the result of accepting conflicting views as truth. It is based on a different logic from Unschuld's own understanding, where either *this* or *that* is true, not both. Patterned knowledge of Chinese

---

[15] The term 'Patterned Knowledge,' is found in the following references; Unschuld, P. U. 1985, *Medicine in China A History of Ideas.* University of California press, Berkeley and Los Angeles, California; Unschuld, P. U. 1986, *Nan Jing The Classic of Difficult Issues* - translation, University of California Press Ltd; Unschuld, P. U. 1992, Epistemological Issues and Changing Legitimation: Traditional Chinese Medicine in the Twentieth Century, in *Paths to Asian Medical Knowledge*, C. Leslie & A. Young, eds., University of California Press, California, pp. 44–61; Unschuld, P. U. 1987, Traditional Chinese Medicine: Some Historical and Epistemological Reflections, *Social Science & Medicine*, vol. 24, no. 12, pp. 1023–1029. Unschuld states that he no longer refers to this idea and is now interested in exploring *fa* 法 variously translated as law, method, rule, way, Buddhist teaching (personal communication 2009).

medicine texts allows for both to be true, even when they contradict each other. In such a framework truth is revealed through its usefulness. Unschuld (ibid) further conjectured that Chinese medicine practitioners may also think in a 'patterned knowledge' way. These six enactments, representing differing epistemological positions (that is, views on what is knowledge) but with points of shared understanding, suggest that Unschuld's conjecture is correct.

The following vignette, by Marian Katz, shows how the local context of social structure and meaning alter understanding (see Vignette 4.3). The analysis she presents draws on data she collected in the early 2000s as part of her PhD dissertation research on Chinese medicine in the United States, which focuses on the practitioner–patient relationship and how local understandings of Chinese medicine are constructed through talk. It also offers an opportunity to see how practitioners are active in the construction of Chinese medicine at any point in time.

VIGNETTE 4.3 ORIENTING TO BIOMEDICINE IN ACUPUNCTURIST[i]–PATIENT INTERACTIONS
MARIAN KATZ

Acupuncturist orientations to biomedicine are sensitive to local contexts of social structure and meaning. An important, but often overlooked, context is the practitioner–patient interaction. Acupuncturists and patients routinely invoke biomedicine in their talk. Here I analyze practitioner responses to patient-initiated talk about biomedicine in three interactional contexts: a complaint, a problem presentation, and a treatment recommendation.

Extract I[ii] is the conclusion of an extended patient complaint about difficulty making a doctor's appointment.

Extract I. Collegial[iii] (5: 5: 478)
PAT = Patient
ACU = Acupuncturist
PAT: So I sent a nasty letter to the doctor himself and said, "Well, I hate to bring that up to you, but this is insane." All I want is an appointment…
ACU: Yeah. That's too bad that he has to give you such a hard time, …usually with appointments I don't think they try to make it so hard.
PAT: Not usually – I have never seen that before.

The acupuncturist responds sympathetically to the patient (line 4), but she also depicts the situation as unusual (lines 5–6). By discouraging the patient's complaining about biomedicine, the acupuncturist displays a collegial orientation toward biomedical doctors.

When a patient's presentation of a skin problem, however, includes her biomedical doctor as a competing medical authority, another acupuncturist responds by asserting his own authority and privileging Chinese medicine. Thus, in Extract 2, the acupuncturist interrupts the patient's talk about the effectiveness of her doctor's prescription by initiating a tongue examination (line 3).

Extract 2. Competitive (7: 5: 81)
PAT: He [the patient's doctor] really helped…the medication really helps…he said…
ACU: Let me see your tongue.

PAT: Is it bad?

ACU: It's not bad it's just that...It's just that there's a lot of dampness and there's alot of dryness both. You know what I mean?

PAT: How can that be?

ACU: Because the dampness and the dryness both basically stem from the fact that your spleen energy isn't transforming [your] fluid metabolism properly. So there's not enough blood, and there's not enough stuff to moisten the skin, an' yet there's plenty...that's what makes that kindah fertile ground for stress blowing through it.

The acupuncturist's diagnosis both justifies his treatment and minimizes biomedicine's authority, by reframing the biomedical cause of the patient's problem, i.e., stress, as a result of the same underlying condition causing the patient's skin problem.

Later in the same visit, the practitioner brings the biomedical assessment back in (Extract 3, line 2), as part of an explanation for changing the patient's herbal prescription.

Extract 3. Parallel systems (7: 5: 366)

ACU: I'm gonna make a change there...I think that overall even though the skin thing is related to stress, it's also related to dryness. So, as much as I can...that your spleen will allow me to, I'm gonna start to build up your blood.

Here the acupuncturist orients to biomedicine as equal to Chinese medicine. The formulation 'even though...it's also' (lines 3–4) constructs biomedicine and Chinese medicine as parallel systems of medicine that can be drawn on selectively according to the needs of a particular situation.

Each of these orientations – collegial, competitive, and parallel system – is produced within a specific interactional context. Thus, understanding acupuncturists' orientations to biomedicine requires understanding the interactional contexts within which they are produced.

i In California, the professional title for practitioners of Chinese medicine is 'licensed acupuncturist', and it is common usage to call Chinese medicine providers acupuncturists.

ii The data presented here are from my dissertation research on the practice of Chinese medicine by locally, English-language trained acupuncturists in Southern California. For a more detailed analysis, see Katz, Forthcoming 2010, *Chinese Medicine in the US: Culture, Interaction, and the Construction of Patient-Centered Care*.

iii For readability and space constraints, the transcripts have been simplified from the conventions developed by G. Jefferson, as described in the Appendix to Sacks, H., Schegloff, E.A., and Jefferson, G. 1974. A Simplest Systematics for the Organization of Turn-Taking in Conversation. *Language* 50:696-735.

Unschuld further proposes that this attitude of 'as well as' knowing is uniquely East Asian,[16] and that this differentiates Chinese medicine from bio-medicine. This approach is in contrast to 'either/or' knowing, which holds that there is only one valid truth, as exemplified in Enactment Three, 'Biomedicine – the facts.' This 'either/or' knowing, Unschuld hypothesizes, arises as a result of the influence, in the West, of the Judeo-Christian legacy of believing in only

[16] It certainly extends well beyond Asia; see Paulo Wangoola's vignette earlier in this chapter (Vignette 2).

one God.[17] Following on from this, with the acceptance of one God there can then logically be only one truth. The data from this study do not support such an East–West divide: practitioners from China and various Western countries make up these enactments. As practitioners taking part in this study all show some correlation with each of the enactments, they are clearly interacting, admittedly to varying degrees, in a 'patterned knowledge'; in other words, they adopt an 'as well as' way. Integration will bring constraints on practice, and these necessarily alter practice, so that an adapted Chinese medicine would once again emerge, this time prioritizing parts that can be validated by a biomedical understanding, with a moratorium on other practices.

Back now to Unschuld's 'either/or' view. Early on in the research process, when practitioners of Chinese medicine were asked how biomedicine influences their practice,[18] the majority held the view that using biomedicine and Chinese medicine together will provide a clearer picture of the whole. In so doing, they assume that there is one whole picture to be known. Thus, by integrating the two systems, the 'true' picture can emerge. Such a view is a widely accepted realist one, based on what Unschuld calls an 'either/or' Western logic (ibid). It ignores power differentials, such as seen in Vignette 3 above, and the process of enacting realities that I have shown in this chapter. This attitude is particularly evident in Enactments One, Three and Six. Since the initial *majority* view was that biomedicine and Chinese medicine together make up a clearer picture, this implies that these three enactments wield greater power than the others, simply because they receive more support. As such, these three enactments will be more widely practiced, funded and otherwise supported by society. Second, descriptions of the remaining enactments bear testament to the ability of the method used to give voice to minority views; although these viewpoints may not dominate Chinese medical practice, they nevertheless exist. Accessing the knowledge of these relatively hidden practices may prove as useful when researching Chinese medicine as when seeking consensual views.

CONCLUSION

Rather than being competing versions of what is the real Chinese medicine, the various enactments can be seen to encompass different types of knowledge that coexist, each being drawn upon to some extent by most practitioners when useful. This is seen through the existence of distinct enactments that nevertheless share points of similarity; all overlap to some extent with each other. Furthermore, and it is beyond the scope of this article to explore this more fully, at the level of the individual everyone connects with these enactments in a particular way: some are strongly associated with one view and are relatively independent of the others, whereas others show strong affiliations with several enactments. The concept of patterned knowledge, mentioned above, describes such a process. However, we can see that this practice

---

[17] The phrase 'Judeo-Christian monotheism' is that used by Unschuld throughout his writings on this topic; however, this is itself a contested subject which is beyond the scope of the paper. It can be engaged with through, for example, *Early Christianity in Context*, ed. J. M. G. Barclay., *Library of New Testament Studies*: Sheffield Academic Press, London 2005. I am indebted to Mary Dobbins and Felicity Moir for pointing this out.

[18] Interviews were the source of the majority of statements that participants ranked.

is not limited to East Asians as previously supposed (Unschuld 1986): it is also adopted by Westerners.

The implications are, first, that the context within which Chinese medicine is to be integrated or researched needs careful defining. Second, – as new contexts will undoubtedly continue to shape practice – rather than querying what Chinese medicine is being integrated, a more important question arises: what will Chinese medicine become through integration? In each and every practice, practitioners can also ask such questions of themselves, both in the macro sphere of their place in healthcare provisions – how government policies or NICE[19] guidelines influence what they do – to the micro level of daily practice and encounters with different patients holding different conceptions of illness.

Every new context of practice will stimulate the emergence of new forms of Chinese medicine that will reflect the values and beliefs of the local culture, hence an array of dynamic and emergent practices will always exist (Hsu 2001; Scheid 2002). The process of integration, like the process of taking part in research, will inevitably alter how Chinese medicine is practiced. Careful examination of the assumptions that practitioners bring to their own practice can lead to a richer, more accurate understanding of Chinese medicine. In turn, this can help to inform researchers and other stakeholders involved in the task of integrating the practice of Chinese medicine into modern healthcare settings.

[19] National Institute for Clinical Excellence.

REFERENCES

Hsu, E., 2001. Innovation in Chinese Medicine. Cambridge University Press, Cambridge.

Karchmer, E.I., 2010. Chinese medicine in action: on the postcoloniality of medical Practice in China. Med. Anthropol. 29 (3), 1–27.

Kitzinger, C., 1984. The Constructing of Lesbian Identities.

Kuriyama, S., 1999. The Expressiveness of the Body and the Divergence of Greek and Chinese Medicine. Zone Books, New York.

Law, J., 2004. After Method Mess in Social Science Research. Routledge, Abingdon.

McKeown, B., Thomas, D., 1998. Q Methodology. Sage, California.

Mol, A., 2002. The Body Multiple: Ontology in Medical Practice. Duke University Press, Durham and London.

Pickering, A., 1992. Science as Practice and Culture. University of Chicago Press, Chicago.

Scheid, V., 2002. Chinese Medicine In Contemporary China: Plurality & Synthesis. Duke University Press, Durham.

Unschuld, P.U., 1985. Medicine in China A History of Ideas. University of California press, Berkeley and Los Angeles, California.

Unschuld, P.U., 1986. Nan Jing The Classic of Difficult Issues—Translation. University of California Press Ltd.

Unschuld, P.U., 1987. Traditional Chinese medicine: some historical and epistemological reflections. Soc. Sci. Med. 24 (12), 1023–1029.

Watts, S., Stenner, P., 2005. Doing Q methodology: theory, method and interpretation. Qual. Res. Psychol. 2, 67–91.

Wiseman, N., 2001. The transmission of Chinese medicine: chop suey or the real thing? Clin. Acupunct. Orient. Med. 2 (1), 36–49.

Standardization and its discontents: four snapshots in the life of language in Chinese medicine

Sonya Pritzker

Language, including translation methods and terminology organization, has been central in efforts to integrate Chinese medicine into a global, mainstream medical framework. Several international organizations, including the World Health Organization (WHO) and the World Federation of Chinese Medical Societies (WFCMS), have become involved in these efforts, placing a great deal of attention on the need to standardize the terminology of Chinese medicine in both Asian languages and English. As it stands, there is still no authoritative standard for the English translation of the key terminology in Chinese medical texts. The result is a host of English-language textbooks, teaching materials and research protocols, all of which use different nomenclature to translate basic Chinese medical concepts. In some circumstances, this leads to confusion when it comes to developing databases, insurance forms and other tools of an integrated health system. The atmosphere surrounding terminology standardization is quite contentious, however, with arguments erupting over how to decide on a standard, how to enforce that standard, and what exactly standards mean. There are also those who argue that terminology standards are fundamentally unethical. Debates worldwide have therefore been quite heated, especially in the last five to ten years. In both Western and international debates, issues of power, authority and the market amplify theoretical discrepancies, making the situation of standardization in Chinese medicine especially volatile at the levels of policy development as well as daily application.

At the same time, language and nomenclature have also proven critical in efforts to integrate Chinese medicine into personal frameworks of meaning. For students and practitioners learning Chinese medicine in translation, terminology becomes a personal issue, one that greatly affects learning on a daily basis. For these individuals, standardization is a complicated notion with the potential to change the way they learn. Sometimes such measures seem useful, even helpful, especially when confusion about terms results in poor communication between teachers, supervisors and students. Other times the possibility of standardization seems absurd, especially when invoked by a distant group of policy makers at the forefront of integration efforts. In this context, personal desires and ideologies of translation combine with communication needs and learning goals to create ambivalence towards the idea of standardization.

In an effort to convey some of these diverse experiences, this chapter offers four 'snapshots' in the life of language standardization in Chinese medicine. Specifically, I show four cases in which the issues of language and terminology come alive in interactive moments where people are participating in the process of talking about, teaching and planning term standards. In this sense, nomenclature in Chinese medicine can be seen as a living entity rather than just a referential tool. The snapshots are derived from extensive, multi-sited ethnographic research conducted over three years in diverse settings, including conferences, schools, and the homes and offices of translators and scholars involved in standardization efforts in both China and the US. The research takes as its starting point Rabinow's apt description that the purpose of anthropological inquiry in a complex contemporary setting is not 'destruction or deconstruction but a reevaluation' (Rabinow 2008, p. 3). The purpose of this chapter is not, therefore, to provide an authoritative account of what standardization in Chinese medicine should or could mean, nor is it to offer a 'solution' to some of the complex debates that surround the issue. Rather, it is to take standardization in Chinese medicine as a complex 'field of practice' (Scheid 2002; Bourdieu 1990) wherein anthropological inquiry 'begins midstream, always embedded in a situation, one both settled and unsettled' (Rabinow 2008, p. 8). Like the work of anthropologist Mei Zhan, this chapter attempts to capture Chinese medicine 'in action' (Zhan 2009, p. 12), presenting a series of images and descriptions that emphasize the human interactions, moral commitments and theoretical stances that comprise the field of language standardization in Chinese medicine.

The hope for such an inquiry is to offer a picture of standardization as an ongoing series of human encounters, a complex web of human networks shaping the ever-changing answers to questions about the motivations behind standardization, the methods used to create standards, and the implications of standards in an increasingly globalized Chinese medicine. This perspective is currently especially vital, when arguments over what is the most authentic or best practice are rampant. For example, when it comes to establishing guidelines for best practice based on an integrated medicine that seeks recognition on the global health scene, there are always both pros and cons to terminology standardization. In all contexts, however, awareness of the human commitments and connections within the debates surrounding this issue can only help in forming and maintaining the relationships that are needed to sustain integrative processes in a way that is most beneficial to patients. This chapter therefore highlights integration as a human process, rather than just a mingling of ideas and actions.

SNAPSHOT ONE: TOKYO, JAPAN, 2005

It is a damp, humid day in Tokyo at the end of June 2005. Experts on language, traditional medicine, science and biomedicine from China, Japan, Korea, Germany and the UK are gathered in a large meeting room at the behest of the World Health Organization, Western Pacific Region (WHO-WPR). They have gathered today for a second time to discuss terminology standardization in traditional Asian medicine. Tensions are running high after a series of presentations from various perspectives have questioned and challenged core principles of translation from Chinese to English, the use of biomedical terminology to translate Asian medical terms, and the blending of Korean, Japanese, Vietnamese and Chinese medicines into one terminology. The experts are currently rearranging their seats in order to break up into groups. Within these groups, they will discuss, debate and argue over specific English translations for thousands of traditional medical terms. Tension will continue to build as speakers with different levels of fluency in English and different perspectives on translation and traditional medicine argue over which terms are appropriate and why. Eventually, several experts will abandon the effort, convinced that the whole attempt is a no-win situation. Most participants will stick it out, however, as they are all equally committed, often for different reasons, to the development of an international standard terminology for traditional medicine in order to further the goal of integrating it into an increasingly globalized international healthcare arena. By the end of the meeting they will have voted on a list of 4200 Chinese terms for inclusion in the international standard. There will be less agreement surrounding the English translations for the terms, but the meeting will be considered a success nonetheless.

This snapshot comes from the second meeting of the WHO-WPR in 2005. The first meeting, held in Beijing in 2004, was instigated by WHO-WPR because of the growing realization that standardization of terminology comprises a first crucial component in efforts to standardize both practice and information sharing within 'traditional medicine', a collective of Asian medicines deriving from ancient China and including traditional Chinese medicine, traditional Korean medicine, Kampo medicine, traditional Vietnamese medicine and others. The official WHO-WPR goal of the development of standards was publicly recognized as integration and 'upgrading' of practice, research and education both locally and globally (WHO 2007, p. 1). Standardization is thus intimately linked to the project of marketing traditional medicine, while at the same time marketing 'Asian cultural traditions' to the mainstream medical world.

Over the course of both meetings, experts from China, Japan, Korea and Macao, as well as two prominent European Chinese medical translators, met to discuss a range of issues, including the development of library browser systems using standardized terminology, the Westward transmission of traditional medicine, and the principles of literal versus free translation. Debates raged over whether to use terms that English speakers were already accustomed to as opposed to creating new ones; whether to use biomedical as opposed to more traditionally focused terminology; whether to privilege native English speakers or native Asian practitioners in the crafting of English terminology for traditional medicine; and whether to emphasize general principles of translation versus debating single, specific terms. By the third meeting, held in Daegu, South Korea, in October 2005, 4000 final terms along with English translations were provisionally agreed upon.

Over the next two years, a draft copy of the terms was circulated among international advisors from the fields of biomedicine, science and traditional medicine. Finally, in June 2007, WHO-WPR published *The WHO International Standard Terminologies on Traditional Medicine in the Western Pacific Region* (IST-WPR) (WHO 2007). This 350-page document includes the final selection of 4000 Chinese terms, understood to represent the most ancient and original language of traditional Asian medicine, along with their English translations and definitions. Among these are various selections of basic theoretical terms, diagnostic terms, disease terms, therapeutic terms, and terms from classic texts. The organization hopes to include the IST-WPR in the upcoming *International Classification of Diseases, Eleventh Edition* (ICD-11), a process that is currently under way. Inclusion in the ICD-11 will further the WHO-WPR's goal of integrating traditional medicine into the global system of medical billing and diagnostic codes, and will therefore be effective in globalizing traditional medicine on a scale previously unknown. The 2007 version of the IST-WPR is, however, only the first step towards such a goal. In it, the authors stress that 'continuous revision' is necessary in order to meet the needs of all potential users (WHO 2007, p. 6). They point out that such efforts are crucial towards promoting international understanding between traditional medical practitioners, students, researchers and consumers.

SNAPSHOT TWO: PHOENIX, ARIZONA, 2006

It is the day before the annual conference of the 2006 American Association of Oriental Medicine, held in Phoenix, Arizona, opens. A pre-conference symposium entitled 'Asian Medical Nomenclature Debates' is in full swing. One after another, Western and Chinese translators of Chinese medical texts step up to the podium and offer their views on everything from the need to develop a standard set of terms for the accurate transmission of Chinese medicine to the need to resist such a standard based on the notion that it limits the Western student's perspective and distorts the depth and flexibility of Chinese meaning. Some audience members listen, mostly quietly, surprised to hear their esteemed teachers and textbook authors arguing over such a seemingly trivial matter as terminology. Other audience members are aware of the debates, as they have been carried out in American journals and in online discussion groups for the past 30 years or more. For those who have been following these debates, today is an exciting first step towards coming together in some form of agreement. For some, the end of the day brings the sense that all the experts are really aiming towards the same thing: an accurate and honest transmission of Chinese medicine to the West. For others, it seems as if the debate participants are as divided as ever, the conference being just a venue for the scholars to advertise their own perspectives and resist hearing anyone else. For still others, the whole thing seems silly and they are eager to move on to the meaty clinical content of the rest of the conference.

This snapshot begins to give us a sense of the American debates over standardization. Since the mid-1990s, there have been heated debates over standardization that have been carried out in journals, informal meetings, internet discussion groups and conferences. These debates are not limited to authors and other scholars. Students, practitioners and teachers also actively participate on a regular basis, although based on a survey conducted at the 2007 American Association of Acupuncture and Oriental Medicine (AAAOM) meetings, terminology standardization has not been a major concern for most of the general population of practitioners in the US (unpublished survey data, 2007).

For the many Americans who oppose standardization, the freedom issue strikes a deep chord. The idea of authors being forced to use a standard not of their own choice seems to go against the freedom that characterizes American culture (Beinfield & Korngold 2001). Opponents of standardization also insist that plurality in translation reflects the plurality of Chinese medical theories in China (Beinfield & Korngold 2001; Shima 2006; Shen 2006; Bensky et al 2006). A related issue is the notion that accurate translation is impossible because of the lack of commensurability between Chinese and Western ways of thinking (Buck 2000). Opponents of standardization further argue that literal translation often leads to terms that are difficult to understand and use (Buck 2000). Another issue related to this particular view is the idea that language is not as important as clinical experience in learning or thinking about Chinese medical ideas (Buck 2000). Finally, critics of standardization argue that the whole debate about language is really about certain publishers and authors seeking to control the textbook market (Deadman 2000).

On the other hand, advocates for standardization argue that, in order to help reverse the culturally based biases that lead to distortions of original Chinese medical ideas, there needs to be clearly delineated source-oriented base standards (Wiseman 2000; Ergil 2001; Ergil & Ergil 2006; Felt 2000, 2006; Flaws 2006). Another big claim for standardization is that, rather than the language of poetry or literature, Chinese medical language constitutes a technical language that should be translated rigorously (Wiseman 2001). Other reasons Western scholars argue for standards include the need for accurate communication across texts and with other scholars and practitioners (Ding 2006); the need to present Chinese medicine to outside parties (Flaws 2006); the need for organized online databases (Flaws 2006); the need to access original source material (Flaws 2006); and finally, the need to be free from the whims of various translators' interpretations (Wiseman 2000).

The first major result of Western standardization efforts includes the 1998 publication of Nigel Wiseman and Feng Ye's *A Practical Dictionary of Chinese Medicine* (Wiseman & Feng 1998). There has also been a major push towards the development of an integrated reference list pegging all the terms used in different English language texts to each other as well as to the Chinese and the WHO-WPR terminology. Recently, several of the scholars working on standardization in the West have teamed with the AAAOM and WHO to try to create a bridge between the terminology that is currently in use in the US and the terminology of the WHO-IST. Underlying all such efforts remains the awareness that in terms of spoken and written use in texts and communications, there is really no way to enforce a single standard.

SNAPSHOT THREE: BEIJING, CHINA, 1997

In 1997, an American anthropologist whose research focuses on the practice of Chinese medicine is sitting in the small, dusty Beijing office of a renowned scholar of Chinese medical history. The American is there because she has been invited by a prominent English-language Chinese medical publisher to write a history of Chinese medicine for Western students. She is hoping that the Chinese scholar will collaborate with her. He is honored, and spends the next few months putting a description together in Chinese. When he emails the proposal to the American professor she is impressed, but comments that she needs the book to be in English. "No problem", the Chinese historian writes back, "I will just get someone to translate it after I write it." The American writes back questioning what type of standard the translator will use for the book. The Chinese scholar is surprised: what standard? Can't we just translate it however we see fit? The American explains the importance of a standard, and suggests they use the standards that the American publisher generally uses. The Chinese scholar is shocked. How come we don't have our own standard for translating Chinese medicine into English? We are, after all, the originators of Chinese medicine, and we should be the ones to decide on standards. He becomes curious about why China has no Chinese medical terminology standards, either in Chinese or in English. This prompts him to contact a Chinese organization responsible for compiling standard terminology in science, asking them why Chinese medicine is not included among the sciences required to have a standard terminology. This leads to a series of discussions between the Chinese scholar and the organization, with the scholar offering to form a committee to develop a standard Chinese and English terminology for Chinese medicine. Over the next ten years, he is so wrapped up in this committee work that he never completes the original book.

This snapshot offers us a glimpse into the many factors influencing peoples' motivations to become involved with terminology standardization. In China, there have been many committees, much like the one described here, formed with the goal of creating both Chinese and English standards for Chinese medical terminology. For the most part, they have formed separately from each other, prompted by different goals and basic assumptions. The two most prominent organizations include the Committee for Terms in Traditional Chinese Medicine (CTTCM), formed in 2000 in association with the China National Committee for Terms in Sciences and Technologies (CNCTST), and the World Federation of Chinese Medical Societies (WFCMS), formed in 2003 in association with the State Administration of Traditional Chinese Medicine (SATCM). The two have worked independently to develop extensive compilations of standard medical terms, in both English and Chinese (CTTCM 2004; WFCMS 2007). Both are also vying to be instituted by the Chinese government as the national standard, and both are jockeying for favor with the WHO-WPR in terms of their credibility to become the international standard.

Outside these official organizations, Chinese scholars all over the country have been far from silent on the issue of standardization. Beginning in May 2003, the well-known and widely circulated *Journal of Chinese Integrative Medicine* started including a monthly section on translation. Major themes in the first group of articles included an emphasis on the importance of Chinese–English translation in the representation of Chinese medicine to the outside world; the need for standards based on scientific research; and the need for scientific principles for accurate translation (Niu 2003; Luo 2004). In recent years, several other journals in China have followed suit, publishing regular articles debating the translation of Chinese medicine according to modern bioscientific standards or traditional cultural practices, and also featuring Chinese and international perspectives on language standardization (Wiseman 2006; CTTCM 2004; WFCMS 2007; Niu 2003; Luo 2004, Xie 2002a, 2002b, 2003).

It is a bright, sunny spring day in Southern California. A group of students in their second quarter of studying Chinese medicine are gathered for diagnosis class in a brightly lit classroom. The room is decorated with posters displaying the body's meridians and acupuncture points, in both Chinese and English, and the reflection of a palm tree is visible in one of the glass frames, swaying gently in the spring breeze. The teacher, an American woman who has little to no training in Chinese, stands before the class discussing various pulse qualities. "Alright" she says, "we're gonna do one more pulse, and then we're gonna take a break, and the reason is this one's kinda gonna make your head spin a little." The students laugh nervously. The reason that their heads will spin, she explains, is because of the words: "This comes down, once again, to nomenclature… Lemme tell ya," she says, "that this whole issue of nomenclature in Chinese medicine just sucks. It really, really sucks. Translation sucks. Comparative nomenclature from book to book sucks. I mean tell me, does this not suck?" She turns to the camera, addressing rhetorically the anthropologist in the room. There is some grumbling from the students, who have started to realize that part of their work in learning Chinese medicine is figuring out the complex and variable terminology in their texts. "It makes our job *so much harder*," the teacher continues, "And the reason for you guys it makes it so much harder is because you have textbooks that the state board relies on to write exams, and very often the nomenclature in those textbooks is misleading and not clinically relevant. So you know, bad for you, you gotta learn things the wrong way, and then you've got to apply them clinically in a completely different way." She goes on to differentiate a 'thready' pulse from a 'thin' pulse, making use of diagrams and rich clinical descriptions. Throughout her lesson, she pays close attention to distinguishing her clinical definitions, and the language they will probably hear being spoken down in the clinic, from the information in the texts, which they have to memorize for tests. The books equate thready, thin, and small, whereas in the clinic they will need to know the difference between all of these. She deems the problem one of 'over-translation.'

This snapshot gives us a sense of how pervasive talk of translation is in the Western classroom. Even though all instruction takes place in English, the issue of translation is constant. Students and teachers are continually reminding each other that this medicine originates in a foreign land, with foreign customs and a foreign language, and that it must be translated into English as well as into an American context. On top of this, students are introduced to the complexities of multiple and varying translations from the very start of their four-year program. From the beginning, then, the students are thinking about translation constantly, and the teachers are always discussing it.

As demonstrated in the snapshot, many teachers in the California context prioritize clinical experience and personal feeling over linguistic accuracy, sometimes going so far as to say that 'the words get in the way' of truly connecting with the meaning. Other teachers build on this notion by emphasizing the sheer difficulty of finding a single English word to capture the rich and complex meaning conveyed in Chinese. In yet other cases, teachers are more rigorous about making their students learn the correct translations and meanings. Like the scholars described above who advocate for terminology standards, these teachers argue that linguistic accuracy is crucial towards developing a strong clinical practice. In most American schools, however, students are only exposed to about ten weeks of Chinese language instruction, if that. This often leaves them more overwhelmed with the recognition of how much they do not learn in English as they begin to get a glimpse into the complexity of the Chinese writing system and linguistic history, not to mention the thousands of texts yet to be translated.

What it often comes down to is their embodied experience, their *connection* with the terms – whether in Chinese or in English. This is often felt as a process of connecting with the 'energy' of the concept. As the students begin to engage with the terms more deeply over the course of their study, this embodied experience of meaning and terminology often shifts, sometimes on a daily basis. Their understanding of terms unfolds through constant interaction with teachers, peers, texts and supervisors, as well as in personal encounters. As they apply the descriptions to their own bodies and those of their families, their learning experiences are not commonly singular or unified. Whereas some students develop a 'visceral' connection to meaning as they learn Chinese characters, for example, others grapple with the quest to apply Chinese medical terms to their personal circumstances. Still others seek to memorize textual definitions only for testing purposes as they plan their careers in acupuncture.

Ideas and feelings about standardization are mapped onto each person's basic experience of the meanings within Chinese medical language. Students' perspectives on standardization are thus complex, textured by the shifting territory inherent in trying to integrate a new language into a personal meaning system. Like the general population in the US, the students resist the notion that such a personal process could ever be mediated by a remote group of 'experts.' At times of frustration and confusion, however, they crave a coherent, quick gloss for terms that seem to have an endless array of definitions and explanations, none of which are clear in English. As they proceed through the program, they begin to get a sense of how much easier communication between practitioners would become if they all spoke a common language. At the same time, they also recognize that something might be lost if such a language were to come at the cost of the multiplicity in translations that gives them a shadowy yet somehow more vivid picture of the richness of meaning in Chinese. In their final years, students often come away with a certain ambivalence towards standardization, a recognition of the ways in which it would help as well as the ways in which it might limit experience. For the American students, however, the issue is never quite as personal as the process of learning how to *use* language in the effort to become an effective and compassionate healer. In the following vignette provided by Elisabeth Hsu, we see that such focus on language use places students in the company of generations of Chinese scholar-physicians, who draw upon techniques of 'situational meaning-making' in order to achieve effective healing as well as maintain social position (see Vignette 5.1).

The imperative to have a standard English translation of each traditional Chinese medical term arises within a certain life world – the bureaucratic one, it would seem. Bureaucracies have always pursued a standardization of terminologies, regardless of whether they were part of what Joseph Needham (1956) called the feudal bureaucracy of Imperial China or of those more recent ones that make up the modern nation-state or transnational organizations. In this sense, the WHO's project on 'International Standard Terminologies on Traditional Medicines' is only to a limited extent a modernist project, and its endeavor to standardize Chinese medical terminology can be conceived as a renewed effort of a longstanding concern that the pre-modern Chinese bureaucracy already embraced. Legal authority, Max Weber [1921] (1980) tells us, takes as premise that 1) any kind of law can be set up; 2) this law is in essence a cosmos of abstract and explicit rules; 3) the typical legal ruler himself also obeys this impersonal order; 4) the one who obeys only obeys 'the law'; and 5) the members of the union are obliged to obey within the domain of assigned, rationally limited and factual competence. Standardized terminologies aim at fostering rationally limited, clearly defined, factual competence within a life world that abides by laws of nature and the science of them.

However, the flowery and almost poetic vocabulary of Chinese medicine is not easily straitjacketed. In some circumstances, it may appear vague and general, pregnant with contradictory meanings; the Chinese medical doctor is then likened to the charismatic quack who, like a demagogue, makes use of words that can mean everything and nothing. In many other situations, however, Chinese medical terms have very clearly bounded, discrete meanings, specific to the context in question. The linguist calls these terms polysemic, i.e., they can have very different, context-specific meanings.

As argued elsewhere (Hsu 2000), I suggest that this polysemic feature of the Chinese medical terminology points to a certain type of authority, namely, Max Weber's patrimonial authority. In contrast to Western biomedicine, which has a highly standardized terminology and which has not only been fostered within but also created some of the largest colonial and postcolonial bureaucracies, and in contrast to the charismatic (folk) healer who appeals to the crowds and masses with words that are ill-defined and general, the physician whose vocabulary is polysemic is ideally suited to provide services in a stratified society, where those in power may use it arbitrarily. If the meaning of the words that the physician uses changes, chameleon-like, in different situations, he may compliment his genteel clientele and he can easily evade being made responsible for what he says he does. Situational meaning-making, which is so characteristic of the scholarly medicines, defies legal authority. It seems to have been brought to perfection in the literate, upper echelons of stratified Asian and East Asian societies, where those who embraced political power could exert it seemingly arbitrarily.

It would be obsolete to conceive of the situation as arising from a tension between modern bureaucrats versus authentic traditional medical practitioners. Rather, the above shows that the different modes of linguistic meaning-making are a constitutive aspect of different socialities within the field of health.

Standardization and its discontents

DISCUSSION

In the introduction to this chapter I argued that adopting a particular 'anthropological' perspective – one that is based on the multi-sited, contemporary work of scholars such as Marcus, Rabinow, Scheid and Zhan, among others – offers us the opportunity to witness standardization in Chinese medicine from a unique vantage point. This is a vantage point that privileges everyday participants, and steps away from merely featuring abstract theoretical arguments. In the present context, viewing the debates and the standardization process through the lenses of these four ethnographic vignettes therefore helps ground some of the theoretical points of contention surrounding standardization in the relationships and commitments that make up the reality of the life of language in Chinese medicine. It is clear from the snapshots that language standardization in Chinese medicine is all about these relationships – relationships between individuals, projected or imagined relationships between China and the West, and relationships between a desired ideal and an experiential self. This vantage point reveals the ways in which language is drawn upon in efforts to control such relationships, as well as to nurture and deepen them.

In each of the above snapshots, as well as in Hsu's vignette, the ways in which language *matters* in the context of Chinese medicine become apparent. It is especially clear how much language matters in efforts to integrate Chinese medicine into the mainstream worldwide healthcare system, into the American medical register and into personal systems of meaning. The many complex arguments surrounding the standardization of terminology in various contexts can be understood not merely as theoretical debates, but as deeply human moral dilemmas that prompt unequally situated participants to think about what kind of terminology best captures the kind of Chinese medicine they want to practice or, in the case of politicians, project onto the world stage. From this perspective, language and terminology are linked to participants' deeply personal and strongly political views on what constitutes 'good medicine' in the contemporary context. As participants navigate this question with regard to terminology, they are involved in webs of interconnected, sometimes overlapping, sometimes conflicting, processes. This highlights the truth that language in Chinese medicine is not merely referential; it also emphasizes the important social dynamics that are involved in a scene where individual students and practitioners with relatively little power beyond their own practice are in dialogue with world leaders attempting to influence international institutions. It shows that for everyone involved, 'meaning' is contingent, emerging and highly personal. Terminology standards are experienced as moral entities, precisely because they are linked to so many core notions of what language is, how meaning is captured and explained, how translation is accomplished, whether translation is even possible, and what Chinese medicine needs to become in a globalized world.

Such notions are not set in stone, and may vary even within individuals. Priorities are clearly different, and, as well as being multiple, they are not always theoretically compatible. For members of the WHO-WPR, the priority of integrating Chinese medicine into the world healthcare system always looms above the particular priorities of any individual. And yet such individual priorities nonetheless continue to exist, making the process fraught with tension. For certain Americans participating in the Western terminology debates, freedom is often prioritized: the right to control one's own experience and not have it controlled by an outside authority. At the same time, the desire for authentic knowledge and clear, open communication is a pressing need that creates ambivalence about standardization in some American students. For many of the Chinese scholars and translators participating in the various Chinese organizations, national pride is a priority, and they thereby maintain the right to develop the language for a medicine that is culturally their own. Simultaneously, communication with the West is crucial, and they must also consider the terms that Westerners will actually use.

From all of this, we witness the heterogeneity of the contemporary 'moral landscape' (Rabinow 2008, p. 79), in the dialogue about standards in Chinese medicine, an arena in which participants have varying ideas about what type of language is good or bad for divergent purposes. Individuals in the context of culture, writes Rabinow 'frequently, perhaps always, employ more than one type and figure of moral discourse' (Rabinow 2008, p. 79). Individuals thus draw upon multiple moral categories to navigate their way through complex, changing fields of practice in ways that defy explanation when we are simply focused on theoretical discrepancies such as those between 'knowledge and practice, text and context' (Zhan 2009, p. 11). The only way to approach such a complex field, Zhan writes, is by approaching it 'in action.' In the words of Rabinow (2008, p. 8), this means stepping in 'midstream,' recognizing that the individuals and organizations involved in standardization are simultaneously embedded in multiple moral discourses.

In this sense, it is helpful to think of 'standardization' in Chinese medicine as a prime example of what Bakhtin would call 'heteroglossia', which he defines as the result of a set of conditions 'that will ensure that a word uttered in that place and at that time will have a meaning different than it would have under any other conditions' (Bakhtin 1981, p. 428). Although the precise meanings, the shifting senses of standardization, might be impossible to resolve from this perspective, we can approach heteroglossic terms and concepts such as standardization with an appreciation for the 'dialogism' inherent in any human notion. Within a dialogic framework, 'Everything means, is understood, as a part of a greater whole – there is a constant interaction between meanings, all of which have the potential of conditioning others' (Bakhtin 1981, p. 426). The web of meanings surrounding standardization, built in and through ongoing and multiple relationships, can thus be approached through an ethnographic method that appreciates the shifting territory of meaning, and recognizes culture as continually emergent in interaction (Scheid 2002; Pickering 1995). Rather than granting us a solution to the 'problem' of language standardization, this view offers us an appreciation for the humanness of it all, the human relationships and experiences behind questions (and constantly shifting answers) regarding the implications of standardization, the pros and cons of standardization, the merits of different methods, and the role of governmental agencies in instituting standards. It gives us an acute 'anthropological' awareness of standardization by asking why, when, and for whom such implications, methods, organizations are valid. Standardization is thus witnessed as a series of human encounters which are deeply personal, overtly political, overwhelmingly social, and clearly economic. In terms of arguments over authenticity and best practice, such a perspective allows us to recognize the contingency of participants' views on what is 'real' or authentic in Chinese medicine, as such opinions are always tied to complex personal, social, political, and economic factors. The perspective offered by a look at language as a living entity further presents the potential to help us move beyond some of the simple theoretical divides that keep us locked into debates that make integration difficult and fraught with misunderstandings.

ACKNOWLEDGEMENTS

This research was funded by The Wenner-Gren Foundation for Anthropological Research, The Jacob K. Javits Graduate Student Fellowship, and the Graduate Division of UCLA. I would like to thank my UCLA advisors, Elinor Ochs, Linda Garro, Yunxiang Yan, Hongyin Tao, and Ka-kit Hui, for their continued support and critical insight. Finally, I would like to thank Volker Scheid, Hugh MacPherson, and Felicity Moir for their invaluable comments on previous drafts of this paper.

REFERENCES

Bakhtin, M.M., 1981. The Dialogic Imagination: Four Essays. Michael Holquist (Ed.) University of Texas Press, Austin.

Beinfield, H., Korngold E., 2001. Centralism vs. pluralism: language, authority, and freedom in Chinese medicine. Clin. Acupunct. Orient. Med. 2, 145–154.

Bensky, D., Blalack, J., Chace, C., et al, 2006. Toward a working methodology for translating Chinese medicine. Am. Acupunct. 37, 14–15.

Bourdieu, P., 1990. The Logic of Practice. Stanford University Press, Stanford, Calif.

Buck, C., 2000. On terminology and translation. J. Chin. Med. 63, 38–42.

Committee for Terms in Traditional Chinese Medicine, (CTTCM), 2004. Zhongyi Yaoxue Mingci (Chinese Terms in Traditional Chinese Medicine and Pharmacy). Kexue Chuban She, Beijing.

Deadman, P., 2000. Book review: a practical dictionary of Chinese Medicine. J. Chin. Med. 62, 54–56.

Ding, W.Y., 2006. Asian Medical Nomenclature Debates. Paper presented at the American Association of Acupuncture and Oriental Medicine Annual Meeting. Phoenix, AZ, USA.

Ergil, M., 2001. Considerations for the Translation of Traditional Chinese Medicine into English. www.paradigm-pubs.com/refs/Translation.html. Accessed February 2011.

Ergil, M., Ergil, K., 2006. Issues surrounding the translation of Chinese medical texts into english. Am. Acupunct. 37, 24–26.

Felt, R., 2000. Reply to Charles Buck. J. Chin. Med. 63, 44–46.

Felt, R., 2006. The role of standards in the transmission of Chinese medical information. Am. Acupunct. 37, 18–20.

Flaws, B., 2006. Arguments for the adoption of a standard translational terminology in the study and practice of Chinese medicine. Am. Acupunct. 37, 16–27.

Hsu, E., 2000. Spirit (shen), styles of knowing, and authority in contemporary Chinese medicine. Cult. Med. Psychiatry 24, 197–229.

Hui, K., Pritzker, S., 2007a. Terminology standardization in Chinese medicine: the perspective from UCLA Center for East-West Medicine, Part 1. Chin. J. Integr. Med. 13 (1), 1–5.

Hui, K., Pritzker, S., 2007b. Terminology standardization in Chinese medicine: the perspective from UCLA Center for East-West Medicine, Part 2. Chin. J. Integr. Med. 13 (2), 152–155.

Luo, L., 2004. Zhongyi Yingyu Fanyi De Yuanze Chutan (A first exploration of the principles of the english translation of Chinese medicine). J. Chin. Integr. Med. 2 (3), 239–240. [in Chinese]

Needham, J., 1956. Science and Civilisation in China. Cambridge University Press, Cambridge.

Niu, C.Y., 2003. Weishenme Yao Yanjiu Zhongyi Yingyu Fanyi (the Importance of Researching the English Translation of Chinese Medicine). J. Chin. Integr. Med. 1 (30), 239–240. [in Chinese]

Pickering, A., 1995. The Mangle of Practice: Time, Agency, and Science. University of Chicago Press, Chicago.

Rabinow, P., 2008. Marking Time: On the Anthropology of the Contemporary. Princeton University Press, Princeton.

Scheid, V., 2002. Chinese Medicine in Contemporary China: Plurality and Synthesis. Science and Cultural Theory. Duke University Press, Durham, NC.

Shen, X.T., 2006. An extra thought about nomenclature. Am. Acupunct. 37, 12–13.

Shima, M., 2006. Asian medical nomenclature debates. Am. Acupunct. 37, 811.

Weber, M., [1921] 1980. Wirtschaft und Gesellschaft. J.C.B. Mohr, Tuebingen.

Wiseman, N., 2000. Reply to Buck and Maciocia. www.paradigm-pubs.com/paradigm/refs/wiseman/JCMAnswer.pdf. Accessed February 2011.

Wiseman, N., 2001. The Extralinguistic Aspects of English Translation of Chinese Medical Terminology. www.paradigm-pubs.com/paradigm/refs/wiseman/extralinguistics.pdf. http://www.paradigm-pubs.com/sites/www.paradigm-pubs.com/files/files/X_2__e_Extralinguistic.pdf (accessed February 2011.).

Wiseman, N., 2006. English translation of Chinese medicine: concerning the use of western medical terms to represent traditional Chinese medical concepts. Chin. J. Integr. Med. 12 (3), 225–228.

Wiseman, N., Ye, F., 1998. A Practical Dictionary of Chinese Medicine, first ed. Paradigm Publications, Brookline, MA.

World Federation of Chinese Medical Societies (WFCMS), 2007. Basic Nomenclature in Traditional Chinese Medicine. People's Medical Publishing House, Beijing.

World Health Organization (WHO), 2007. WHO International Standard Terminologies on Traditional Medicine in the Western Pacific Region. WHO Library Cataloguing in Publication Data, Manila.

Xie, Z.F., 2002a. On standard nomenclature of basic Chinese medical terms (Ii). Chin. J. Integr. Med. 8 (3), 231–234.

Xie, Z.F., 2002b. On standard nomenclature of basic Chinese medical terms III. Chin. J. Integr. Med. 8 (4), 310–311.

Xie, Z.F., 2003. On standard nomenclature of basic Chinese medical terms IV. Chin. J. Integr. Med. 9 (2), 148–151.

Zhan, M., 2009. Other Worldly: Making Chinese Medicine Through Transnational Frames. Duke University Press, Durham and London.

Standardization and its discontents

International standardization of East Asian medicine: the quest for modernization

Christopher Zaslawski • Myeong Soo Lee

Standards development, albeit a relatively new term for East Asian medicine, has been a central feature in the healthcare sector of many countries for several decades. It is only in recent years that countries such as China, Korea and Japan have been actively pursuing standardization of their traditional medical practices in the quest for modernization (Chan & Lee 2002). Currently there are also movements to establish regional and global standards for East Asian medicine that will throw up further challenges and opportunities. There are many factors driving the modernization of East Asian medicine, including the development of new technologies, the growing commercialization of herbal medicine, increasing research activity within the field, and the regulation and integration of traditional medicines into the public and community healthcare sector (Li et al 2008). Coupled with this modernization process has been the globalization of East Asian medicine, which has spread well beyond its Asian boundaries to many countries, including Australia, North America and Europe (Alter 2005). This chapter will explore how the modernization and globalization process has driven the need to standardize as well as evaluate how standardization will affect the practice and future development of East Asian medicine. Standardization has the potential to affect clinical practice, research, policy development and education, and will require extensive consultation and discussion if all stakeholders and interested parties are to achieve suitable outcomes. This raises important questions, such as who should be and who wants to be involved, what aspects of Asian medicine should be standardized, and how consensus can be achieved given the complexity and diversity of opinion from stakeholders. To complicate matters even further, Asian medicine has inherent cultural values, and many stakeholders will need to reflect on their national and regional interests, which will lead them to assert their own priorities.

The term standard is very broad and can be defined as a uniformity of technical specifications, criteria, methods, processes, services or practices. Indeed, the breadth of products and current practices under the umbrella of Asian medicine make the determination of the scope of standardization very complex. Given this diversity and complexity, some standards may generate relatively little argument, whereas standards relating to education, where stakeholder countries may have differing regulatory or legislative requirements, may prove to be very difficult to harmonize and achieve satisfactory consensus for all. Nevertheless, the aim of standardization should not be forgotten in these debates, as when standardization is correctly implemented, it will ensure that the product or service is safe, reliable, and can perform consistently in the way it was intended to. As a corollary of this aim, standards also establish a common language, which often defines safety criteria and quality.

Some standards are regulated by legislation and are mandatory, whereas others can be voluntary. Indeed, many countries have standards that are embedded in legislation ensuring their implementation. Other standards, however, may only provide guidance and may include international standards and joint standards, national standards, codes, specifications, handbooks and guidelines.

Furthermore, some national standards developed in isolation from other countries may need to be harmonized for internationalization because of differing national regulatory or legislative requirements (Dobos et al 2005). In addition, standards developed by other international organizations, such as the World Health Organization (WHO) standards for traditional medicines or other working committees in standardization bodies such as the International Organization for Standardization (ISO) or the International Electrotechnical Commission (IEC), may need to be considered to facilitate harmonization.

HISTORICAL PERSPECTIVE

The concept of standardization is not new to China's traditional medicines. At various points in time efforts have been made to standardize the practice of both acupuncture and herbal medicine. The Song dynasties as well as the Jin-Yuan era provide examples of the attempt to standardize and institutionalize the practice of medicine in imperial China (Unschuld 1986; Goldschmidt 2009). During this time the Imperial Medical Service established medical institutions, systematized medical education, introduced medical examinations and facilitated the dissemination of the newly revised and printed medical literature. This resulted in the standardization and promulgation of medical texts to the outlying prefectures. Another example of a standardizing initiative during this period was the revision of the location of the acupoints by Wang Weiyi, and the publication of his book *Illustrated Manual on the Points for Acupuncture and Moxibustion on a New Bronze Figure*. This task resulted in the casting of the two bronze figures which were used for examination and the standardization of acupoint location (Chen 1987). Although it can be argued that during this period efforts such as these attempted to institutionalize and standardize medical practice, there is very little evidence to suggest this occurred on a widespread basis outside the capital district.

The more recent period of 1957 to 1963 was also a time when China's medical practices were markedly institutionalized and standardized. Under the direction of the Chinese Communist Party, the first sets of edited national textbooks were produced and a comprehensive theory of the medicine was developed to become what is now known as traditional Chinese medicine (TCM) (Taylor 2005). The aim of this movement was to modernize Chinese medicine, which Taylor proposed as 'a means intended to preserve Chinese medicine within a society itself unsure of the medicine's worth.' Standardization, however, is only ever effective if it can be consistently enforced. Given the presence of spaces in Chinese society where this is not the case, non-standard traditional medical practices persist. Hsu (1999), for instance, has demonstrated the ongoing diversity in terms of both the practice and informal education of practitioners in modern China, and Scheid (2002) has written extensively on the plurality of medicine in contemporary China and its causes. Both argue that despite the attempt of the Chinese central government to institutionalize and standardize their traditional medicine education system and the delivery of acupuncture and herbal medicine within the public healthcare system, many individuals and groups successfully operate outside these confines.

The most recent phase of standardization can be traced back to the publication in 1991 of the World Health Organization (WHO) document titled *A Proposed Standard International Acupuncture Nomenclature: Report of a WHO Scientific Group* (WHO 1991). For a number of reasons the development of acupuncture occurred earlier in the West than herbal medicine, so it is to be expected that the first attempts to standardize Chinese medicine involved the English nomenclature of acupuncture. In the standard it was reported that the international group had reached agreement on the proposed international acupuncture nomenclature and that it involved four components:

- The English translation of the Han character name of each channel;
- An alphanumeric code for the acupuncture points;
- The Chinese phonetic alphabet (Pinyin) names of channel and acupoints;
- The Han character names of channels and acupoints.

Shortly afterwards the second edition was published, titled *Standard Acupuncture Nomenclature* (WHO 1993). In this second edition, each of the 361 acupoint entries had three parts:

- The standardized English name of the classic point,
- A brief explanation of the name of the point; and
- A multilingual comparative list of the names of the acupoint.

Also around 1991, the WHO commissioned a report by a Working Group on Auricular Acupuncture Nomenclature. This report detailed the anatomy of the ear and auricular nomenclature. Both of these documents have contributed to the ongoing development of acupuncture. For example, the auricular acupuncture nomenclature report standardized the many conflicting auricular acupoint locations that had been developed by different groups up until that time. Since then, several publications associated with standards and guidelines have been produced by WHO, totaling 22 documents (WHO 2010a).

More recently, the Western Pacific Region of WHO initiated the second wave of standardization. A recent search of their website found 13 documents associated with standardization (WHO 2010b). Published in English, the language most commonly used for international communication, and uploaded onto the internet, they provide guidance for regulatory, academic, professional and industry bodies. Most recently cited publications have been the International Standards Terminologies in Traditional Medicine in the Western Pacific Region (WHO, 2007a) and WHO Standard Acupuncture Point Locations in the Western Pacific Region (WHO 2008).

Meanwhile, China has also embarked on a program of standardization for its traditional medicines. The earliest publication of a TCM standard was in 1988 and concerned TCM pattern diagnosis (*bian zheng* 辨證). It was the first time that China had attempted to develop a comprehensive modern standard for its traditional medicine (Deng 1990). In July 2006 the State Administration of Traditional Chinese Medicine issued an ambitious development plan (2006–2010) to standardize Chinese medicine. Their plan was to develop 500 standards of Chinese medicine, including 50 national and three to five international standards, involving standards for basic, technical, management and ethnic medicine. As of January 2010, 305 TCM standards had been issued, including 47 national standards, 258 at a professional level covering 13 basic standards, 234 technical standards and 49 standards associated with management. In addition, five professional technical national committees have been organized, recruiting experts from national academic associations (Lu 2010).

International non-governmental professional organizations have also instigated standardization activities. In March 2009 the World Federation of Chinese Medicine Societies (WFCMS) convened the 1st International Forum on Chinese Medicine Standardization (World Federation of Chinese Medicine News 2009). WFCMS has also published two standards, one on Chinese – English TCM nomenclature and the other on undergraduate TCM education. Standardization is also on the agenda for the World Federation of Acupuncture and Moxibustion Societies (WFAS). A review of their internet site found a web page dedicated to standardization, confirming that there is a concerted effort directed towards acupuncture standardization. This standardization of Chinese acupuncture–moxibustion is being rapidly developed, with 12 national standards having been issued, including acupuncture-related nomenclature and the locations of acupuncture points. In addition, 11 standards on manipulation of acupuncture needles and moxibustion practice have been developed, and another 14 standards on manipulation are still in the process of development. This flurry of activity resulted, in early 2009, in the submission by the Chinese standards body (Standardization Administration of China – SAC) to the International Organization for Standardization (ISO) of a proposal to establish a technical committee for the development of standards in TCM.

Japan has also been setting an agenda for the standardization of its traditional medicine practices. In May 2005, several societies and institutions organized a summit where they established the Japanese Liaison of Oriental Medicine (JLOM). Since its formation, JLOM has represented Japan (for both Kampo and acupuncture organizations) at several international standardization meetings, and the Japan standards national body (Japanese Industrial Standards Committee – JISC) has appointed JLOM as the mirror committee for the newly established international standards Technical Committee for traditional Chinese medicine (TC 249). Japan has consistently been active in regulating and establishing its own standards nationally, such as the standard for the acupuncture needle, the regulation of Kampo medicines and the practitioner licensing system.

The other major Asian country pursuing a program of standardization for its traditional medicines has been South Korea. As in China, historical examples also exist of attempts by Korean physicians to standardize their traditional medical system. Around the early 1600s the royal physician Heo Jun published the Donguibogam, which was an attempt to synthesize and standardize the then current medical practices. This text, as Dr Ahn points out in his vignette below, was a virtual encyclopedia of the medical knowledge of that time and a synthesis of the various schools of medicine then existing (see Vignette 6.1).

More recently, the Korean Institute of Oriental Medicine (KIOM), located in Daejeon, was instrumental in organizing a number of international

Donguibogam is an encyclopedia of medical knowledge and treatment techniques compiled in early 17th century Korea. A synthesis of diverse schools of medicine in East Asia, *Donguibogam* was officially promoted and incorporated into the system of public health and preventative medicine during the Chosun Dynasty of Korea. As an encyclopedia of East Asian philosophy and practice, and as an early embodiment of the concept of public health services, the importance of *Donguibogam* in standardizing Korean traditional medicine was immeasurable.

Since the 12th century, diverse medical theories have emerged in Asia based on centuries of empirical and clinical observation. Although various compilations of these theories and texts had been published, *Donguibogam* successfully collated and systematized the traditional medical knowledge and clinical experiences with the competing theories of the time in a single collection of volumes.

For example, *Naegyeong* is a volume in *Donguibogam* that provides a general introduction and explanation of basic theories associated with the human body. It standardized the current theories and understanding of the human body of the time in addition to identifying the essential viscera and tissues. Along with the physiology and pathology of the five viscera and six bowels, the volume also includes information relating to health-promoting and life-nurturing strategies and activities to promote a longer and healthier life for the common people. This was symbolic of an egalitarian approach to health maintenance at the time, as the *Donguibogam* was not intended solely for the royal family or aristocratic class, but also for the ordinary majority.

Since the publication of *Donguibogam*, most research on traditional Korean medicine has used it as a reference. Even the *Sasang* Medicine, which was devised by Doctor Lee Je-ma (~1900) and known as the 'Constitutional Medicine,' references *Donguibogam* and its theories. For instance, the initial concepts of constitutional medicine in *Donguibogam* were classified as fat, thin, white and black hue types.

According to research by Han et al (2009), who conducted a systematic review of the 213 published papers relating to *Donguibogam*, 58 papers were related to prescriptions, 48 to theoretic concepts and 40 on the physiology and pathology of *Donguibogam*. These studies have increased markedly in number over the last decade, reflecting the importance of *Donguibogam* today as traditional Korean medicine research.

The fact that *Donguibogam* remains a fundamental reference for research and development in traditional Korean medicine, and that it is widely referenced in clinical practice today, reflects the success of the government of the time standardizing the contemporary medical knowledge and its inherent usefulness.

non-governmental forums to develop a standard for the single-use disposable acupuncture needle, in order to develop a strategy to align acupuncture needles for single use with WHO traditional medical standards. The objective of these forums was to obtain the agreement of several countries regarding specifications for single-use acupuncture needles over the period of three years. To

International standardization of East Asian medicine

this end the International Network for developing Standards for Acupuncture (INSA) was established at the 3rd International Forum (February 2009) as an informal network for Asian traditional medicine devices, specifically the single-use acupuncture needle. The objectives of INSA were to develop a working committee for Asian traditional medical devices and to publicize any international standards associated with them. In May 2009, INSA, along with non-governmental organizations from America, Australia, Japan, Korea, New Zealand and Vietnam, via the Korean Agency for Technology and Standards (KATS), also proposed to ISO a new field of technical activity called Asian Traditional Medicine Devices. The scope of this technical committee was to standardize methods of testing and specifications applicable to the materials, instruments, appliances and equipment used in the practice of acupuncture and its associated practices. These standards would be applicable to materials and the specifications of the single-use acupuncture needle, moxibustion materials, cupping devices, auricular needles, indwelling needles and dermal hammers. However, the submission of this proposal coincided with that from China (SAC), and a decision was made to merge the two submissions to form a single committee.

The submissions to the International Organization for Standardization (ISO) to develop international standards were a significant event. ISO is the world's largest non-governmental organization that develops standards. Established in 1947, it has published in excess of 180 000 standards ranging from agriculture and mechanical engineering through to medical devices and information technology. Currently ISO has 163 members and includes both developed and developing nations. Its role is to develop standards in a transparent and equitable manner that has global relevance. The development of a new standard is usually initiated in response to a 'stakeholder' or an industry sector request. Once accepted by participating members of ISO and confirmation from the ISO Technical Management Board, a technical committee is formed consisting of experts from the member national bodies who have requested the standard or intend to use them in the future.

SO WHAT DO WE MEAN BY A STANDARD?

Wikipedia defines a standard as an 'established norm or requirement. It is usually a formal document that establishes uniform engineering or technical criteria, methods, processes and practices.'

Standards Australia (SA) define a standard as 'published documents setting out specifications and procedures designed to ensure products, services and systems are safe, reliable and consistently perform the way they were intended to.'

The ISO define a standard as a 'document, established by consensus and approved by a recognized body that provides, for common and repeated use, rules, guidelines or characteristics for activities or their results, aimed at the achievement of the optimum degree of order in a given context.' They further note that, 'Standards should be based on the consolidated results of science, technology and experience, and aimed at the promotion of optimum community benefits.'

From these three definitions one can see that a standard is a formal document; it can refer to products and processes, and has to do with reliability of performance and attempts to ensure safety. Four major categories of standard can be identified:

- Fundamental standards. These concern terminology, conventions, signs and symbols. An example of this type would be the recent WHO International Standards Terminologies on Traditional Medicine in the Western Pacific Region (WHO 2007a).
- Test methods and analysis standards. These measure characteristics such as temperature or chemical composition. The WHO Guidelines for Assessing Quality of Herbal Medicines with Reference to Contaminants and Residues (WHO 2007b) is an example of a standard for test measures.
- Specification standards. These define the characteristics of a product or service and their performance thresholds, for example factors such as interchangeability, health and safety, or environmental protection. The national standards for the acupuncture needle developed in China, Japan and Korea are examples of this type of standard.
- Organization standards. These describe the functions and relationships of a company, as well as elements such as quality assurance, maintenance, or production management. Documents such as WHO Guidelines on Safety Monitoring of Herbal Medicines in Pharmacovigilance Systems (WHO 2004) reflect such an organizational standard.

FORCES DRIVING STANDARDIZATION

So why has the drive for standardization increased so markedly over the last decade? One possible reason relates to politics and professionalization. In China, Korea and Japan, where their traditional medicine professions are either integrated into the public healthcare system or regulated by the government, the need to justify funding is increasingly reliant upon evidence that these national traditional services are both efficacious and cost-effective. Proponents of traditional medicines are being asked to 'show proof' in order to maintain government support or continue funding at their current levels. Furthermore, in countries such as Australia and the United Kingdom, where the practice of Chinese medicine is yet to be fully integrated into the healthcare system, there is a strong desire to professionalize. If Chinese medicine is to compete in the diverse medical fields that exist in many countries, the pressure to professionalize and demonstrate the effectiveness of practice will increase. The first step in integrating into mainstream healthcare throws up many challenges and will require standardization in several areas, such as diagnostic standards for medical records and quality standards for herbal medicines.

In a recent article, Professor Seung-Hoon Choi, the former regional advisor in traditional medicine for the WHO Western Pacific Region, identified four major challenges facing traditional medicine: the varying degree with which TCM is recognized by governments; the lack of scientific evidence concerning the efficiency of many of its therapies; the difficulties relating to the protection of many of its therapies; and problems in ensuring its proper use (Choi 2008).

Choi argues that WHO will only be able to overcome these obstacles by adopting a policy of 'standardization with evidence based approaches.' He further states that the role of standards in traditional medicine is to raise levels of quality, safety, reliability, efficacy and interchangeability.

It is very difficult to disagree with improving quality and safety. Practitioners require assurance that the acupuncture needle they use is sterile and will not break off in the skin, or that the herbal medicines they are dispensing have no or negligible levels of pesticide residue. The identification and enforcement of safety requirements is an essential aspect of standardization and will lead to the development of greater technical skill and less potential for adverse events during practice.

Clinical researchers in herbal medicine would also argue strongly for the need to standardize (Zhang et al 2009). Commercially developed products that include herbal substances grown in different regions need to contain similar levels of active ingredients and be of a certain quality if they are to be consistently effective. Without such assurance, herbal medicine research results will be unpredictable. In addition to phytochemical standardization, the issue of the traditional aspect of quality in herbal medicine must also be considered.

A recent paper by two well known and respected herbal researchers has argued that although the high-tech quality control measures 'satisfy the modern scientific requirements for identity, purity and quality in the assessment of chemical drugs, they are not suitable for handling the complex chemical nature of Chinese medicine, whose multifunctional components and inherent holistic activities are frequently unknown and hence not adequately analyzed by these methods. In order to assess properly and meaningfully the identity and quality of complex Chinese herbal medicines, additional measures that can retain the traditional aspect of Chinese medicine need to be included. This requires a basic understanding of traditional Chinese medicine' (Xie & Leung 2009). This highlights some of the difficulties for Chinese herbal medicine if it is to be standardized for the purpose of commercialization.

ADVANTAGES OF STANDARDIZATION

So what does the drive for standardization mean for clinicians, researchers and educationalists? Depending on the situation and perspective, there are both advantages and disadvantages.

One basic problem that is slowly being resolved is TCM terminology. Without standardized clinical terms the documentation and portability of medical records is restricted. A number of recent researchers have explored this issue with regard to the English terminology associated with TCM pulse nomenclature, diagnostic tongue characteristics and TCM pattern names.

A recent review (Walsh and King 2008) found a variety of English terms used for the majority of the 28 traditional pulse qualities. However, whereas standardizing these terms may be relatively easy, the issue of operationally defining the 28 pulse qualities is not easily achieved. This is likely to be due to the particular pulse qualities that were described in the medical classics as metaphors or images. In Chapter 3, Judith Farquhar explores some of these issues, including the subjective nature of the pulse and the need for a focus on its clinical significance. Other researchers have also found a similar problem when cross-referencing the English literature for the different Chinese patterns terms associated with the biomedical diseases. Berle (2008) found that many authors used different pattern nomenclatures, leading to confusion. This was also the case when another researcher reviewed the English literature for various tongue characteristics and their equivalent English terms used by English and Chinese authors (Kim 2003).

In all three situations differing, and in some cases ambiguous, terms are used, making communication and understanding unclear. If the terminology in the medical record is ambiguous, this can make things difficult when referring patients to other practitioners. Clinicians need to be able to communicate accurately and clearly for patient safety. Standardized terminology is also important for education. Educators also need standardized technical terms, to enable good educational practice and satisfactory student learning. For clinical facilities and hospitals the need to maintain standardized medical records is paramount. For example, the outpatient clinic at the University of Technology, Sydney, Australia, has an electronic database of clinical data on all patients attending the acupuncture outpatient clinic (Meier & Rogers 2006). The advantages of mining the database are enormous, but if a need arises to integrate and expand into other such clinical databases there would be great difficulties. Certain technical terms used in the database are unique to the platform, and the alignment of diagnostic terms, including pattern names and tongue and pulse descriptions, would be problematic. From an international perspective, integrating various databases presents additional problems, such as heterogeneity of data formats, cultural and linguistic differences, and the lack of standard terminology. Data sharing will be key to advancing Asian medicine in the digital age, and the ability to standardize will be important in promoting data harmonization (Cheung & Chen 2010).

One area of standardization that has been successful concerns devices, especially the filiform acupuncture needle. Currently China, Korea and Japan all have a national standard for the acupuncture needle. The Chinese standard (GB 2024–94), which was developed in 1987 includes documentation for a number of criteria for the filiform acupuncture needle. These include physical dimensions (diameter and length of the needle), shape and profile, properties such as rigidity, tensile strength around the needle root, sharpness of the tip or apex, and surface roughness; test methods specifying their methods and sampling rules and packaging and storing requirements, including primary and secondary packaging and labeling.

The Japanese standard JIST 9301 is more recent, having been developed in 2005. Similar in content to the Chinese standard, it documents and describes the needle standard in terms of a variety of criteria, including scope, normative references terms and definitions, physical requirements, chemical requirements, assurance for sterility, endotoxin test, tolerance of dimensions, configuration, needle tip, performance and packaging and labeling.

The newest needle standard is the Korean KSP 730, which is the only one of the three needle standards that has been developed specifically for the single-use disposable filiform needle. This standard also documents and describes the needle standard in terms of a variety of criteria, including scope, normative references terms and definitions, physical requirements, chemical requirements, assurance for sterility, biological and physical tests, tolerance of dimensions, configuration, needle tip, performance and packaging and marking.

These three national needle standards demonstrate similar content and the potential to develop an international standard. Given the complexity associated with standards development for East Asian medicine, it behoves standard developers to give thought to practicality and the level of cooperation needed for standardization. Indeed, projects for developing standards for devices such as the filiform needle may be the easiest to achieve and have the most potential to gain agreement from all stakeholders.

ISSUES FOR DEVELOPING STANDARDS

One criticism of standardization is that it promotes the 'flattening' of diversity. As stated earlier, many would argue that traditional Chinese medicine today is already a standard system of knowledge that was developed for teaching in China's newly constructed Chinese medicine colleges in the 1950s. Many practitioners worry that standardization may restrict many clinical practices and lead to failure to improvise and innovate. From a clinician's perspective this may be very important. East Asian medicine is based on the central tenet of individualization of treatment, and standardization threatens this. Scheid (2002) makes a very good argument for maintaining diversity of practice based on historical grounds. His research has demonstrated that the practice of medicine in ancient China was intrinsically diverse and a heterogeneous tradition (Scheid 2002). He argues that East Asian medicine is a living tradition that is evolving and constantly developing, and that it was this flexibility that ensured its survival and also its effectiveness over time. Scheid points out that unlike Western medicine, East Asian medicine 'locates effectiveness in the practitioner and not the medicine.'

Another concern associated with standardization is the fear that the process will lead to the biomedicalization of Asian medicine. As Garvey points out in her vignette, there is always the prospect that traditional medical concepts could be reconceptualized during the standardization process, for example the translation of traditional Chinese disease terms into modern biomedical disease nosology in preference to retaining their traditional meaning (see Vignette 6.2). The retention of the essential features and characteristics of East Asian medicine will be paramount if the standardization process is to be successful.

One form of standardization that has been increasingly used in biomedicine and affects the individualistic practice of East Asian medicine is the development of clinical practice guidelines (CPG). These aim to guide decisions and criteria regarding diagnosis, management and treatment in specific areas of healthcare. Such documents have been in use for thousands of years during the entire history of medicine: indeed, many of the classics of Chinese medicine can be seen as examples of this approach. However, in contrast to previous approaches, which were often based on tradition or authority, modern medical guidelines are more commonly based on an examination of current evidence within the paradigm of evidence-based medicine.

As part of China's 20th-century drive to modernize Chinese medicine, revisions aimed at standardizing education and training were extended to terminologies, theoretical principles and therapeutic content. Textbook content had to be adjusted in its representations of Chinese medicine concepts to demonstrate their connections with Western medical (biomedical) terms and categories, and all the new textbook content had to be standardized to comply with the centralized training curriculum.

Consequently, Chinese medicine textbooks of Chinese and Western origin today are able to present structured frameworks for the learning and application of traditional medical theories that have been revised to suit the contemporary climate and reader. These texts usually do not locate or contextualize traditional concepts or their revisions within the classic, biomedical or research literature; and translations, technical language and terminology to date have been largely interpretive, idiosyncratic and difficult to cross-reference.

For a discipline whose discourses and methods have been developing over many centuries, standardization offers a number of benefits. It improves communication for education and medical practice; it gives the discipline a firm foundation for education and clinical learning; and it improves the interexaminer reliability of Chinese medicine practice and research. The biomedical standardization of Chinese medicine's content and categories allows clinicians and researchers to apply these therapies to biomedical diagnoses.

Unfortunately, and particularly when guided by a biomedical agenda, standardization also simplifies thousands of years of diversity and reduces the tradition's inbuilt flexibility.

"Chinese medicine has lately been engaged in fixing its elements in increasingly immutable signifying relations. This arrangement would then be a suitable candidate to be investigated epistemologically along Western lines. But it would not much resemble the more processual, contingent and pragmatic approaches to illness of an earlier Chinese medicine (Farquhar 1987, p. 1018).**"**

On the standardization of terminology, for example, the uncritical translation of traditional-to-biomedical terminologies is fraught with Eurocentric biases and leads to a false sense that traditional Chinese medicine is essentially similar to biomedicine (Waldram 2000). It removes their original contexts and meanings and uncouples them from the Chinese medical archive – their conceptual histories and contexts. The biomedical standardization of terms and concepts disrupts Chinese medicine's internal coherence, and dismantles it as a system of medicine.

In Australia, quality assurance and minimum training standards are required for public safety and best practice. Quality markers and safety standards are applied to therapeutic instruments, technologies, herbal substance production and manufacturing processes. In this context, and when combined with the sweeping changes wrought by standardization, acupuncture techniques and herbal substances are easily reconceptualized as technologies and active constituents independent of their traditional context, allowing their assimilation into biomedical practice and research.

International standardization of East Asian medicine

Biomedical clinical practice guidelines aim to identify, summarize and evaluate the best evidence and provide the most up to date information about prevention, diagnosis, prognosis and therapy, including dosages, risk/benefit and the cost-effectiveness of a particular medical condition. They define the most important questions related to clinical practice and identify all possible decision options and their outcomes. Some guidelines contain decision or computation algorithms to be followed based on an evaluation of the best current evidence on disease management. They attempt to integrate the identified decision points and respective courses of action to the clinical judgment and experience of practitioners. Many guidelines place treatment options into different hierarchical categories to help providers in deciding which treatment to use. Where research-based evidence is not available, expert consensus forms the basis of the guideline. This 'consensus by expert' is seen as representing the lowest form of evidence for developing clinical practice guidelines and is used where there is a lack of quality evidence. This may especially be the case where clinical practice guidelines are to be developed for Asian medicine where there is a relatively short history of research, and underdevelopment of evidence, compared to biomedicine. Consensus methods, as pointed out by MacPherson, are not without their limitations (see Vignette 6.3).

VIGNETTE 6.3   CONSENSUS OR NONSENSUS? CONCERNS REGARDING METHODS USED TO GENERATE STANDARDS
HUGH MACPHERSON

Consensus methods are commonly used to agree standards. In the field of East Asian medicine they have been used to agree nomenclature and terminology, point locations and clinical guidelines. The very need for consensus stems from a lack of consensus. Why involve so many people in consensus-related activities if consensus already exists? Moreover, it is precisely where there is a lack of good evidence that consensus methods are being used. Typical approaches include the Delphi method and the Nominal Group Technique (Black et al 1999). Although the outcomes of these processes can appear beguilingly acceptable, the reality behind them can raise more questions than answers. So what are the key concerns about consensus methods?

The first concern relates to the representativeness of participants contributing to the consensus and the transparency of the process by which they were selected. The inherent tension between choosing participants likely to satisfy the desire for consensus and the willingness to open up to diversity is not always explicit. The more careful the selection, the easier it is likely to be to achieve consensus. Token dissidents might be included, but their contrary views are unlikely to be reflected in the published outcome. The implicit rationale behind the relative breadth and narrowness of the selection process is not always made clear.

The second concern relates to the transparency of decision making. Whereas on the surface a consensus group may be made up of individuals who each have an equal opportunity to contribute, the actual processes that bring together consensus are not always reported. This may be because of behind-the-scenes power-brokering, or where trade-offs are agreed in order to reach an acceptable compromise. These hidden processes may not be seen as acceptable for public consumption, which may explain cases where transparency is limited.

The third concern relates to the different contexts that participants may bring to the table. Acupuncture is practiced in such different ways in different countries, and even within the same country, that it is questionable whether a consensus is possible without the influence of power-brokering. Moreover, it is questionable whether a consensus is useful in terms of applicability when it might be seen as irrelevant in areas where it does not reflect the local context.

Fourth, because consensus methods are used precisely where evidence is lacking, participants need to make judgments based on both their personal and their community opinion. The problem here is highlighted by the apocryphal story of the old Chinese method of consensus that was used to settle the question of the length of the Emperor's nose (Skrabanek 1990). As no one was allowed to see the Emperor's nose, direct measurement was not possible. So instead, experts from around China were consulted and, because they were experts, all provided an estimate. Then these answers were averaged. Assuming enough data were collected, the standard error of the mean was found to be low and the estimate precise! The point here is that although a consensus will reflect majority opinion, this may or may not be a reflection of reality. Therefore, it is important to consider the extent that such methods lead to a nonsensus consensus.

Chen and Jiang (2009) conducted a review of 11 Chinese CPGs that had been developed for Chinese medicine. They found that there was an inadequate standardization of guideline development and a lack of high-grade evidence to support the guidelines. Although there has been some integration of acupuncture and herbal medicine into CPGs in Western countries (Ravindran et al 2009), there is yet to be published in the English language a CPG specifically for Chinese medicine. Until the level of quality research reaches a sufficient threshold, the publication of an East Asian medicine-specific CPG will not be achieved.

Finally, it should be evident that some standards may be easier to develop than others. For example, broad agreement for less contentious technical standards for needle production would be easier to achieve than the development of international standards for education, where there are likely to be competing international interests and regulatory constraints. Other standards, for example for herbal medicine quality, may be so complex as to require widespread consultation and extensive research evaluation over several years until informed consensus can be reached (Dobos et al 2005; Wang et al 2009).

FURTHER DEVELOPMENTS

Whereas the standardization projects and documents mentioned so far have all been primarily national or regional, there have been recent moves to establish international standards for Chinese medicine through the International Organization for Standardization (ISO). On 24 August 2009, 41 technical experts and representatives from the four National Standards bodies of China, Korea, Japan and Australia met for a preliminary discussion on the establishment of a technical committee for Chinese medicine under the governance of ISO. Shortly afterwards, based on the recommendations from this meeting, the Technical Management Board of ISO voted for the establishment of a technical committee (TC 249) for Chinese medicine. This committee will be charged with developing international standards across a range of areas for Chinese medicine. Currently there are 20 participating member countries and ten observer countries associated with the committee. The participating countries are China, Korea, Japan, Australia, United States of America, Canada, France, Finland, India, Israel, Germany, Ghana, Mongolia, Netherlands, Norway, Spain, South Africa, Thailand, Tunisia and Vietnam. It should be noted that although there are only 20 participating countries, all 163 ISO national member countries have the opportunity to be involved, either participating or observing. As with any international standard it is to be expected that different nations will have differing perspectives, and that disagreement may be common. This may especially be the case for TC 249, where it is likely that cultural, political and national interests may be at play. Fortunately, there are many benefits to the ISO standardization process: ISO has established protocols for achieving consensus and policies to ensure equitable representation of all stakeholders. These include a code of ethics, rules for decision making and policies for dealing with intellectual property rights. Policies such as these will ensure a fair and equitable process for all stakeholders, including the practice of 'one country one vote.' Furthermore, each participating country is required to establish a 'mirror' committee which will be responsible for developing, debating and eventually agreeing on their national perspective. A member from the mirror committee would then represent the national opinion regarding the particular standard at the larger international ISO Technical Committee meeting. Each national mirror committee also has requirements for membership, including a broad representation of all interests and adherence to committee protocols and procedures. Committee members representing education and research institutes, professional practitioner bodies, appropriate government regulators, consumers and industry groups will ensure a broad and diverse opinion. In addition, ad-hoc groups of experts can be selected by the committees (both the international and the national mirror committee) who are interested and willing to contribute to and evaluate international proposals. Finally, there is the opportunity to develop formal liaison agreements with international organizations such as WHO.

With the development of standards it is also important to ensure that, where appropriate, the best available evidence and technical expertise be obtained to inform discussion and standard development. The ISO process of developing national mirror committee perspectives will facilitate wide-ranging consultation and feedback into the international decision-making process. Finally, if during the voting, the national position is one of opposition and a negative vote is returned, it is essential that this be supported by clearly expressed technical comment to the International Technical Committee, ensuring a transparent and open process.

Standardization has much to offer Asian medicine and acupuncture. It has the potential to improve the quality and safety of devices such as needles or electrostimulators. Herbal medicine will also benefit by ensuring safe and effective products for both clinical practice and research. Communication will be enhanced for both education and research, and the integration of meaningful clinical information into databases will be possible. However, this comes with a caveat: care must be taken to ensure that any standard developed accords with traditional and authentic traditional medicine practices and does not restrict the creativity, innovation and diversity of clinical practice.

As stated in the 2008 Beijing declaration adopted by the WHO Congress on Traditional Medicine:

'The knowledge of traditional medicine, treatments and practices should be respected, preserved, promoted and communicated widely and appropriately based on the circumstances in each country.'

We need to ensure that any standardization process does not limit or restrict the practice of acupuncture and herbal medicine, yet at the same time have the ability to achieve its aims of safety, reliability and therapeutic efficiency. CZ and MSL are both members of their local national mirror committees for TC 249 in Australia and South Korea respectively.

REFERENCES

Alter, J.S. (Ed.), 2005. Asian Medicine and Globalization. University of Pennsylvania Press, Philadelphia.

Beijing Declaration, 2008. Adopted by the WHO Congress on Traditional Medicine. Beijing, China, 8 November. http://www.wpro.who.int/NR/rdonlyres/A0AB4D18-5B18-4513-BC4C-2FF15369C6FE/0/TRM_BeijingDeclarationEN.pdf (accessed 18.01.10).

Berle, C., 2008. The effect of acupuncture on people with hepatitis C virus: a randomized controlled pilot study. MSc Thesis. University of Technology, Sydney.

Black, N., Murphy, M., Lamping, D., et al., 1999. Consensus development methods: a review of best practice in creating clinical guidelines. J. Health Serv. Res. Policy. 4 (4), 236–248.

Chan, K., Lee, H. (Eds.), 2002. The Way Forward for Chinese Medicine. Taylor and Francis, London.

Chen, K.J., Jiang, Y.R., 2009. Current status and problems in developing clinical guidelines for Chinese medicine and integrative medicine. Zhong Xi Yi Jie He Xue Bao 7 (4), 301–305.

Chen, X.N. (Ed.), 1987. Chinese Acupuncture and Moxibustion. Foreign Languages Press, Beijing.

Cheung, K.H., Chen, H., 2010. Semantic Web for data harmonization in Chinese medicine. Chin. Med. 5 (2).

Choi, S.H., 2008. WHO traditional medicine strategy and activities standardization with evidence based approaches. J. Acupunct. Meridian Stud. 1 (2), 153–154.

Deng, T.T., 1990. Standardization of Traditional Chinese Medicine Syndromes. Guangdong Scientific and Technical Publishers (Chinese), Guangzhou.

Dobos, G.J., Tan, L., Cohen, M.H., McIntyre, M., Bauer, R., Li, X., et al., 2005. Are national quality standards for traditional Chinese herbal medicine sufficient? Current governmental regulations for traditional Chinese herbal medicine in certain Western countries and China as the Eastern origin country. Complement. Ther. Med. 13 (3), 183–190.

Farquhar, J., 1987. Problems of knowledge in contemporary Chinese medical discourse. Soc. Sci. Med. 24 (12), 1013–1021.

Goldschmidt, A.M., 2009. The Evolution of Chinese Medicine: Song Dynasty, 960–1200. RoutledgeCurzon Press, London.

Han, C., Park, S., Kwon, O., et al., 2009. Systematic review on the Donguibogam in the Korean Medicine Journal. The J. Korean Med. Hist. 22 (2), 7–13.

Hsu, E., 1999. The Transmission of Chinese Medicine. Cambridge University Press, Cambridge.

International Organization for Standardization, http://www.iso.org/iso/home.htm (accessed 18.01.10).

Kim, M., 2003. Traditional Chinese tongue inspection: an examination of the inter and intra practitioner reliability for specific tongue characteristics. MSc Thesis, University of Technology, Sydney.

Li, W.F., Jiang, J.G., Chen, J., 2008. Chinese medicine and its modernization demands. Arch. Med. Res. 39 (2), 246–251.

Lu, A., 2010. TCM research and standards in China and its impact worldwide. Presentation handout at International Seminar on TCM Standardization.

Beijing, People's Republic of China, 25–26 January.

Meier, P.C., Rogers, C., 2006. Reporting traditional Chinese medicine morbidity — A University of Technology, Sydney, project with an emphasis on developing standards for testing and reporting data. J. Altern. Complement. Med. 12 (6), 529–534.

Ravindran, A.V., Lam, R.W., Filateau, M.J., et al., 2009. Canadian network for mood and anxiety treatments (CANMAT) Clinical guidelines for the management of major depressive disorder in adults. V. Complementary and alternative medicine treatments. J. Affect. Disord. 117 (Suppl. 1), S54–S64.

Scheid, V., http://www.volkerscheid.co.uk/ index.php/clinical_practice/east_asian_ medicine/ (accessed 18.01.10).

Scheid, V., 2002. Chinese Medicine in Contemporary China. Duke University Press, Durham.

Skrabanek, P., 1990. Nonsensus consensus. Lancet 335 (8703), 1446–1447.

Standards Australia, http://www. standards.org.au/cat.asp?catid=2 (accessed 18.01.10).

Taylor, K., 2005. Chinese Medicine in Early Communist China 1945–1963: A Medicine of Revolution. Routledge, New York.

Technical Committee 249-Traditional Chinese Medicine, http://www.iso.org/ iso/standards_development/technical_ committees/list_of_iso_technical_ committees/iso_technical_committee. htm?commid=598435 (accessed 07.02.10).

Unschuld, P.U., 1986. Medicine in China. A history of pharmaceutics. University of California Press, Berkley.

Waldram, J.B., 2000. The efficacy of Traditional medicine; current theoretical and methodological issues. Med. Anthropol. Q. 14 (4), 603–625.

Walsh, S., King, E., 2008. Pulse Diagnosis: a Clinical Guide. Churchill Livingstone, Edinburgh.

Wang, J.S., vander Heijden, R., Spruit, S., et al., 2009. Quality and safety of Chinese herbal medicines guided by a systems biology perspective. J. Ethnopharmacol. 120, 31–41.

Wikipedia, http://en.wikipedia.org/wiki/ Standardization (accessed 18.01.10).

World Federation of Acupuncture and Moxibustion Societies (WFAS) standardization, http://www.wfas.com. cn/en/list.asp?men=8&class=317&li

ststate=1&Position=Acupuncture%20 Standardization (accessed 18.01.10).

World Federation of Chinese Medicine News No. 1, July, 2009. http://www .wfcms.org/uploads/20090903/ WFCMS_NEWS_No.1.pdf (accessed 18.01.09).

World Health Organization, 1991. Proposed standard international acupuncture nomenclature. Report of a WHO scientific group. World Health Organization, Geneva.

World Health Organization, 1993. Standard Acupuncture Nomenclature. WHO Regional Office for the Western Pacific, Manila.

World Health Organization, 2004. WHO Guidelines on Safety Monitoring of Herbal Medicines in Pharmacovigilance Systems. World Health Organization, Geneva.

World Health Organization, 2007a. WHO International Standards Terminologies on Traditional Medicine in the Western Pacific Region. WHO Regional Office for the Western Pacific, Manila.

World Health Organization, 2007b. WHO Guidelines for Assessing Quality of Herbal Medicines with Reference to Contaminants and Residues. World Health Organization, Geneva.

World Health Organization, 2008. WHO Standard Acupuncture Point Locations in the Western Pacific Region. WHO Regional Office for the Western Pacific, Manila, Manila.

World Health Organization, 2010a. Western Pacific Region publications listing. http://www.wpro.who.int/internet/ templates/INF_Pub_Listing.aspx?NRM ODE=Published&NRNODEGUID=%7b6 82D9AD8-F889–43E8–9F81–14B369B52F5 7%7d&NRORIGINALURL=%2fpublicati ons%2fpublications%2ehtm&NRCACHE HINT=Guest (accessed 12.04.10).

World Health Organization, 2010b. Geneva publications listing. http://apps.who. int/medicinedocs/en/cl/CL1.1.1.3.1/ clmd,50.html#hlCL1_1_1_3_1 (accessed 12.04.10).

Xie, P.S., Leung, A.Y., 2009. Understanding the traditional aspect of Chinese medicine in order to achieve meaningful quality control of Chinese materia medica. J. Chromotogr. A 1216, 1930–1940.

Zhang, Y.T., Zhang, Y., Guo, Y., et al., 2009. Overview of quality standardization for traditional Chinese medicine. China Standardization March 2009 Issue.

Standardizing tongue diagnosis with image processing technology: essential tension between authenticity and innovation**

Sean Hsiang-lin Lei 雷祥麟 • Chiao-ling Lin 林巧玲
Hen-hong Chang 張恆鴻

TONGUE IMAGE VS TONGUE PERCEPTION

It was an important event, followed with great interest by countless observers, when Sun Yatsen 孫中山 (1866–1925), the founding father of the Republic of China (1911–) and a modern-trained physician, deliberated over whether to use traditional Chinese medicine to save his own life that was being threatened by liver cancer. To many of Sun's comrades and progressive intellectuals, the very act of taking Chinese medicinals was no less than a public betrayal of the notion of modernity: a modernity that Sun himself personified, since he had led the revolution to overthrow the Qing dynasty and establish the first Republic in East Asia. According to the account provided by Lu Xun 魯迅 (1881–1936), one of the fathers of modern Chinese literature and once a student of modern medicine, the dying Sun in the end reasoned this way: "While some Chinese medicinals might be effective, [reliable] diagnosis is lacking [in Chinese medicine]. How can one take drugs without a trustworthy diagnosis? There is no need to take [Chinese drugs]" (Lu 1973). Like the statement by Liang Shuming 梁漱溟 cited by Scheid in Chapter 2, this episode reveals that, ever since the dawn of medical modernity in East Asia, one of the greatest barriers to recognizing the efficacy of traditional medicine has been its methods of diagnosis, at least to modernizers such as Lu Xun, Liang Shuming and others.

Indeed, traditional diagnosis had many drawbacks, especially in the context of tongue diagnosis. First, the traditional four diagnoses all took place in the split moment of the clinical encounter between doctor and patient. There was almost nothing that could be stabilized and recorded as tangible, objective

** This article is based on Lin Chiao-ling's Master Thesis "Capturing Tongue Perception with Tongue Image: A Study of Chinese Tongue Diagnosis with Image-Processing Technology in Taiwan's Chang Gung University," (2004) Institute of History, National Tsing-hua University, TAIWAN. We would like to thank Volker Scheid and Hugh MacPherson for their experimentalism, encouragement, and very valuable suggestions, and Dr Sabine Wilms for her editorial inputs.

© 2012 Elsevier Ltd.

evidence in this method of diagnosis. Partially as a result of this, the system of apprenticeship became a necessity. The only way for a student to learn to see the varieties of tongue dispositions was to sit beside the master and have the opportunity to see the 'same' tongue as the master, even though the disciple might still have problems recognizing what the master perceived effortlessly. In this sense, the introduction of tongue imaging into Chinese medicine is a revolutionary effort to create tangible and visible evidence for Chinese medical diagnosis.

It seems quite natural that modern researchers became interested in standardizing tongue diagnosis with image processing technology. Among the traditional four areas of diagnosis –inspection (*wang* 望), listening and smelling (*wen* 聞), inquiring (*wen*問), and palpation (*qie*切) – inspection, and tongue diagnosis in particular, involved the most abstract of the senses. Especially compared with pulse diagnosis (Li 1994; Maciocia 2004), tongue diagnosis appeared to be relatively objective and therefore most promising in rendering a publicly shared image of the diagnostic process. Because of this relative objectivity, when proponents of Chinese medicine endeavored to integrate Chinese medical diagnosis with modern biomedical diagnosis in the early 20th century, tongue diagnosis became a popular focus of such efforts. In 1920, Cao Bingzhang 曹炳章 (1878–1956) published *Bian she zhinan* 辯舌指南 (*Manual for Differentiating the Tongue*), which included not only an anatomical illustration of the tongue but also 117 color drawings of pathological tongues (Liang 2004; Holroyde-Downing 2005). The central players of the present paper, the Taiwanese research team from the medical school of Chang Gung University 長庚大學, have followed the same valuation of visual objectivity, but replaced the drawings with photographs, thereby further increasing the objective value of the visual representation. If they succeed in creating a system of standardized images of tongues, their research has the potential to become the first widely used visual image library for clinical diagnosis in Chinese medicine.

Nevertheless, it could be argued that this kind of standardization constitutes a betrayal of the authenticity of Chinese medicine. As medical historian Shigehisa Kuriyama has argued, whereas nowadays the Chinese term *se* is often used as the translation of the English 'color,' the meaning of *se* in *wangse* 望色 (lit. 'inspecting color,' one of the major aspect of the diagnostic method of inspection) cannot be equated with color or hue (Kuriyama 1999). Moreover, the etymology of *wang* suggested the act of a person stretching to see something that is difficult to make out or not there yet. In this sense, the very idea of *wang* demands the viewer's active participation in making sense of something that is not readily comprehensible. As a specific style of looking, *wangse* is very different from the idea of mirroring the reality out there without any involvement of human subjectivity.

From this point of view, the very idea of standardizing tongue diagnosis with image processing technology is no less than a 'research oxymoron' (see Vignette 7.1). Anyone who values the authenticity of Chinese medicine will realize how much loss of knowledge will result from such apparently reasonable efforts. It was in the face of this classic dilemma that the Taiwanese research team started conceiving its own project. Judging from the proposal

There are many studies that have aimed for objectivity and quantification in tongue diagnosis as part of the clinical modernization of Traditional Chinese Medicine (TCM) (Cui et al 2001; Han & Yu 1993; Liu et al 2003; Pang et al 2004; Wei et al 2002; Zou et al 2003). These studies seek to legitimize tongue diagnosis as a diagnostic tool by adapting it to fit a biomedical understanding of science, whereby what can be seen when looking at the tongue is reduced to that which can be measured. Such research aims to overcome the perceived limitations attributed to this method of diagnosis:

'due to its qualitative, subjective and experience-based nature, traditional tongue diagnosis has a very limited-application in clinical medicine'

Pang et al 2004.

I take one such study aiming at objectification (Gareus et al 2005) and consider what underlies it. In this study, tongues were photographed and doctors asked to describe their color. Parameters (such as lighting) were standardized to allowed good-quality (standardized pixels) images to be produced. Leaving aside the irony that only 'experienced' doctors of TCM were chosen to take part, there were several assumptions at play: first, that bodily signs – markers of a possible pathology – can be extracted from the person displaying them; and second, that objective value-free observation is possible. What was found was that different doctors saw different colors in the same tongues, and the same doctor saw different colors at different times. How can this be possible from the standpoint of the assumptions mentioned above?

Does looking at the color of a tongue involve seeing pixel-defined color alone? A historical and linguistic look at the Chinese term for color challenges the relevance of research aiming for objectivity. The main aspect of the looking diagnosis in Chinese medicine is 'gazing upon color – wangse – 望色' (Kuriyama 1999). The original meaning of se is not simply or directly designating hue but rather the look on a person's face. This term later came to be used for the realm of appearance (in the Buddhist sense of 'being itself'). The character wang of wangse is made up of a picture of someone stretching forward to catch a glimpse of the distant moon. Its etymology springs from two characters meaning to be absent and obscure, hence to gaze expresses the effort of seeing something difficult to make out. Practitioners of Chinese medicine develop their use of color from reading faces, and this was a learned skill dependent on the looker's experience and ability to perceive the subtle. What could be seen was dependent on who was seeing: it is open to interpretation. The most advanced doctors were those believed to be able to diagnose through looking alone.

Looking at the tongue involves an interpretation of hue, shimmer, moistness, movement and so on. The reported 'objective' research is limited in matching the skills of practitioners; its design therefore falls short as a method of tongue diagnosis. Instead, such research can be seen to shape and create a new object that may provide significant new knowledge, as Lei argues in this chapter, but can never replace the interpretation of the subtle.

Standardizing tongue diagnosis with image processing technology the team submitted to the funding agency, this project looked not that different from other typical efforts to standardize Chinese medicine. However, as the team became aware of the dilemma between authenticity and standardization, they carefully set up their objective to find a way out of this paradox that has troubled the reformers of traditional East Asian medicine since the latter half of the 19th century. To highlight this difficult situation, Professor Chang Hen-Hong 張恆鴻, the Director of Chang Gung University's Graduate Institute of Traditional Chinese Medicine and the leader of the research team for 'Standardizing Tongue Diagnosis with Image Processing Technology,' explicitly differentiates two kind of *shexiang* (Chang 2007). Although both varieties are pronounced identically, they consist of different characters in Chinese and have distinctively different connotations. The first kind of *shexiang* 舌像 ('tongue image') refers directly to the image of the tongue that is captured with image processing technology. In contrast, the second kind of *shexiang* 舌象 refers to the perceptual experience that a doctor forms in his or her mind during the process of tongue diagnosis. While the first *shexiang* can be produced with a camera in an automatic fashion, the subjective involvement of the perceiver is the defining element of the second *shexiang*. By way of coining two different terms, Professor Chang thus made clear that his research team was keenly aware of the difference between the two and thereby emphasized the fact that their research objective was never to substitute one for the other. On the contrary, their exploration started from the recognition of this essential tension between the tongue image and the process of tongue perception.

By documenting Professor Chang's team's efforts to create new possibilities out of the apparent opposition between authenticity and innovation, we would like to use their research as a window to shed some light on the constraints, possibilities, innovative strategies and limitations as they tried to go beyond this structural opposition. Hopefully, our insights will be useful to researchers involved in similar projects of integrating East Asian medicine into the contemporary healthcare system.

RECONNECTING WITH HISTORY

One of the major motivations for developing tongue diagnosis imaging technology was 'to improve the objectivity and precision of tongue diagnosis' (Chang et al 2005). There are a few reasons why tongue diagnosis imaging can increase the objectivity of tongue diagnosis. First, perhaps with the exception of pulse diagnosis, tongue diagnosis imaging would be the first evidence to come directly from the patient's body, with minimal participation – and hence potential distortion – from the observer. The image-taking process is so mechanical and automatic that it feels as if the researchers just 'let nature speak for itself,' and the images created hereby are therefore free from the corruption of human deliberation. Starting with the simple premise that the human eye works just like a camera, the researchers decided to use image processing technology to record the image of the tongue as created during diagnosis. As these images are stabilized, standardized, classified and multiplied, they can serve as valuable tools in the contexts of documentation, education, classification and even data mining and further research and analysis. Moreover, instead of just erasing subjective judgments from the diagnostic process, these standardized images could help construct an objective baseline that could then be used to identify practitioners who possess an unusual perceptive capability in tongue diagnosis. In other words, instead of aiming to 'reduce' the clinical encounter of tongue diagnosis into a mechanical, and hence objective, process of image-taking, tongue diagnosis imaging is specifically designed to assist in identifying those practitioners who possess an unusual, above-average 'subjective sensory capability' in diagnosis.

Nevertheless, the research team soon became aware of the crucial weakness of the metaphor of the camera. They realized that what they valued and wanted to record was not really the image of the tongue, but the perception of the tongue by experienced practitioners as they conducted tongue diagnosis. Instead of a high-quality camera capable of capturing the most minute details of the tongue, what these doctors possessed was highly specialized 'seeing eyes' that were trained to recognize the specific patterns informed by the theory of Chinese tongue diagnosis. Let me elaborate on this difference with the example of moisture. From an outsider's point of view, the moisture on the surface of the tongue is bound to cause reflection and therefore blurs much of the image. As a result, experts in image processing technology consider this reflection as noise and try to eliminate it by technical means. From the viewpoint of the experienced practitioner, however, this moisture holds crucial information for evaluating a patient's health. For example, a red tongue implies heat (re 熱) in the patient, but if that is the case, the red appearance should be companied by a lack of moisture. If instead an abundance of moisture is found, the experienced doctor will question whether the cause of the patient's suffering is indeed genuine heat. Once the researchers recognized the informative role played by moisture, or fluid (jinye 津液) in the language of Chinese medicine, they no longer treated moisture as noise but as a valuable source of information that had to be preserved in the image. Moreover, as they strove to capture the valuable information that experienced practitioners unconsciously acquired during tongue diagnosis, the researchers were forced to reflect upon and make explicit what exactly this valuable information consisted of and, more importantly,[1] to explore new ways of stabilizing, standardizing and capturing these details by innovatively micro-adjusting the system of their image technology.

The whole project rested on the crucial assumption that there is valuable knowledge created in the traditional, face-to-face clinical encounter of tongue diagnosis. The key to image formation was not to represent the tongue as it objectively existed 'out there', but to capture the subjective perception of senior practitioners. The slogan was never 'what you see is what you get,' but rather, to use Professor Chang's words, to "capture what is deposited within the brains of the senior doctors" (Chang 2007). To help make explicit these senior doctors' perceptual, and hence often tacit, knowledge, Professor Chang asked them to delineate the most salient and significant structures of the tongue (on the picture) as they made judgments about its color, texture,

---

[1] In other words, while the traditional *wang* is an unconscious, in-a-blink and holistic pattern recognition, the research team was forced to make the theory and recognizing process behind it conscious in order to re-inscribe these informative features into the settings of image-processing technology.

luster and shape. In this sense, these tongue images could then be used as a tool for making the perceptual knowledge of tongue diagnosis explicit, comparable, and thus communicable.

More than just making this knowledge explicit, the research team further strove to re-inscribe this knowledge-laden perception onto the image of the tongue and to create a network[2] for the circulation of these images. To achieve this first goal, they reproduced, as far as possible, the exact setting in which senior doctors conducted tongue diagnosis. The idea behind this effort was that by reading and studying the images thus produced, students might learn to train their eyes to perceive in the way that senior practitioners do. In other words, these images of tongue diagnosis could help novice practitioners to become connected with the historically developed repertoire of visual experience, represented both by the medical canons and by the senior practitioners. To put it more bluntly, the objective of developing tongue diagnosis imaging was to reconnect the practitioners with history and thereby to make the transmission of traditional diagnostic skills more effective.

Let us again take moisture as an example. Given that moisture is a valuable visual clue, the question then becomes how to best represent it in the images so that one can use it to form a clinical diagnosis in the way that senior doctors do. Technically speaking, there are a number of different ways to simultaneously capture the moisture and reduce the reflection in an image. One way is to adopt the technology of 'diffraction of light sources', that is, using a few soft sources of light coming from different directions, so that the phenomenon of reflection will be reduced. As one can imagine, the intended objective would not be to completely eliminate any reflection, since senior practitioners during tongue diagnosis must have also encountered a certain amount of reflection caused by the moisture. The trick lies in reducing reflection to the appropriate level. Therefore, the question now becomes what we mean by appropriate level? The solution is again to rely on human judgment. The research team from Chang Gong University decided to leave it up to the trusted practitioners to decide which one among a spectrum of images adjusted with diffraction of light sources was closest to the diagnostic experience that they had during conventional tongue diagnosis. Because of the valuation of history, instead of purging every possible involvement of human intervention, the researchers actually inscribed human judgment into the specific configurations of the instrumentation, as represented by the appropriate level of reflection.

The research team was very much aware that the core objective of their project was history and human perception. As Professor Chang put it, 'in any efforts of innovation, we should always stick to/connect with our senses, and then try to stretch from there and extend their scope.' The same concern informed their design of a standardizing protocol for image taking: for example,

[2] The concept of network is borrowed from the actant network theory developed by science studies scholars Bruno Latour and Michel Callon. Instead of rigorously following this theory, here I just use its most important insight that no scientific artifact (in this case a tongue image) can function by itself but always needs a stable network, which associates various humans and objects with each other, to enable its functioning. I use this notion to emphasize that although in appearance Dr Chang's team was just working with two kinds of images and practices (tongue image vs tongue perception), in fact they had to do much more than that, for example by building a professional association. For a concise and readable introduction to this theory see Latour (1999).

the appropriate distance between the viewer and the machine, the brief time span of the viewing process, and so on.[3] Being very much aware of the fact that traditional *wangshe* takes places in just one blink of the eye, the standardizing protocol specifies that 'the tongue is extended to expose the full tongue body and the image is captured immediately', and that 'extension time should not exceed five seconds' (Chang et al 2005). The tension between the two different meanings of *shexiang* required the research team to at once achieve two seemingly contradictory objectives: on the one hand, their research objective was to preserve and to stabilize the traditional tongue perception that required subjective involvement; on the other hand, they also aimed at converting these tongue perceptions (*shexiang* 2 舌象) into standardized tongue images (*shexiang* 1舌像) and thereby creating a standardized network in which different people would be able to exchange, understand and make use of these images with ease. To realize both objectives, the research team had to standardize a series of environmental settings and activities that had in the past been left to individual practitioners' discretion, such as the way that patients present their tongues or the material setting of image-taking, especially the arrangement of lighting. Moreover, it was also crucial to standardize the perceptive capability of the individual practitioners involved.[4] Instead of focusing on teaching written knowledge, the objective was to 'bring back what was experienced by the senses of these senior doctors', or in other words, to re-establish the sensory knowledge as the center of teaching traditional Chinese medicine. As a result, the researchers introduced into their research protocol the 100-hue test, which allowed practitioners to improve their ability of differentiating colors by arranging the color orders of the objects. In addition to this material tool, a social institution was built to help standardize the perceptual capability of practitioners, or in other words, to train the standardized 'seeing eyes.' In March 2004 Professor Chang led the way in establishing The Formosan Association of Clinical Diagnosis in Traditional Chinese Medicine; in future the society will issue certificates to those practitioners who have received the training and passed the examination.

MAPPINGS OF THE TONGUE

The most serious challenge in constructing a network of 'tongue perception/ image' turned out to be the following question: Whose perception, experience and judgment was trustworthy to serve as representative of both history and

---

[3] The research team was very aware of the difference between (1) looking at an image of the tongue and reading from one area to another and (2) looking at the tongue in one blink of the eye. At this moment, they insist on creating images that replicate the second situation. However, as they are given the new possibility to gaze at an image of the tongue, read it from one area to another, and often with the optional function of amplification, these scientists have begun to wonder whether the traditional way of viewing in a blink is a result of constraints that can now be lifted or whether it is indeed an essential way of knowing that should be preserved as much as possible.

[4] In other words, they strove to re-inscribe the perception of tongue diagnosis back into a standardized network of instrumentation. However, since not every valuable piece of information can be re-inscribed back to this network, the team tentatively decided to sacrifice the information related to the "spirit of the tongue" (*sheshen* 舌神) since the image only captures a fixed moment rather than the dynamic movement through which the tongue manifests its "spirit."

experienced practitioners? This problem arose precisely because the research team did not aim at producing just an 'image of tongue diagnosis' in the pursuit of what historians of science have called 'mechanical objectivity.' According to historians of science Lorraine Daston and Peter Galison, the notion of objectivity, which nowadays can be used to mean so many things from empirical reliability to procedural correctness to emotional detachment, has a very complicated and multilayered history. The common feature shared by all forms of objectivity is their negative character: each of the several components of objectivity opposes a distinct form of subjectivity. Rising to prominence in the last two-thirds of the 19th century, mechanical objectivity was indifferent to the subjectivity of personal idiosyncrasies, but 'combated the subjectivity of scientific and aesthetic judgment, dogmatic system building, and anthropomorphism' (Daston & Galison 1992). In the name of 'letting nature speak for itself,' scientists developed this objectivity through a set of instrumentalities that minimized human intervention and valorized mechanically created images. One of the best representatives of this valuation of mechanical objectivity is the use of photography to replace hand-crafted drawings of scientific objects.

It is useful here to spell out the brief history and concept of mechanical objectivity because Professor Chang's team subscribed to a closely related but radically different idea. Although the team certainly valued the images of tongue diagnosis for their results of providing empirical evidence, enhancing communication, and thereby increasing objectivity, they nevertheless did not consider it their goal to pursue 'mechanical objectivity', which aims to minimize, if not eliminate completely, human participation. Instead, what they assumed to be most valuable and thus in need of being preserved was precisely the senior doctors' perceptual experience. With this historically situated notion of mechanical objectivity serving as comparative background,[5] we can get a clearer sense of how the research team conceived the complicated, even dialectic, relationship between tongue image and tongue perception, especially in the way they managed the potentially dangerous but valuable contribution of subjectivity by the senior practitioners. To say the least, while they aimed at capturing senior doctors' tongue perception, the tongue images they

---

[5] I would like to take this opportunity to point out that the history of objectivity is just one of many occasions that practitioners and researchers of traditional East Asian medicine might find useful in the field of science studies, including history of science. By way of revealing the diversity and contingency of the many components that make up the current concept of objectivity, historians of science offer valuable resources to improve our understanding of questions like whether scientific knowledge is objective and thus pave the way for better answering the related question of 'how to improve the objectivity of traditional East Asian medicine.' Most importantly, as practitioners and researchers gain a more nuanced understanding of science, or objectivity in this case, they are in a better position to negotiate the sometimes necessary modification of scientific methodology as they conceived their research design with regard to traditional East Asian medicine. For example, after the dominance of mechanical objectivity, in the 20th century a new form of objectivity arose that valued the judgment of the researchers' experience and 'interpreted image', both of which were rigorously guarded against by mechanical objectivity. This new objectivity can serve as a useful inspiration, even a conceptual allay, for Dr Chang's efforts in constructing a productive and dialectical relationship between tongue perception and tongue image (Galison 1998). Another good example in the field of East Asian medicine is Ted J. Kaptchuk's efforts to historicize placebo control and to turn the difficulty he encountered in studying Chinese medicine into a tool for transforming the mainstream conception of the placebo effect (Kaptchuk 1988).

created nevertheless provided a valuable common ground for practitioners to communicate with each other and thus build consensus.

Instead of taking standardization simply as an end-result, the research team regarded the objective of creating standards as an active tool for generating consensus. It is a well-known fact that different masters of Chinese medicine can have very different ways of both perceiving and characterizing the tongue. Since masters rarely get together to view the same patient and the same tongue at the same time, almost no shared basis exists for comparing their different diagnoses. Practitioners simply do not know to what extent their diagnoses differ from each other. Nevertheless, the introduction of images for tongue diagnosis, no matter how primitive and unsatisfactory it may be, created a shared common ground, or, to use Professor Chang's language, a platform (*pingtai* 平台). On the individual level, these images allow practitioners to compare the different diagnoses they made at different times, to reflect upon and make conscious the exact features behind their judgments, and to detect their own inconsistencies in judging the same image. More importantly, on the interpersonal level, these images allow different practitioners to made judgments about the same tongue image and to exchange ideas and interact with each other.

This might sound rather ironic: whereas image-processing technology was meant to serve as a tool for building consensus and standardization, the first and foremost manifested effect of its introduction has been the exposure of huge differences in terms of individual judgments. To exaggerate somewhat, image-processing technology has thus become a tool for making visible the remarkable discrepancy in senior doctors' judgments. Whereas some practitioners of Chinese medicine might find this kind of discrepancy embarrassing and prefer to shy away from it, Professor Chang's research team decided to confront this problem face-on.

Let us take for example their investigation of the areas of the tongue that correspond to the viscera (*zang-fu* 臟腑). Traditional Chinese medicine postulates that the tongue can be separated into distinctive areas and that each one of these areas connects to and reveals the situation of aspecific viscera. For such a fundamental feature of tongue diagnosis, in a group of 17 respected practitioners from Taiwan and mainland China (Fig. 7.1) Chang's team discovered seven different ways of 'mapping' the tongue.

In their attempt at integrating these 17 mappings by means of computer-aided drawing software, the research team found almost no overlapping area shared by all the mappings. This result reveals how little consensus exists in traditional tongue diagnosis,[6] at least in terms of relating the subdivision of the tongue with specific internal organs. In order to build consensus from

---

[6] Very interestingly, Nancy Holroyde-Downing has noticed the remarkable homogeneity of contemporary tongue diagnosis. Holroyde-Downing, *Mysteries of the Tongue*, pp435 and 56. Since the senior practitioners recruited in the Chang Gung research team included both Taiwanese and mainland Chinese practitioners, and the former had not attended the Academies of Traditional Chinese Medicine established in the 1950s in China, this phenomenon could lend support to her hypothesis that the homogeneity of tongue diagnosis, especially in comparison to pulse diagnosis, was largely the result of the creation of these academies and their standardizing efforts.

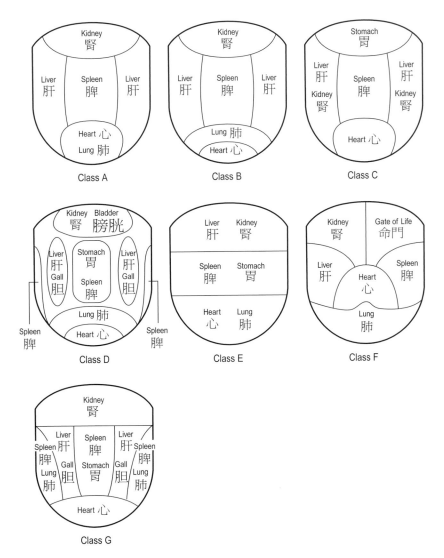

FIG. 7.1 Division of the tongue according to the viscera.

such individual differences, the team decided to adopt the mapping that was shared by 85% of all participating practitioners.[7]

It is worth pointing out that the mapping thus created is distinctively different from all the original 17 mappings created by the practitioners. For example, all 17 mappings included the boundary on both sides of the tongue. As participating practitioners related these two areas to different viscera – from

---

[7] There may be a simple reason for this apparent lack of congruence: the different doctors can be seen as operating within different frameworks that are not necessarily contradictory because Chinese medicine physicians are able to operate using diverse models of the body at the same time. Hence the Liver may be located both in the lower burner (the root of the tongue), the left side, both sides, and so on, without one view contradicting the other. This means that the standardization attempted here may also reduce effectiveness in that it substitutes a fixed reality with an emergent one. We would like to thank Volker Scheid for this elaboration.

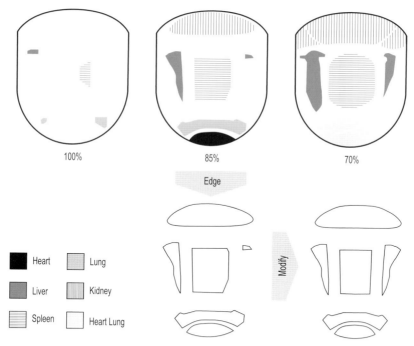

100%	85%	70%

Edge

■ Heart	▨ Lung
■ Liver	▥ Kidney
▤ Spleen	□ Heart Lung

Modify

FIG. 7.2 Integration of the 17 mappings by means of computer-aided drawing software.
Note: "Edge" means outlining the images and "Modify" means "making the image into a symmetric one.

liver, kidney, stomach to spleen – in the end these two areas were not included in the final mapping (Fig. 7.2) that represented the result of an 85% consensus. This difference suggests that the research team was not aiming at creating a final, standardized mapping of the tongue but was in the process of finding the most cost-effective way to construct a working hypothesis. Instead of trying to impose this mapping as the sole standardized characterization of the tongue, their objective was to create a 'platform' in which senior practitioners could start to interact with one another. The research team could then conduct further research to discover if any correlation existed between pathological development of any viscera and the postulated tongue changes in the corresponding area. Since this kind of research has the potential to expose the errors and problems of this tentative working framework, it will provide evidence for re-evaluating which practitioners' mappings are indeed more valuable and trustworthy. Instead of being a zero-sum game, in Professor Chang's conceptualization the relationship between the two types of *shexiang* can hence be mutually complementary and continuously constitutive.

While the research project at Chang Gung University started from the assumption that valuable information was stored in the way in which senior doctors perceived the tongue during traditional diagnosis, it nevertheless has the potential to self-rectify this assumption. Given the fact that tongue diagnosis is so crucial for the Warm Disorder School (*wenbing* 溫病) of Chinese medicine, for example (Liang 2004), it would be very problematic if a practitioner's tongue perception did not change at all after the patient had taken a formula designed according to the doctrine of this school. With the help of tongue imaging, it becomes more feasible to conduct this kind of evaluation, since it only takes a careful comparison of two or more images of the tongue. In fact, preliminary studies indicate that no systematic changes in the tongue can be associated with the development of diabetic mellitus and osteoporosis, for example (Chang et al 2005). On the other hand, Professor Chang has pointed out that there might be a certain correlation between the changes in tongue perception and the pathological development from chronic hepatitis, the 'national disease of the Taiwanese', into liver cirrhosis (Chang et al 1999). If this correlation can be substantiated scientifically with the help of tongue images and epidemiological studies, tongue perception can be of value not only to Chinese medicine, but to modern biomedicine as well. Practitioners can start using tongue changes to diagnose biomedical problems and to use traditional formulas that were used to treat symptoms defined by way of tongue perception to help patients suffering from hepatitis. In this sense, tongue imaging can do much more than preserve and standardize traditional Chinese medical diagnosis. Rather, it will allow contemporary researchers to re-evaluate and create new values of tongue diagnosis for us in the process.

CREATION OF VALUES

Efforts to integrate traditional East Asian medicine and modern biomedicine have been ongoing in China for more than a century; their different approaches are reflected in the names that the proponents of each movement adopted, such as 'communication between Chinese and Western medicine' in the late 19th century, 'systematization' and 'scientization' of Chinese medicine in the 1920s, and 'integration' of Chinese and Western medicine in Communist China in the 1950s. Despite their differences, these efforts often faced a dilemma similar to the one that puzzled Dr Chang when he conceived the project of standardizing tongue diagnosis. The dilemma lies in the difficulty of pursuing two seemingly contradictory objectives at once: on the one hand, to make traditional medicine more standardized, systematic and objective, and thereby to validate its efficacy; on the other hand, to preserve its specific features and strengths, which developed in the historical context and are often not in congruence with the presumptions of modern science. As many scholars have pointed out, when the presumptions of the applied research methodology fundamentally contradicted those of traditional East Asian medicine, a mechanical and unreflexive application of that methodology often led to the denunciation of traditional medicine (Adams 2002).

In light of Dr Chang's innovative efforts in research design, we should by now be able to see that the two conventional positions – 'respect and preserve the authenticity of traditional medicine' and 'dissolve traditional medicine through scientific integration' – were just the two polarized extremes. Between these two mutually exclusive positions, a whole spectrum of possibilities exists for integrating East Asian medicine within contemporary healthcare systems, possibilities that I would characterize as the 'creation of values.'[8]

---

[8] I fully develop the idea of 'creation of values' in my study of Taiwan's first PhD of medicine and the prominent scientist Tu Tsungming 杜聰明 (1893–1986; Du Congming in Pingyin system) (Lei 2010).

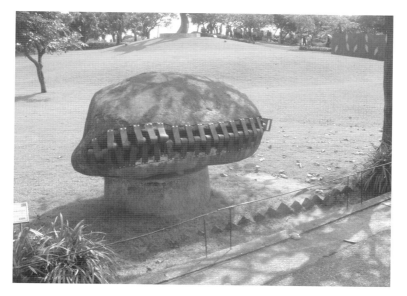

FIG. 7.3 Sculpture by Ju Jun.

Allow us to adopt an unconventional approach by elaborating on this idea with a visual image. The sculpture in Figure 7.3 was created by the Taiwanese artist Ju Jun朱雋and is displayed in the outdoor sculpture museum in Wanli, Taiwan, which was established by his father, the internationally famous sculptor Ju Ming 朱銘 (1938–). Apparently, this piece of art is also about integration: a zipper is absorbed into a solid rock. Nevertheless, this is not the kind of integration we normally think of when we use the term, in the sense of a single element being absorbed and becoming part of a larger whole, while the absorbing entity goes through no change except the mere addition of one new element. In sharp contrast, the image of the rock has been completely transformed by the addition of the zipper. It is transformed from a hard, solid rock into something like a leather purse with a soft and light touch. Moreover, when one of the authors (Sean Lei) asked his daughter, who is in second grade, if this sculpture looked like a purse, she responded resolutely, "Not at all. It looks like a monster's head." Look closely! We think she has a good point. If we try to see the zipper as its teeth, the rock ceases to be hard and static: it appears to be a living creature, which is about to open its mouth towards us. In order to recognize this lively creature and its threatening look, however, we have to ignore the carefully crafted pull-tab, which is one of the most distinctive features of the original zipper. Only when we are willing to make this kind of 'sacrifice' do we become capable of seeing a threatening monster. In the end, to see is to not see; creating implies destroying.[9]

Using this sculpture as a metaphor, we would like to point out three features of value-creating integration:

[9] Scheid made similar points in terms of the paired concepts of emergence and disappearance (Scheid 2002, pp52–3).

First, appreciation, (*shangshi* 賞識) the researcher should be able to appreciate the value of the traditional elements (i.e. the zipper in this example). Appreciation implies both knowledge and attitude. The researcher has to possess the relevant knowledge and commitment to recognize additional potential values of this element – values that can potentially be realized in a brand new context (the teeth of a monster).

Second, translation and sacrifice: the researcher has to be able to translate this element and thereby use it in a new context, transforming it into a different thing (teeth). The key word here is not preservation but use. This kind of transformative use sometimes does involve a salient sacrifice such as transforming the carefully crafted pull-tab into a meaningless appendix.

Third, this kind of integration should not be unidirectional. By way of creating something that did not exist before the act (the leather purse, or the

VIGNETTE 7.2 MAKING HYBRID MEDICAL INSTITUTIONS
JONGYOUNG KIM

Korean medicine, a local adaptation of Chinese medicine, has actively integrated science, technology and biomedicine since the 1990s. In laboratories, scientists and Korean medical researchers work together to verify the scientific effects of herbal medicine and acupuncture (Kim 2006, 2007, 2009). Not only advanced technologies such as functional magnetic resonance imaging (fMRI), high-performance liquid chromatography and DNA microarray, but also state-of-the-art laboratory systems, are implemented for this scientific integration. For example, acupuncture studies via fMRI have attracted Korean medical researchers and scientists alike and they have collaborated in laboratories exchanging their knowledge and skills. In this 'trading zone' (Galison 1997), mobilizing instruments play a significant role in the scientific interpretation of acupuncture. Instrumentation functions to legitimize alternative medicine's scientific project, and researchers attempt to 'tune' these instruments with diverse concepts and experimental procedures. Eventually, these processes are intended to objectify Korean medicine's clinical efficacy, which is currently regarded as subjective and episodic. I have characterized this translation of Korean medicine as 'the movement and readjustment of elements from the clinical setting to the laboratory setting' (Kim 2007).

In clinics, various hybrid medical practices have been formulated through the collaboration between Korean medical doctors and biomedical doctors. For example, the East–West Medical Center in Kyung Hee Medical Center, where I conducted extensive fieldwork, has implemented hybrid medical settings where a biomedical doctor and a Korean medical doctor see and treat the same patients together. The hospital also uses diverse instruments to create fusion therapies. In the clinic, there are two computers for each doctor. The whole medical center is a sort of digital hospital. Except for the patient chart, all medical information is transferred to personal computers through the central controlling system. For example, MRI and X-ray films are transferred by a picture archiving system, and doctors see them through their personal computers. Because of this digital system, one does not see nurses delivering MRI and X-ray films. Two doctors share a large table during medical interviews, and a female nurse supports various activities, such as admission processes, blood pressure examinations and the removal of needles after acupuncture.

The biomedical doctor diagnoses patients' illnesses and diseases in terms of biomedical concepts. S/he also orders various biomedical examinations such as X-rays, MRI scans or blood tests. In addition, s/he prescribes medicine to patients through a computerized order communication system . On the other hand, the Korean medical doctor uses four examination methods. After a clinical interview, s/he conducts acupuncture therapy in a treatment room connected to the clinical room. S/he also prescribes a herbal formula through the order communication system. In this setting, we can find the instrumentation of diverse devices in a hybrid medical setting.

It should be noted that hybrid medical institutions are actively constructed through continuous conflicts, negotiations and achievement between diverse instruments, concepts, practitioners and organizations. Through these tedious and complex processes, Oriental medicine's diversity and multiplicity emerges (Scheid 2002). From ancient times to the recent past, Oriental medicine has had constant exchanges with other medical traditions. For traditional doctors, other medical traditions including biomedicine and science have functioned as resources that can enrich the plurality of Oriental medicine. The traditional doctor's agency synthesizes these diverse practices and, in consequence, new hybrid medicines have been created. By highlighting the emergent property of new practices, it can be argued that the synthesis cannot be reduced to previous medical structures or systems. The combinations of different skills and techniques are usually 'partial connections' because a new hybrid practice does not encompass all aspects of previous medical practices. In this process, multiple formations of Oriental medicine compete, coexist, and co-evolve.

monster's head), this integration can, at least sometimes, change not only the absorbed element but also the absorbing system as well, thus resulting in a mutual transformation, even if it is local and thus limited (see Vignette 7.2).

Because Dr. Chang *appreciated* the sensory basis of Chinese medicine, his research did not aim at using image-processing technology to reduce the process of tongue perception to a mere tongue image. Instead, he foregrounded this essential tension and strove to realize the potentially complementary relationship between tongue image and tongue perception. On the other hand, as his team committed themselves to improving the relevance of traditional tongue diagnosis in contemporary healthcare, medical education, scientific communication and objectivity, they were willing to make some *sacrifice* with regard to Chinese medicine, at least tentatively, by way of the introduction of image-processing technology into tongue diagnosis. As Andrew Flower points out (Vignette 7.3), this technology is designed to work with images and thus has the risk of reducing tongue perception to tongue imagery and disrupting the contextuality of traditional tongue diagnosis. Instead, Dr Chang's research design managed to *translate* the tongue images into tools for tongue perception, making the perceptual knowledge of traditional tongue diagnosis explicit, comparable, communicable, and hence more robust and trustworthy. Finally, Dr Chang's team strove whenever possible to validate the knowledge of Chinese tongue diagnosis, which has previously been difficult for the mainstream scientific community to accept, such as the correspondence between the divisions in the tongue and the viscera. Because of this research objective

When exploring methods to standardize the process of tongue diagnosis it is important to appreciate that this is only one of the classic four pillars of East Asian medical diagnosis. The other methods relate to questioning, palpation, smelling and tasting, and other forms of looking such as face or body diagnosis. This makes tongue diagnosis both partial and highly contextual. As one part of a whole diagnostic system, tongue diagnosis should only be considered as one possible indicator of disease. Clinically, in some instances, changes in the tongue might presage a disease that has yet to manifest symptomatically. The clearest example in my clinical experience was the peeling of tongue fur in the area related to the lung in an asymptomatic HIV patient two weeks before the onset of a dry cough and night sweats that was eventually diagnosed as TB. As a peeled coat can relate to a depletion of Yin, and TB is classically diagnosed as lung Yin deficiency, this was a highly appropriate early indicator of this disease.

However, the opposite is also true. A patient may report a fixed stabbing pain of many months' duration that corresponds to a diagnosis of blood stagnation. Yet the tongue may not have any of the classic purple discoloration or congested sublingual veins that relate to this condition. In these instances it is still valid to treat the symptoms even if they are not reflected in the tongue. This partiality of tongue diagnosis is an important caveat that needs to be acknowledged in attempts to standardize both the process of imaging and the systems used for its interpretation.

The contextuality of tongue diagnosis is a subtler but equally important caveat. In practice, tongue diagnosis usually takes place after an in-depth process of questioning and observation. Rather than taking a whole picture of the tongue, the practitioner is more likely to look for signs that either confirm or refute a process of diagnostic analysis that is already under way. These expectations will have an effect on the gestalt of the tongue, and subtle features or changes on the tongue relating to the condition being assessed will be foregrounded and acquire greater significance than those with less clinical relevance. This is an important part of the 'art' of tongue diagnosis that is contingent upon the clinical experience of the practitioner involved and cannot be standardized.

and design, Dr Chang's work has the potential to teach something new to medical scientists, thereby transforming some basic assumptions of modern biomedicine.

Even though Chang's project aims at creating values in integration, there is absolutely no guarantee that these efforts will succeed. Besides, what is perceived to be the value of Chinese medicine would keep changing as time move on. Nevertheless, this kind of research opens the door for us to think of integration not in terms of two mutually exclusive objectives, namely authenticity and standardization/scientization, in a logical deadlock that has confounded reformers since the 19th century, but rather in terms of appreciation, translation and sacrifice, and most importantly in terms of values (epistemic, clinical and socioeconomic). At times we might still have to sacrifice some valuable elements, such as the carefully crafted pull-tab, but at least we will be painfully aware of this loss of values and therefore feel compelled to compensate for this sacrifice with some new and valuable contributions. Finally, in order to better appreciate traditional medicine, researchers should treat traditional medicine the way that the most creative scientists treat their research subject, namely as what philosopher of science Rheinberger (1997) calls an 'epistemic thing', so that they will always strive to learn something unexpected and surprising from traditional East Asian medicine.

REFERENCES

Adams, V., 2002. Randomized Controlled Crime: Postcolonial Technoscience in Alternative Medicine Research. Soc. Stud. Sci. (32), 659–90.

Chang, Hen-Hong Chang 張恆鴻, Lin, I-Hsin Lin 林宜信, Heish, Po-chow 謝伯舟, 2005. The Instrumentation of Tongue Diagnosis in Traditional Chinese Medicine. In: The 13th International Congress of Oriental Medicine. Exco, Daegu.

Chang, Hen-hong 張恆鴻, 2007. *Shexiang* (舌像) and *Shexiang* (舌象). In: The 77th National Medicine Day Conference. China Medical University, Taichung.

Chang, Hen-Hong 張恆鴻, et al., 1999. Manxing B Xing Ganyan Huanzhe Shexia Luomai Chutan 慢性 B 形肝炎患者舌下絡脈初探 (An exploration of the Luomai underneath the tongue in patients with chronic hepatitis). Zhongguo Yiyao Xueyuan Zazhi 中國醫藥學院學誌 (Chin. Med. Col. J.) 8 (2), 7–12.

Cui, M.G., Xu, B.Y., Huang, S.J., 2001. '(Quantitative study on tongue diagnosis in stroke patients)'. Zhongguo Zhong. Xi.Yi Jie.He.Za Zhi 21 (9), 670–673.

Daston, L., Galison, P., 1992. The image of objectivity. Representation 40, 81–128.

Galison, P., 1997. Image and Logic: A Material Culture of Microphysics. The University of Chicago Press, Chicago.

Galison, P., 1998. Judgment against objectivity. In: Jones, C.A., Galison, P. (Eds.), Picturing Science, Producing Art. Routledge, London.

Gareus, I.K., Tan, L., et al., 2005. Introducing a computer assisted, digital tongue-imaging device to standardise and evaluate traditional Chinese tongue diagnosis. Focus Altern Complement Ther 10 (1), 20–21.

Han, X.M., Yu, Y.M., 1993. (Quantitative analysis of 200 human tongue pictures). Zhongguo Zhong. Xi. Yi Jie. He. Za Zhi 13 (2), 110–111, 70.

Holroyde-Downing, N., 2005. Mysteries of the tongue. Asian Med. 1 (2), 432–461.

Kaptchuk, T.J., 1988. Intentional ignorance: a history of blind assessment and placebo controls in medicine. Bull. Hist. Med. 72, 389–433.

Kim, J., 2009. Transcultural medicine: a multi-sited ethnography on the scientific-industrial networking of Korean medicine. Med. Anthropol. 28 (1), 31–64.

Kim, J., 2007. Alternative medicine's encounter with laboratory science: the scientific construction of Korean medicine. Soc. Stud. Sci. 37 (6), 855–880.

Kim, J., 2006. Beyond paradigm: making transcultural connections in a scientific translation of acupuncture. Soc. Sci. Med. 62 (12), 2960–2972.

Kuriyama, S., 1999. The Expressiveness of the Body. Zone Books, Cambridge.

Latour, B., 1999. Give me a laboratory and I will raise the world. In: Biagioli, M. (Ed.), The Science Studies Reader. Routledge, New York and London.

Lei, Sean Hsiang-lin 雷祥麟, 2010. Du Congmin de danyiyao Yanjiu zhi Mi: Jianlun chuangzhao jiazhi de zhenghe yixue yanjiu (The Enigma Concerning Dr. Tsungming Tu's Reserach of Traditional East Asian Medicine: On the Creation of Values in Integrative Medicine) 杜聰明的漢醫藥研究之謎：兼論創造價值的整合醫學研究. Keji Yiliao yu Shehui 科技、醫療與社會 (Technoscience, Medicine and Society) .

Li, Naimin 李乃民, 1994. Zhonguo Shezhen Daquan Z中國舌診大全 (Collections of Tongue Diagnosis in China). Xueyuan Chubanshe, Beijing.

Liang, Rong 梁嶸, 2004. 1949 Nian yiqian Zhongyi Shezhen Xueshu Fazhan Licheng De Tanjiu (Probing into the academic evolution of tongue Inspection in TCM before 1949) 1949年以前中醫舌診學術發展歷程的探究. Zhiran Kexueshi Yanjiu (Stud. Hist. Nat. Sci.) 自然科學史研究 23 (3), 257–273.

Liu, Q., Yue, X.Q., Deng, W.Z., Ren, R.Z., 2003. (Quantitative study on tongue color in primary liver cancer patients by analysis system for comprehensive information of tongue diagnosis). Zhong. Xi. Yi Jie. He. Xue. Bao 1 (3), 180–183.

Lu, Xun 鲁迅, 1973. Ji wai ji 集外集 (A Collection Outside of Collection). Renming Wenxue Chubanshe, Beijing.

Maciocia, G., 2004. Diagnosis in Chinese Medicine: A Comprehensive Guide. Church Livingstone, London.

Pang, B., Zhang, D., Li, N., Wang, K., 2004. Computerized tongue diagnosis based on Bayesian networks. IEEE Trans. Biomed. Eng 51 (10), 1803–1810.

Rheinberger, H.J., 1997. Toward a History of Epistemic Things: Synthesizing Proteins in the Test Tube. Stanford University Press, Stanford.

Scheid, V., 2002. Chinese Medicine in Contemporary China: Plurality and Synthesis. Duke University Press, Durham and London.

Wei, B.G., Shen, L.S., Wang, Y.Q., Wang, Y.G., Wang, A.M., Zhao, Z.X., 2002. (A digital tongue image analysis instrument for Traditional Chinese Medicine). Zhongguo Yi Liao Qi Xie Za Zhi 26 (3), 164–166, 169.

Zou, J.P., Wang, W.D., Li, G.X., 2003. (Study on relationship between quantitative data of tongue picture and state of illness in 224 patients with severe acute respiratory syndrome). Zhongguo Zhong. Xi. Yi Jie. He. Za Zhi 23 (10), 740–743.

Efficacy, effectiveness and efficiency

Claudia M. Witt • Hugh MacPherson
• Ted J. Kaptchuk • Ayo Wahlberg

INTRODUCTION

That interventions should be based on evidence has been a consistent rallying cry from the evidence-based medicine movement. Within this movement, the results from randomized controlled trials are considered to be high on the list of what constitutes good evidence. The results of such trials are often synthesized in systemic reviews and meta-analyses, leading to an authoritative summary of whether the evidence for particular interventions is strong or not. In turn, these data are used to inform policy and practice, with implications for patients on whether interventions for particular conditions are covered by state funds or insurance-based reimbursement. In this chapter we focus on the way that randomized controlled trials are used to establish efficacy, effectiveness and efficiency. We explore some of the controversy around these methods of collecting evidence in general, and situate these specifically in the context of the evaluation of East Asian medical practices. In doing so, we highlight some of the underlying assumptions that drive the process of generating evidence, setting out the advantages and disadvantages of different approaches. Our chapter also provides insights into how evidence can be used in different ways to influence policy and practice. To set the scene we first introduce the historical development of randomized clinical trials and the role of placebo.

THE HISTORY OF THE RANDOMIZED CONTROLLED TRIAL AND THE ROLE OF PLACEBO

The Euro-American tug-of-war between what were, at the time, orthodox and unorthodox medicines that began about 200 years ago is critical for understanding the development of the randomized controlled trial. Orthodox medicine became dominant in part because it has been aligned with cultural and scientific norms and continues to be vigilant in maintaining hegemonic control (Warner 1987; Rothstein 1972). In the West, unorthodox medicine that did not conform to the dominant approach has been, by definition, the rebellious medicine. When the conflict became intense, as it often did, both sides resorted to a rhetoric of demonstration and evidence. Usually, the unorthodox schools, given the 'deviance' of their beliefs, were required to provide higher standards of demonstration than required for orthodoxy (Kaptchuk 1998). Ironically, this demand for more stringent evidence fostered many of the innovations that after World War II created the modern placebo-controlled randomized controlled trial.

The first placebo experiments were performed in 1784 by the Royal Commission headed by Benjamin Franklin and Antoine Lavoisier in efforts to debunk the claim that 'mesmeric energies' (to be renamed 'psychic energy' by later generations) could cure illness (Kaptchuk 2006; Kaptchuk et al 2009; McClenon 1984). Franklin's team reported that fake treatments worked as well as the real treatments and any effect of mesmerism was due to the 'imagination.' Not surprisingly, supporters of mesmerism also resorted to placebo-controlled experiments and found that only the genuine therapy affected patients and that fake therapy was a dud. Inspired by the mesmerism controversy, by the middle of the 19th century opponents and advocates of homeopathy had adopted placebo-controlled experiments (Dean 2000). In turn, in the early 20th century these experiments inspired the use of placebos by mainstream pharmacologists testing stimulants (Kaptchuk 1998).

In order to strengthen masking, random assignment to treatment exposure was adopted in many early mesmerism and homeopathic experiments. However, the main impetus for formal randomization procedures came from the telepathy controversies at the end of the 19th century, well before Fisher proposed such methods to test fertilizers for potatoes in 1926 (Hacking 1988; Box 1980). After World War II, British medical researchers combined placebo controls and random assignment with the emerging methods of the British Statistical School to create the modern randomized controlled trial (Kaptchuk & Kerr 2004). What was once a method primarily used to adjudicate between orthodox and irregular, thus became a normative method within orthodox medicine. Not by coincidence, the historical link to alternative medicine was forgotten.

In the early 1970s, when East Asian medicines began their migration to the West, researchers adopted the randomized controlled trial to investigate acupuncture without generally being aware that these methods had a long history in alternative medicine. Not surprisingly, the same kind of impetus as existed in earlier historical periods once again inspired acupuncturists to seek a higher level of rigor and refinement. For example, whereas only between 2% and 7% of biomedical clinical trials test the success of blinding (Hrobjartsson et al 2007; Fergusson et al 2004), assessment of the credibility of blinding, as well as measures of baseline expectation and belief, have become almost routine in randomized controlled trials of acupuncture (Linde et al 2007). Whereas mainstream medicine tolerates controversy concerning proper placebo controls (de Craen et al 1997; Golomb 1995; Collier 1995), the quest for optimal placebo controls in acupuncture has spurred an entire literature vastly larger than in all mainstream medicine (Kaptchuk 2002; Dincer & Linde 2003; Vickers 2002; Langevin et al 2006). As this volume itself suggests, the need for the highest quality research has stimulated acupuncturists to critically examine the theoretical assumptions of the randomized controlled trial and the advisability of dividing therapies into 'more than placebo' versus 'placebo' (Paterson & Dieppe 2005; Mason et al 2002; Kaptchuk 1996, 2001).

RANDOMIZED CONTROLLED TRIALS: WHAT IS THE CONTROVERSY ABOUT?

Randomized controlled trials generate considerable controversy in the field of East Asian medicine. For example, these methods have been shown to exacerbate the inequalities between biomedical pharmaceutical research and traditional medical practitioners in Tibet to the point that they have been labeled by one anthropologist as 'randomized controlled crime' (Adams 2002). Some criticisms may be fully justified, for example where trials are poorly conceived and badly implemented, but at other times it can be misplaced. Trials that are well designed can answer important questions that might otherwise be impossible to answer. In this context it may be useful to focus on two questions: Why are randomized controlled trials needed at all, and what are their limitations? To address these questions, a few of the key features of randomized controlled trials will be outlined next.

For many, the reason for conducting randomized controlled trials is to establish what is known as 'causality.' Can one isolate a specific cause (treatment) and show this is unequivocally associated with an effect (outcome)? The stronger the association between cause and effect, the higher the 'internal validity' is said to be. Trial designs with this mechanistic aim are said to be 'explanatory' (Schwartz & Lellouch 1967). However, for others, the rationale for conducting randomized controlled trials is to determine whether there is an overall effect compared to some other treatment or standard of care. This more practical aim can lead to decision-making, whether by patients or by policy makers, some of whom may have to decide on the allocation of potentially limited resources for healthcare. This latter type of trial is called a pragmatic trial (Schwartz & Lellouch 1967; MacPherson 2004).

Whether explanatory or pragmatic, the central design feature of randomized controlled trials is the random allocation of patients to different arms of a trial, in each of which patients receive different interventions. The most valuable benefit of this form of allocation is that changes due to the natural history of a disease (for example the possibility that all patients might tend to recover over time) are controlled for, so that these factors do not influence the comparison between interventions. As a result, differences between the groups are associated with different treatments, and this enhances internal validity.

In explanatory randomized trials, a placebo (or sham) arm is often used to further enhance internal validity by giving patients in the treatment group and patients in the placebo group an experience that is as closely identical as possible. This makes it possible to identify more precisely which specific aspect of treatment (which is not delivered within the sham intervention) causes the effect. If a specific aspect can be identified in this way, there is said to be evidence of 'specificity.' Randomized controlled trials designed along these lines are often described as the 'gold standard.'

Although randomized controlled trials clearly have a useful role in answering certain types of research question, they have also been criticized in several ways. For example, such trials only detect an average effect on the particular condition under investigation across a population. Explanatory trials often have a more homogeneous population than would be expected in usual practice. In reality, patient groups are often heterogeneous with more complex conditions, for example with comorbidities that create complicating factors. To reduce variability, explanatory trials often exclude patients who have multiple pathologies, are receiving concurrent treatments, or have strong preferences about treatment. Caution must be used in applying the results of such explanatory trials to everyday populations. The more confidence one has in generalizing the results of a trial, the stronger the 'external validity' is said to be.

Another complicating factor is that many East Asian medical practices could be described as complex interventions (Paterson & Britten 2004), and therefore do not suit the gold standard randomized controlled trial, where ideally the intervention is in the form of a single component, as is the case in drug trials. Complex interventions may have many components, and indeed it may not be clear which of these are 'active' therapeutically and which are not. In such cases, setting up a placebo-controlled trial is not usually feasible. And, even if such trials are attempted, the impact of synergistic effects (interactions that enhance the overall effect) between multiple components cannot be ruled out (Paterson & Dieppe 2005). For example, acupuncture treatments are often dependent on the relationship between the practitioner and the patient (MacPherson et al 2006), and if this is a positive relationship then patients are more likely to engage in self-care activities that are designed to enhance acupuncture treatment effects (MacPherson & Thomas 2008). Accordingly, care must be taken when extrapolating the results of trials using standardized treatments to contexts where treatments are individualized in routine practice.

To conclude, randomized controlled trials offer us an important way of controlling for certain complicating factors, including the common situation where patients tend to get better anyway. Careful consideration of how well the randomization is conducted, and ensuring that allocation to groups is concealed from anyone who might subvert this process, will help reduce the likelihood of bias compromising internal validity. Even so, such trials may have limitations, and – depending on the way the trial is designed and implemented – may be less able to answer the research question. Paying attention to both the patients in the trial and the type and quality of the treatment provided will help determine how well results can be generalized, and can lead to a better assessment of external validity. Finally, it should be noted that the randomized controlled trial is not the only way to develop the evidence base for East Asian medical treatments. Some research questions are better answered by other non-randomized research designs, such as surveys or observational studies (McKee et al 1999). Moreover, the single case study has historically had a central role in the development and dissemination of evidence within East Asian medicine (see Vignette 8.1).

VIGNETTE 8.1 CONSTELLATIONS, SIGNIFICATIONS, METHODS: CASE HISTORIES IN LATE IMPERIAL CHINA
VOLKER SCHEID

In the hierarchy of evidence that proponents of evidence-based medicine take to be natural and self-evident, evidence from individual cases is placed close to the bottom. It does not count for much. Chinese medicine has historically taken the opposite view. Objective knowledge and statistically significant effects were of little significance to Chinese physicians and their patients. What mattered to them, above all, was the single case. There are many reasons for this; too many, in fact, to outline here in detail. To some historians they indicate an entire cultural orientation. To others they merely reflect the social organization of medicine in late Imperial China.

Thinking in cases is not a definitive feature solely of Chinese medicine or specialised activities in China. It also characterizes the practice of specialists in the West, including those of physicians in modern high-tech hospitals. Like inductive reasoning or modes of classification thinking in cases can be considered one of several distinct 'styles of reasoning' that historians and philosophers of science see as being linked to distinctive contexts of practice (Forrester 1996). Case histories in Chinese medicine are not unchanging in terms of format or style. The discursive case of a Ming physician outlining the characteristics of their style of practice with regard to local competitors differs considerably from the terse poetic lines of a Qing case, intelligible only within a series of similar such cases and often only with significant interpretive effort. Yet, there is nevertheless something distinctive about the Chinese medical case that makes it immediately recognizable as belonging to that tradition (Furth et al 2007).

Discussing the case histories of the Ming dynasty physician Wan Quan 萬全 (1500-1585?) the historian Barbara Volkmar shows the typical case to be formulated according to a tripartite structure that can be applied to most other cases before and since (Volkmar 2006). The first of these elements is the specific constellation (*zheng* 證) of symptoms, signs, pulse, disease, personal data and other relevant information that mark out the case. As Volkmar points out, *zheng* 證, which can be translated as 'evidence' or 'sign,' is a term that is historically related to the astrological reading of constellations in the sky indicating the condition of the cosmos at any moment in time. The various elements that make up a constellation of relevant data in the medical case similarly reveal the condition of the human body to those able to read them. Not only can each additional sign change the constellation as a whole or even turn it upside down, it is also critical to know which piece of information counts as part of the pattern and what is simply noise.

The second element of the case is the significations (*yi* 意) that the constellations reveal to the physician. The significations may include the pathodynamic of a disorder (*bingji* 病機), its cause (*bingyin* 病因), its momentum (*shi* 勢), and treatment plans. Given that these significations are not simple cause-and-effect chains but apprehensions of complex dynamic relationships, these significations often remain implicit or are merely hinted at in the published case. Yet, like a poem, they are nevertheless intelligible to those in the know.

The final element of the case is the method of treatment (*fa* 法): a formula, a list of herbs or acupuncture points, a method of manipulation, dietary and life style advice, and so on. Often, the method alone can provide information as to the significations and even the constellations. In any case, it is usually assumed that the reader will have sufficient knowledge and ability to interpret the linkage between these various elements and to fill in all the information that appears missing to the uninitiated.

Reading and thinking in cases is thus revealed as both a reflection of Chinese medical practice and as an intrinsic aspect of it. The goal of that practice is to grasp the significations of each new case based on a knowledge of possible constellations and methods already at hand.

EXAMPLES FROM ACUPUNCTURE RESEARCH FOR EXPLANATORY AND PRAGMATIC TRIALS

The randomized controlled trial is not a simple model; instead, it consists of a complex family of methods. A good example in the field of East Asian medicines is acupuncture, because both explanatory trials determining its efficacy and pragmatic trials evaluating its effectiveness have been published. As discussed above, the aim of pragmatic clinical trials is to inform decisions about routine practice, and to make this possible they use fewer narrow inclusion and exclusion criteria, a less standardized treatment protocol and more patient-centered outcomes. In Table 8.1, and with a layout guided by reporting guidelines for pragmatic clinical trials (Zwarenstein et al 2008), the key differences for both types of randomized trial are outlined using the example of chronic low back pain.

Table 8.1	*Example from acupuncture research*	
	Explanatory randomized controlled trial of low back pain (Brinkhaus et al 2006)	Pragmatic randomized controlled trial of low back pain (Thomas et al 2006)
Question	Is acupuncture more efficacious in reducing pain than sham acupuncture or no acupuncture in patients with chronic low back pain?	Does referral of primary care patients with persistent low back pain to acupuncturists lead to clinical benefits and, if so, are these cost-effective?
Setting	30 well-trained study centres in primary care all over Germany	Three private acupuncture clinics, with referrals of patients from 39 general practitioners working in 16 primary care practices in York, UK
Participants	Aged 40–75 years, clinical diagnosis of chronic low back pain, disease duration > 6 months, average pain intensity of 40 mm or more on a 100 mm VAS during previous 7 days, use of oral non-steroidal anti-inflammatory drugs for pain treatment only in the 4 weeks prior to acupuncture treatment. In addition, 12 exclusion criteria	Aged 18–65 years, non-specific low back pain, disease duration 4–52 weeks, assessed as suitable for primary care management by their general practitioner
Intervention	Semistandardized acupuncture developed in a expert consensus, 12 treatments of 30 min duration in 8 weeks	Up to 10 individualized acupuncture sessions, the acupuncturist determined the content and the number of treatments according to patient need
Outcomes	Visual analogue scale for pain (0–100)	Short Form 36 (SF-36) Bodily Pain dimension
Relevance to practice	Indirect: patients and clinicians are highly selected and it is not clear how widely applicable the results are	Direct: results reflect usual care and can be used for decision making by patients and policy makers

It is clear that both studies use randomization to evaluate acupuncture in patients with chronic low back pain. However, the studies were also designed to answer different research questions. This emphasizes the point that the study design is driven by the research question, and not vice versa. This is the reason why an explanatory study was used to evaluate an acupuncture point specific effect and a pragmatic clinical trial was used to evaluate the effectiveness of acupuncture treatment in routine care.

Nevertheless even in pragmatic trials that reflect routine medical care the intervention can be predefined. Although the treatment protocol is not developed by the researchers themselves, it is influenced by professionals (e.g. practitioner associations or individuals) who may for various reasons, some of which are discussed in other chapters, routinize or standardize how acupuncture is performed in usual care.

EXPLANATORY VERSUS PRAGMATIC TRIALS: STRENGTHS AND LIMITATIONS

As outlined above, explanatory trials and pragmatic randomized controlled trials are similar in some ways, in that they both control for spontaneous recovery due to the natural history of the condition being investigated. These trial methods can be contrasted because they are designed to answer different research questions. Explanatory trials answer questions about whether a specific component of an intervention can be said to cause an effect ('efficacy', see Box 8.1). Such trials are based on what has worked in the development

---

BOX 8.1 Definitions

'Efficacy' refers to 'the extent to which a specific intervention is beneficial under ideal conditions' (Last et al. 2001). It concentrates primarily on the causal effects of a treatment, e.g. by comparing an intervention to a placebo.

'Explanatory trial' is a randomized controlled trial designed with the purpose of measuring 'efficacy' under experimental (ideal) conditions. For example, inclusion and exclusion criteria are usually used to select patients without any comorbidity and who are expected to have excellent compliance.

'Effectiveness' is a 'measure of the extent to which an intervention when deployed in the field in routine circumstances does what it is intended to do for a specific population' (Last et al. 2001). In other words 'effectiveness' reflects whether a treatment is beneficial under conditions close to those of routine care, and effectiveness studies use a more 'pragmatic' approach.

'Pragmatic or practical clinical trial' is a randomized controlled trial designed with the purpose of informing decisions about routine practice. Pragmatic trials are designed to find out about how effective a treatment actually is in everyday practice, and this design is of relevance to complementary medicine (MacPherson 2004; Witt 2009). Guidelines have been designed to improve the reporting of pragmatic trials, which include a focus on applicability (Zwarenstein et al 2008).

'Efficiency' is a measure of the relation between resource inputs (costs) and health outcomes and providing evidence on whether healthcare resources are being used to get the best value for money.

---

of drug therapies, where early testing of a potentially 'active' compound is tested against a placebo which should match the drug in all aspects except the active ingredient. If properly conducted, such trials will have high internal validity as they should provide an unequivocal association between a clearly defined 'cause' and 'effect.'

The dominance of the methodology of evidence-based medicine in bio-medicine has led to a widespread, though not unanimous, acceptance among physicians, regulators, the pharmaceutical industry and researchers that explanatory trials that provide evidence of specific effects are a prereq-uisite before a new therapy can become accepted. Their argument is that internal validity trumps external validity, and that whatever other evidence is available – whether from observational studies or pragmatic randomized controlled trials – until there is explanatory trial evidence of a specific effect then we continue to have 'no evidence of an effect.' As a consequence, it is argued, such interventions that have not been proved against a placebo should not be made more widely available or supported by insurance funds or national health services.

There are counter arguments to the reductionist approaches described above. Initiated by patient advocates, practitioners of East Asian therapies, university-based social scientists and health service researchers, there has been a focus on a broad range of research questions, only one of which leads to the explanatory trial to assess efficacy. As stated above, research methods need to be driven by research questions, not the other way around, and dif-ferent research questions are best answered by different research designs (see Fig. 8.1). For those stakeholders interested in establishing the overall benefits of a therapy, as provided in its normal clinical setting, the prag-matic clinical trial (MacPherson 2004) is the design of choice to assess 'effec-tiveness' (see Box 8.1) . Such a trial can not only establish the evidence on whether the overall 'package of care' is beneficial or not, it can also estimate cost-effectiveness ('efficiency'). For this reason, pragmatic trials can pro-vide the evidence that will help policymakers to choose between potentially competing interventions. This design is of special value where insurance funds or national healthcare services have limited resources and decisions have to be made about whether to increase or reduce resources for a particu-lar intervention. In reality, explanatory (efficacy) trials and pragmatic (effec-tiveness) trials exist across a spectrum, and hybrid trials may incorporate

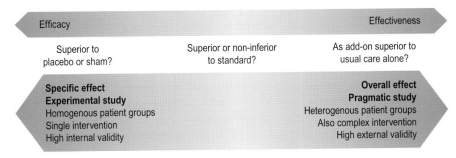

FIG. 8.1 The spectrum of efficacy and effectiveness research.

both explanatory and pragmatic aspects in the same design (see Fig. 8.1) (Thorpe et al 2009).

Explanatory trials have their limitations, as intimated above. First, the explanatory trial was designed for the context of drug development, and applying such a methodology to complex interventions such as East Asian medicines is inherently problematic. The most difficult aspect when evaluating a complex intervention with multiple components is knowing in advance what precisely are the active components (Medical Research Council 2000). Of equal concern is the fact that any separation of components – in order to test these in isolation from the others – could lead to an irretrievable loss in synergy between those components (Campbell et al 2000). The potential synergy is an interaction effect where the whole is more effective than the sum of the parts. There are other challenges regarding explanatory trials associated with the selection of an ideal patient group, i.e. one deemed beforehand as expected to respond best to the intervention. Clearly there could be limitations associated with this narrowing down, especially when one wants to generalize the results of the trial. Thus, whereas internal validity is a strength of explanatory trials, the downside is that external validity may be compromised.

Pragmatic trials also have their limitations. First, it is not precisely clear what the active components of the intervention are, unlike a well-conducted explanatory trial with a standardized intervention. In a pragmatic trial the 'cause' of any putative change is less well defined, and therefore the internal validity will be reduced. As discussed above, East Asian medical practices are often complex, and we are usually not certain which aspects of the intervention are active and which are not. As a result, we have less clarity about the nature of the 'cause' of any putative change in 'effect.' Indeed, critics of complementary therapies are usually quick to point out that there may be no 'specific' effect, but rather the overall effect could be all 'non-specific.' Non-specific effects are those associated with contextual factors, such as the empathy of the practitioner and the ambience of the treatment room. Where strong contextual effects are assumed, then the next logical step for many scientists and physicians is to argue that these contextual effects should be imported into mainstream medicine, while at the same time they often argue that the practice of East Asian medicines should be considered redundant, if not perhaps fraudulent, on the basis that the effect is all placebo. Nevertheless, the initial point that was raised above holds true, namely that research designs should reflect the research question. If a specific effect was not sought, but rather an overall effect, then it is not appropriate to criticize a pragmatic trial for not answering a question it was never designed to answer in the first place.

DECISION-MAKING BASED ON ACUPUNCTURE TRIALS IN THE UNITED KINGDOM

One of the points of conducting research is to affect policy. From the point of view of health services research, such decisions could lead to the provision of interventions that are shown to be effective and the withdrawal of those shown to be ineffective. Where there are limited resources, issues of cost-effectiveness also become important. In the UK, where there is a National Health Service that provides free healthcare at the point of delivery, judgments about introducing or withdrawing interventions are made by the National Institute for Health and Clinical Excellence, known as NICE.

Two full-scale acupuncture trials with pragmatic designs have been conducted in the United Kingdom funded by the Health Technology Assessment programme. As these trials were designed to answer questions about overall effectiveness as well as cost-effectiveness, they were ideally suited to help NICE in its decision-making. The results of the first of these trials, conducted by Vickers et al., were published in the *British Medical Journal* in 2004 and focused on clinical effectiveness (Vickers et al 2004) and cost-effectiveness (Wonderling et al 2004) of acupuncture for chronic headache. This research team found that headaches were reduced as a result of a course of 12 sessions of acupuncture provided over a three-month period, and that benefits at three months were sustained at 12 months. While NICE has yet to conduct a review of treatments for headaches, the British Association for the Study of Headache published guidelines in 2007 (http://216.25.88.43/upload/NS_BASH/BASH_guidelines_2007.pdf). Interestingly, no mention was made of the Vickers trial, or any other trial of acupuncture for headache, and the guideline simply stated that 'The role of acupuncture is unproven but worth trying in the absence of other options.'

The second full-scale acupuncture trial from the UK focused on chronic low back pain. Some of its design features are set out in Table 8.1. Two papers were published in the *British Medical Journal*, one on clinical effectiveness (Thomas et al 2006) and another on cost-effectiveness (Ratcliffe et al 2006). This trial involved comparing 10 sessions of acupuncture plus usual care to usual care alone. Follow-up of patients continued until 24 months after randomization, at which point the results favoured acupuncture in terms of both clinical and economic benefits. The results of this trial did feed into the NICE decision-making process. NICE commented that:

'This study shows that acupuncture for low back pain in primary care confers a modest health benefit for a modest increase in costs. The base case estimate is £4241 per QALY gained. Sensitivity analysis showed acupuncture to have a more than 90% chance of being cost effective at a £20,000 cost per QALY threshold. Including patient costs and the costs of lost productivity further strengthens the economics of acupuncture: that is, using a societal costing perspective acupuncture costs less and is more effective than usual care.'

Rothstein 1972. See http://www.nice.org.uk/nicemedia/pdf/CG88fullguideline.pdf

The cost-effectiveness data from this trial were central to decision-making for the clinical guideline, leading NICE to state, 'Consider offering a course of acupuncture needling comprising up to a maximum of 10 sessions over a period of up to 12 weeks' in the context of 'taking patient preference into account.'

To summarize, provided a number of factors are in place, policy can be influenced. Clearly, the condition being considered needs to be of sufficient priority to the national health service or insurance fund to be assessed, perhaps in terms of burden to the population. Next, the accumulated evidence needs to show a clinically meaningful effect, ideally across a number of trials that are reasonably representative. And finally, there must be a well-conducted evaluation of the cost-effectiveness of the intervention, which shows that the intervention provides value for money.

DECISION MAKING BASED ON ACUPUNCTURE TRIALS IN GERMANY

In October 2000, the German Federal Committee of Physicians and Health Insurers recommended that special 'model projects' on acupuncture (*Modellvorhaben Akupunktur*) be developed in order to determine the evidence-based role of acupuncture in the treatment of certain illnesses. These programmes were initiated after the German Federal Committee of Physicians and Health Insurers determined that the scientific evidence supporting the use of acupuncture was not sufficient to justify routine reimbursement within the German healthcare system. The intention was that the results from these model projects would aid the further decision making on the reimbursement of acupuncture treatment.

Efficacy and effectiveness studies were performed side by side using comparable outcome measures (Cummings 2009). This dual project provides a good example in order to discuss how they were used in decision making. In total, eight randomized controlled trials were designed as explanatory trials with the aim of evaluating the acupuncture point specific effects. A superficial needling technique at non-acupuncture points (penetrating sham) was the main control group. Four of these trials included a third arm of conventional standard treatment (Endres et al 2007; Haake et al 2007; Diener et al 2006; Scharf et al 2006) and in the other four studies a waiting list control arm was included (Brinkhaus et al 2006; Linde et al 2005; Melchart et al 2005; Witt et al 2005).

Across all these trials, it was not possible to determine a general acupuncture point specific effect. The effect in the penetrating sham acupuncture group appeared to be comparable to that in the acupuncture group. However, sham acupuncture, in the form of minimal off-point needling in a therapeutic context, is unlikely to be an inactive placebo. Nevertheless there were unexpected results: acupuncture for both low back pain and osteoarthritis of the knee showed clinically relevant improvements that were better than conventional standard treatment.

Six other trials following on from these German model projects evaluated the effectiveness and cost-effectiveness of additional acupuncture treatment and were mainly designed to inform decision makers. These studies used the design of a pragmatic clinical trial, and their main results showed that additional acupuncture treatment was more effective for all six diagnoses (chronic low back pain, neck pain, headache, osteoarthritis, allergic rhinitis and dysmenorrhoea) than usual care alone. In addition, acupuncture in routine care appears to have acceptable cost-effectiveness (Witt et al 2006, 2008a,b, 2009; Willich et al 2006).

In April 2006, based on the above mentioned efficacy studies, the German health authorities decided that acupuncture would be included for routine reimbursement by government health insurance funds for two diagnoses: chronic low back pain and chronic pain due to osteoarthritis of the knee. It is notable that the discussion within the health authorities' board responsible for this decision was based solely on the efficacy studies. The rationale behind the decision that only these two conditions were to be reimbursed was that, for both conditions, acupuncture was shown to be more efficacious than standard treatment. Those studies that were designed to inform decision making by evaluating the effectiveness and cost-effectiveness of an additional acupuncture treatment were not included in the decision-making process.

COMMENT OF POLITICAL ASPECTS OF DECISION MAKING IN BOTH COUNTRIES

As we saw earlier, the emergence of the randomized controlled trial has been historically linked to political struggles around the monopolization of medical practice, exposing fraud in a context of competing (orthodox and unorthodox) claims, therapies and patent medicines, as well as increasing demands for safety and quality control of industrialized pharmaceuticals (Kaptchuk 1998; Wahlberg 2008). Although these aspects certainly persist, today's clinical trials and the evidence-based medicine movement have become embroiled in yet another form of political wrangling – namely, processes of health rationing in a context of 'exploding healthcare costs.' Determining the efficacy, effectiveness and efficiency of a medicine or therapy has become a matter of health economics: Why should a national health delivery system or private health insurance company pay for a treatment or medicine that does not work, or is 'only' as effective as a placebo treatment, or is inferior to other available treatments?

As we saw above, in Germany, the German Federal Committee of Physicians and Health Insurers initiated a series of trials to determine the efficacy and effectiveness of acupuncture in the treatment of six diagnoses. In the UK, the Health Technology Assessment programme of the National Institute for Health Research (which is a part of the National Health Service) funded two trials to determine the effectiveness of acupuncture in the treatment of two conditions, headache and low back pain. In both cases their objectives were similar: 'to provide appropriate evidence for future NHS purchasing decisions' in the UK, and to 'aid further decision making on the reimbursement of acupuncture treatment' in Germany. An evidence base is required to justify reimbursement/purchasing decisions.

This raises two important questions: What is being paid for? and How are decisions reached about what should be paid for? At first glance, the answer to the first question seems obvious, namely acupuncture treatment for a given condition. However, if we take a closer look at the study designs and conditions involved, it quickly becomes apparent that it is treatment of chronicity (e.g. chronic lower back pain, neck pain, headaches and osteoarthritis) rather than cure that is at stake. That is to say, what you are paying for is an improvement of an individual patient's life, as measured by how patients rate the intensity and amount of pain they experience, their quality of life, their ability to function independently/participate socially or their emotional state, before, during and after acupuncture treatment. A successful treatment outcome is therefore not defined by absence of a condition, but rather by an improvement in the way in which a patient experiences his or her life (Wahlberg 2008, 2009). As discussed above, critiques of randomized controlled trials in the context of East Asian medicine have most often focused on how the standardized diagnoses and standardized treatments required by randomized controlled trials clash with the individualized and holistic approach of East Asian medicines. In comparison, the standardized rating scales used to measure trial outcomes have received relatively little critical attention, which is perhaps all the more surprising given that it is these rating scales that will ultimately value a particular treatment, i.e. affect decisions about whether it is appropriate to pay for it.

The second question concerns the workings of such institutions as the National Institute of Health and Clinical Excellence (NICE) in the UK, and the Federal Joint Committee (*Gemeinsamer Bundesausschuss*) in Germany. It is these institutions which are responsible for providing guidance on which medicines and therapies should be eligible for reimbursement via national health insurance. Such institutions bring together clinicians, hospital representatives, patient representatives, health insurance organizations and others to examine 'available evidence', and on this basis to recommend which indications (if any) a certain drug, device or therapy should be prescribed and ultimately reimbursed for. As such it has become an important research question for social scientists to understand how consensus on recommendations and guidance is achieved through negotiation and debate between assessment committee members (Moreira 2005; Sjogren 2008; Timmermanns & Berg 2003; Wahlberg & McGoey 2007). Although NICE argues that in situations where there is 'confusion or uncertainty over [a treatment's] value... our advice ends the uncertainty and helps to standardize access to healthcare across the country' (http://www.nice.org.uk/aboutnice/whatwedo/abouttechnologyappraisals/about_technology_appraisals.jsp), social science studies of how such committees make their decisions have shown how knowledge about the efficacy, effectiveness and efficiency of medicines or therapies 'is routinely ambiguous and uncertain... mak[ing] it necessary to negotiate a coherent and decision-able knowledge – rather than merely compile it, as posited by rational choice-based models' (Sjogren 2008). It is a process that 'entails contrasting and combining pragmatic and political concerns with epidemiological statistical calculations' (Moreira 2005). This can, in part, explain national differences in the ways that decisions are made. In the acupuncture research discussed above we saw how the German Federal Committee based its decision solely on evidence of specific effects, whereas in the UK there was a primary emphasis on cost-effectiveness. We might see these differences in terms of competing concerns of medicine and health economics, respectively. Further studies into how the compositions, mandates and working practices of the German Federal Committee and NICE can influence the ways in which 'best available evidence' is collected and discussed would shed further light on how decision making is simultaneously both scientific and political.

REFERENCES

Adams, V., 2002. Randomized controlled crime: postcolonial sciences in alternative medicine research. Soc. Stud. Sci. 32, 659–690.

Box, J.F., 1980. R.A. Fisher and the design of experiments, 1922–1926. Am. Stat. 34, 1–7.

Brinkhaus, B., Witt, C.M., Jena, S., et al., 2006. Acupuncture in patients with chronic low back pain—a randomised controlled trial. Arch. Intern. Med. 166, 450–457.

Campbell, M., Fitzpatrick, R., Haines, A., et al., 2000. Framework for design and evaluation of complex interventions to improve health. BMJ 321, 694–696.

Collier, J., 1995. Confusion over use of placebos in clinical trials. BMJ 311, 821–822.

Cummings, M., 2009. Modellvorhaben Akupunktur—a summary of the ART, ARC and GERAC trials. Acupunct. Med. 27, 26–30.

Dean, M.E., 2000. A homeopathic origin for placebo controls: 'an invaluable gift of God'. Altern. Ther. Health Med. 6, 58–66.

de Craen, A.J., Tijssen, J.G., Kleijnen, J., 1997. Is there a need to control the placebo in placebo controlled trials? Heart 77, 95–96.

Diener, H.C., Kronfeld, K., Boewing, G., et al., 2006. Efficacy of acupuncture for the prophylaxis of migraine: a multicentre randomised controlled clinical trial. Lancet Neurol. 5, 310–316.

Dincer, F., Linde, K., 2003. Sham interventions in randomized clinical trials of acupuncture—a review. Complement. Ther. Med. 11, 235–242.

Endres, H.G., Bowing, G., Diener, H.C., et al., 2007. Acupuncture for tension-type headache: a multicentre, sham-controlled, patient- and observer-blinded, randomised trial. J. Headache Pain. 8, 306–314.

Fergusson, D., Glass, K.C., Waring, D., et al., 2004. Turning a blind eye: the success of blinding reported in a random sample of randomised, placebo controlled trials. BMJ 328, 432.

Forrester, J., 1996. If p, then what? Thinking in cases. History of the Human Sciences 9 (1), 1–25.

Furth, C., Zeitlin, J.T., Hsiung, P., 2007. Thinking with Cases: Specialist Knowledge in Chinese Cultural History. University of Hawai'i Press, Honolulu.

Golomb, B.A., 1995. Paradox of placebo effect. Nature 375, 530.

Haake, M., Muller, H.H., Schade-Brittinger, C., et al., 2007. German Acupuncture Trials (GERAC) for chronic low back pain: randomized, multicenter, blinded, parallel-group trial with 3 groups. Arch. Intern. Med. 167, 1892–1898.

Hacking, I., 1988. Telepathy: origins of randomization in experimental design. Isis 79, 427–451.

Hrobjartsson, A., Forfang, E., Haahr, M.T., et al., 2007. Blinded trials taken to the test: an analysis of randomized clinical trials that report tests for the success of blinding. Int. J. Epidemiol. 36, 654–663.

Kaptchuk, T., 1996. Complementary medicine: efficacy beyond the placebo effect. In: Ernst, E. (Ed.), Complementary Medicine: An Objective Appraisal. Butterworth Heinemann, Oxford, pp. 42–70.

Kaptchuk, T.J., 1998. Intentional ignorance: a history of blind assessment and placebo controls in medicine. Bull. Hist. Med. 72, 389–433.

Kaptchuk, T.J., 2001. The double-blind, randomized, placebo-controlled trial: gold standard or golden calf? J. Clin. Epidemiol. 54, 541–549.

Kaptchuk, T.J., 2002. Acupuncture: theory, efficacy, and practice. Ann. Intern. Med. 136, 374–383.

Kaptchuk, T., 2006. Vitalism. In: Micozzi, M.S. (Ed.), Fundamental of Complementary and Integrative Medicine, third ed. Saunders, St. Louis, pp. 43–52.

Kaptchuk, T.J., Kerr, C.E., 2004. Commentary: unbiased divination, unbiased evidence, and the patulin clinical trial. Int. J. Epidemiol. 33, 247–251.

Kaptchuk, T.J., Kerr, C.E., Zanger, A., 2009. Placebo controls, exorcisms, and the devil. Lancet 374, 1234–1235.

Langevin, H.M., Hammerschlag, R., Lao, L., et al., 2006. Controversies in acupuncture research: selection of controls and outcome measures in acupuncture clinical trials. J. Altern. Complement. Med. 12, 943–953.

Last, J., Spasoff, R.A., et al., 2001. A Dictionary of Epidemiology, fourth ed. Oxford University Press, Oxford.

Linde, K., Streng, A., Jürgens, S., et al., 2005. Acupuncture for patients with migraine —a randomized trial (ART Migraine). JAMA 293, 2118–2125.

Linde, K., Witt, C.M., Streng, A., et al., 2007. The impact of patient expectations on outcomes in four randomized controlled trials of acupuncture in patients with chronic pain. Pain 128, 264–271.

McClenon, J., 1984. Deviant Science: The Case of Parapsychology. University of Pennsylvania Press, Philadelphia.

McKee, M., Britton, A., Black, N., et al., 1999. Methods in health services research. Interpreting the evidence: choosing between randomised and non-randomised studies. BMJ 319, 312–315.

MacPherson, H., 2004. Pragmatic clinical trials. Complement. Ther. Med. 12, 136–140.

MacPherson, H., Thorpe, L., Thomas, K., 2006. Beyond needling—therapeutic processes in acupuncture care: a qualitative study nested within a low-back pain trial. J. Altern. Complement. Med. 12, 873–880.

MacPherson, H., Thomas, K., 2008. Self-help advice as a process integral to traditional acupuncture care: implications for trial design. Complement. Ther. Med. 16, 101–106.

Mason, S., Tovey, P., Long, A.F., 2002. Evaluating complementary medicine: methodological challenges of randomised controlled trials. BMJ 325, 832–834.

Medical Research Council, 2000. A framework for development and evaluation of RCTs for complex interventions to improve health. MRC, London.

Melchart, D., Streng, A., Hoppe, A., et al., 2005. Acupuncture in patients with tension-type headache—a randomised Trial. BMJ 331, 376–382.

Moreira, T., 2005. Diversity in clinical guidelines: the role of repertoires of evaluation. Soc. Sci. Med. 60, 1975–1985.

Paterson, C., Britten, N., 2004. Acupuncture as a complex intervention: a holistic model. J. Altern. Complement. Med. 10, 791–801.

Paterson, C., Dieppe, P., 2005. Characteristic and incidental (placebo) effects in complex interventions such as acupuncture. BMJ 330, 1202–1205.

Ratcliffe, J., Thomas, K.J., MacPherson, H., et al., 2006. A randomised controlled trial of acupuncture care for persistent low back pain: cost effectiveness analysis. BMJ 333, 626–628.

Richter, S.H., Garner, J.P., Wurbel, H., 2009. Environmental standardization: cure or cause of poor reproducibility in animal experiments? Nat. Methods 6, 257–261.

Rothstein, W.G., 1972. American Physicians in the Nineteenth Century: From Sects to Science. Johns Hopkins University Press, Baltimore.

Scharf, H.P., Mansmann, U., Streitberger, K., et al., 2006. Acupuncture and knee osteoarthritis: a three-armed randomized trial. Ann. Intern. Med. 145, 12–20.

Schwartz, D., Lellouch, J., 1967. Explanatory and pragmatic attitudes in therapeutical trials. J. Chronic. Dis. 20, 637–648.

Sjogren, E., 2008. Deciding subsidy for pharmaceuticals based on ambiguous evidence. J. Health. Organ. Manag. 22, 368–383.

Thomas, K.J., MacPherson, H., Thorpe, L., et al., 2006. Randomised controlled trial of a short course of traditional acupuncture compared with usual care for persistent non-specific low back pain. BMJ 333, 623–626.

Thorpe, K.E., Zwarenstein, M., Oxman, A.D., et al., 2009. A pragmatic-explanatory continuum indicator summary (PRECIS): a tool to help trial designers. CMAJ 180, E47–E57.

Timmermanns, S., Berg, M., 2003. The Gold Standard: An Exploration of Evidence-based Medicine and Standardization in Health Care. Temple University Press, Philadelphia, PA.

Vickers, A.J., 2002. Placebo controls in randomized trials of acupuncture. Eval. Health Prof. 25, 421–435.

Vickers, A.J., Rees, R.W., Zollman, C.E., et al., 2004. Acupuncture of chronic headache disorders in primary care: randomised controlled trial and economic analysis. Health Technol. Assess. 8, 1–50.

Volkmar, B., 2006. Die Fallgeschichten des Arztes Wan Quan (1500–1585?). Medizinisches Denken und Handeln der Ming-Zeit. Urban & Fischer Bei Elsevier.

Wahlberg, A., 2008. Above and beyond superstition—western herbal medicine and the decriminalizing of placebo. Hist. Hum. Sci. 21, 77–101.

Wahlberg, A., 2009. Serious disease as kinds of living. In: Bauer, S., Wahlberg, A. (Eds.), Contested Categories: Life Sciences in Society. Ashgate, Aldershot, pp. 89–112.

Efficacy, effectiveness and efficiency

Wahlberg, A., McGoey, L., 2007. An elusive evidence base: the construction and governance of randomized controlled trials. BioSocieties 2, 1–10.

Warner, J.H., 1987. Medical sectarianism, therapeutic conflict, and the shaping of orthodox professional identity in antebellum American medicine. In: Bynum, W.F., Porter, R. (Eds.), Medical Fringe and Medical Orthodoxy. Croom Helm, London, pp. 1750–1850.

Willich, S.N., Reinhold, T., Selim, D., et al., 2006. Cost-effectiveness of acupuncture treatment in patients with chronic neck pain. Pain 125, 107–113.

Witt, C., Brinkhaus, B., Jena, S., et al., 2005. Acupuncture in patients with osteoarthritis of the knee: a randomised trial. Lancet 366, 136–143.

Witt, C.M., 2009. Efficacy, effectiveness, pragmatic trials—Guidance on terminology and the advantages of Pragmatic Trials. Forsch. Komplementärmed. Klass. Naturheilkd. 16, 292–294.

Witt, C.M., Jena, S., Selim, D., et al., 2006. Pragmatic randomized trial of effectiveness and cost-effectiveness of acupuncture for chronic low back pain. Am. J. Epidemiol. 164, 487–496.

Witt, C.M., Reinhold, T., Jena, S., et al., 2008a. Cost-effectiveness of acupuncture treatment in patients with headache. Cephalalgia 28, 334–345.

Witt, C.M., Reinhold, T., Brinkhaus, B., et al., 2008b. Acupuncture in patients with dysmenorrhea: a randomized study on clinical effectiveness and cost-effectiveness in usual care. Am. J. Obstet. Gynecol. 198, 166–168.

Witt, C.M., Reinhold, T., Jena, S., et al., 2009. Cost-effectiveness of acupuncture in women and men with allergic rhinitis: a randomized controlled study in usual care. Am. J. Epidemiol. 169, 562–571.

Wonderling, D., Vickers, A.J., Grieve, R., et al., 2004. Cost effectiveness analysis of a randomised trial of acupuncture for chronic headache in primary care. BMJ 328, 747.

Zwarenstein, M., Treweek, S., Gagnier, J.J., et al., 2008. Improving the reporting of pragmatic trials: an extension of the CONSORT statement. BMJ 337, a2390.

Constructing an evidence base for East Asian medicines

9

Andrew Flower • Volker Scheid • George Lewith

Evidence does not just appear or passively await discovery. It is deliberately constructed and utilized within specific socioeconomic, political and epistemological contexts. The current evidence-based medicine movement began in earnest in the 1980s (Claridge & Fabian 2005) and has since transformed the understanding, practice and teaching of biomedicine. East Asian medicines have their own tradition of gathering and presenting evidence. However, evidence based medicine is now the global currency of medical legitimization and has already had a significant impact on these traditional practices. This chapter offers a brief critique of the current state of evidence-based medicine and then discusses ways in which East Asian medical practices may be able to integrate conventional approaches to the principles of evidence-based medicine and its production without fatally compromising their integrity.

EVIDENCE-BASED MEDICINE (EBM) IN CONTEXT

Sackett's often quoted definition of evidence-based medicine (EBM) as 'the conscientious, explicit, and judicious use of current best practice in making decisions about the care of individual patients' (Sackett & Rosenberg 1996) has an apparently unassailable logic to it. However, the high ideal that Sackett described differs in several important ways from the practical reality of EBM as it has developed over the past 30 years.

The current practice of EBM is predicated upon the randomized controlled trial (RCT) as the 'gold standard', which compares the effect of an active treatment with a suitable control and uses randomization and (ideally) blinding to eliminate bias and reduce confounding influences. Standardized and validated outcomes measures are employed to generate quantitative data that can be statistically analyzed to reveal the 'true' effect of an intervention. The synthesis of related RCTs into systematic reviews and meta-analyses is designed to swell this trickle of evidence into an irresistible flood of scientific fact that can be used to accurately and definitively assess a medical intervention and provide a rational basis for evidence-based treatment guidelines. The logic appears impeccable; the reality, unfortunately, is deeply flawed.

Criticism of EBM emerges from two main sources. The first is 'in house' and can be seen in the response by supporters of EBM to increase its rigor, to reduce various sources of bias, to broaden its range of reference and increase its clinical relevance. The second is a less sympathetic critique that exposes the limitations of the scientific epistemology of EBM and identifies the social, economic and political vested interests behind the EBM movement.

139

If we compare current practice to Sackett's ideal outlined above, it becomes apparent that there is a large gap between the two. In the original article in the *British Medical Journal*, good doctoring required the use of 'both individual clinical expertise and the best available external evidence, and neither alone is enough,' for 'without clinical expertise, practice risks becoming tyrannized by evidence, for even excellent external evidence may be inapplicable or inappropriate for an individual patient' (Sackett & Rosenberg 1996). The development of practice guidelines and treatment algorithms ends up elevating simplified population-based data over the complexity of an individual case. This is frequently unsatisfactory for both patient and medical practitioner, and it is hardly surprising that compliance with clinical practice guidelines is notoriously poor (Cabana et al 1999).

EBM is also compromised by an over-reliance on the RCT. The classic experimental RCT was designed to evaluate the impact of a drug by assessing 'the average effect of a standardized intervention on a homogeneous population with a single condition' (MacPherson et al 2009). This is a highly artificial and idealized version of medical practice that fails to take into account the complexities of comorbidity, multidrug regimens, and diversity in socioeconomic status, ethnicity, gender and age. In addition, the quantitative data produced by RCTs to allow statistical comparison often does not accurately reflect the lived experience of patients, and in some instances may actually contradict qualitative reports on the same intervention (Campbell et al 2003). Although the maths may be precise, the ability of RCTs to truly record, evaluate and predict the impact of a medical intervention on an individual is at best crude. For these reasons, the traditional hierarchy of research evidence, with RCTs and systematic reviews at the apex and qualitative research and case histories disregarded at the base, is now increasingly being seen as overly reductive. Sir Michael Rawlins, chairman of the UK's National Institute of Health and Clinical Excellence (NICE) – which recommends the introduction or withdrawal of a medical intervention into the UK National Health Service on the basis of a rigorous consideration of the available evidence – has described the over-reliance on RCTs and systematic reviews as 'inappropriate' and 'illusory', and ideally something that should be replaced by 'a diversity of approaches that involve analysing the totality of the evidence base' (Rawlins 2008).

These limitations are relatively minor stumbling blocks to the rapid progress of EBM. However, the broadening of what is considered as valid evidence could have important implications for how we research East Asian medicines. Before we leap (or tentatively step) through this window of opportunity, we need to take a deeper look at some of the shortcomings of EBM that are more difficult to refute.

EBM is based on a positivist philosophy that believes in an objective, material, 'factual' reality that can be apprehended and verified through the scientific method. Positivism does not acknowledge that the practice and dissemination of science is partial, influenced by the beliefs, assumptions and personal interests of scientists, and like any other human activity, shaped by political, economic and social forces. This naive belief in science has been challenged in recent decades by an entire literature of detailed ethnographic and historical case studies that explore how science is actually done (Biagioli 1999) and how scientific practices are oriented by distinctive 'ways of knowing' (Pickstone 2001) or 'epistemic virtues' (Daston & Galison et al 2007). Observations are increasingly recognized as being conditioned by the prevailing theory of the observers and potentially subject to 'multiple interpretations' (Goldenberg 2006) that resist the attempt to use 'objective' standardized and validated means of measurement. DeVries (2004), for example, provides a fascinating account of how vested interests and entrenched belief systems led two teams of researchers to collect different data as the basis for completely opposing evaluations of the Dutch home birth maternity service. The current controversy over the interpretation of data relating to homeopathy, acupuncture and herbal medicines where, for example, the non-specific effects of an intervention that may arise from various aspects of the therapeutic relationship are used to dismiss the specific value of the therapy being scrutinized (Colquhoun 2009), are instances of subjectivity in science that are closer to home. As one philosopher of science has noted: 'The appeal to the authority of evidence that characterizes evidence based practice does not increase objectivity but rather obscures the subjective elements that inescapably enter all forms of human inquiry' (Goldenberg 2006).

Such criticism acquire additional weight when placed in the context of attempts by EBM to evaluate medical practices such as Chinese medicine that contain their own ideas regarding the relationship between evidence, effectiveness and good practice. For, unless these are dismissed *a priori* as not worthy of consideration, they present a serious challenge to the universalist claims of EBM to constitute the sole arbiter of what counts as truth and, by implication, of what is real and what is not. Historians and philosophers such as Jullien (1995) or Hall and Ames (1995), for instance, demonstrate that there exist irreconcilable differences between dominant discourses on effectiveness in ancient China and Greece that remain relevant for culturally inflected practice even today. Given that EBM's notions of truth and bias are direct descendants of Platonic epistemology, and that Chinese medicine orients itself even more clearly towards the past, the import of these differences on medical practice becomes relevant in any serious discussion of how the interface between EBM and East Asian medicines might be constructed.

Needless to say, the existence of such difference does not exclude the possibility of finding common ground, of dialogue, and of eventual synthesis. For just as there exists a strong empiricist tradition in East Asian medicines that seeks to objectify knowledge, the enduring importance of the single case (Montgomery 2006) in biomedicine attests to a pragmatic orientation whose concerns are consistently different from the positivist attempts to ground actions in objective truths outlined above.

In addition to epistemological blind spots, EBM is also disingenuously silent on the socioeconomic forces that influence its practice. These social processes are less 'innocent' than the philosophical shortcomings of current EBM and relate to the way EBM has been manipulated to suit the interests of the pharmaceutical industry. New drugs have to pass through increasingly expensive phases of clinical research to ensure their safety, efficacy and product consistency. It has been estimated that it costs somewhere between $1 billion (DiMasi et al 2003) and more recently a staggering $3.8 billion (Munos 2009) to license a new drug successfully. Older drugs have to be able to demonstrate a rationale for their continued place in the health marketplace. The pharmaceutical industry spends vast sums of money on product development and is also the driver in most of the research conducted to assess these products. This means that EBM has become a self-referential movement that only validates the kind of knowledge that it has the means and expertise to produce.

In addition, the pharmaceutical industry is adept at manipulating and distorting the production and dissemination of evidence to suit its own interests. This is apparent in the delayed reporting of drug side effects (e.g. Seroxat (Giles 2004) or Cox 2 inhibitors (Jørgensen et al 2010)), the failure to report negative outcomes from clinical trials (Chalmers 1990; Bodenheimer 2000), and the three to four times greater likelihood of industry-sponsored trials reporting positive results than from non-commercial trials (Bekelman et al 2003). The integrity of clinical trials is further undermined by reports that up to 11% of articles reporting drug trials published in six leading academic journals used ghost writers before being credited to more respectable academic authors (Flanagin et al 1998). The very process of evidence-based research and peer-reviewed publication, set up to provide unbiased scientific evidence, is deeply compromised by the covert influence of corporations with powerfully vested interests in certain economically desirable outcomes.

The economic interests that drive the research into pharmaceutical products have less incentive to investigate East Asian medical practices, which frequently involve several therapeutic modalities, such as dietary and lifestyle advice, and offer individualized rather than standardized treatments. This resistance to the production of a simple marketable product reduces the incentive for commercial funding or leads to the development of standardized products that may not reflect the best practice of East Asian medical traditions.

The EBM movement has been developed and marketed as a tool to offer a rational and effective medical service. However, like any tool, its value and function are determined by who uses it and for what purpose. If EBM maintains its over-reliance on RCTs and systematic reviews, it will marginalize the vast majority of non-pharmaceutically sponsored medical practices. This process of marginalization has vital implications for the allocation of resources, legal and professional status, and the availability of non-sanctioned methods of healthcare. Evidence is now inextricably linked to power. A lack of acceptable evidence means a lack of power and increasing marginalization. In the EU at the time of writing, the status of East Asian medical practitioners and their ability to access their materia medica is currently in the balance. For these reasons there is a powerful argument to actively engage with the demands of EBM. The question is whether it is possible to enter into a constructive relationship with the current form of EBM, or whether the process of subjecting East Asian medicine to the kind of scrutiny designed to suit biomedical interventions will also contribute to its destruction.

GATHERING EVIDENCE IN EAST ASIAN MEDICINES

In East Asian medical traditions disease is viewed as a dynamic process of disequilibrium. Evidence of this is gathered from information provided by the patient and from the observations of the practitioner, derived from visual inspection (e.g. of the tongue, face and skin); palpation (e.g. of the pulse, channels and internal organs); and smell (e.g. body odor and breath). Although they have an objective existence, the interpretation and classification of these empirical observations retain a high degree of subjectivity.

These data are then used by the practitioner in a process that usually involves a synthesis of several different systems of diagnosis that have emerged from the long history of East Asian medicines. Symptoms, for example, may be categorized according to the 12 channels, the eight principles, the six external pathogenic factors, the five phases, the four levels, the three *jiao* or according to syndromes or patterns of diseases of the internal organs. A weeping eczema around the ear may, for example, be considered an Exterior excess (eight principles) condition of Damp Heat (six pathogens) affecting the Gall Bladder channel with an internal deficiency of the Spleen and stagnation of the Liver organs. This diagnosis will then typically be used to help formulate an individualized herbal prescription for a patient that will try and strike a balance between treating the symptoms (表 *biao*) and addressing the underlying constitutional dysfunction (*ben* 本). The herbal prescription will usually be a modified version of one or more classic recipes that may have a recorded use of several hundred years. As the patient's condition changes so the diagnosis will alter and the prescription be adapted to the new set of clinical circumstances.

Although standardized preprepared treatments are available, best practice in East Asian Medicine is characterized by diagnosis and treatment that is individualized and adaptable (Bensky & Gamble 1986; Farquhar 1994). The analysis of diagnostic patterns and the precise nature of the therapeutic intervention are highly contingent upon the training of the practitioner, their clinical experience, and the subjectivity of their empirical observation of a patient. Although objective measures derived from conventional medical diagnosis such as blood pressure, blood assays and scans are increasingly incorporated into the East Asian medical consultation process, the principal determining factor in the delivery of East Asian medicines remains the skill of the practitioner and their relationship with the patient.

This emphasis on practitioner skill and individualized treatment means that best practice in East Asian medicines conforms to a different hierarchy of evidence from conventional medicine. Rather than eliminating the subjective biases of individual practitioners by randomization and blinding, it is precisely these 'biases' that are seen as essential mechanisms of effective practice. Research methods that clarify and permit modeling of the decision-making processes of experienced practitioners are held in high esteem. In this inverted hierarchy of East Asian medicines, RCTs that test standardized preformulated herbal prescriptions have a lesser value than detailed case studies or case series that provide a degree of insight into the way a practitioner manages a particular condition. It seems that there are two incompatible approaches to evidence gathering. Is it possible that a way can be found to allow them to be successfully integrated into a meaningful but more inclusive framework?

Before we can do this we need to take a closer look at the range of research methods available to us, and instead of locating them within a hierarchy according to progressive elimination of bias, we need to consider them functionally. What kind of contribution to the evidence mosaic can each methodology make? What are their relative strengths and weaknesses? How should these methods be prioritized with regard to the evidence requirements of East Asian medicines?

RANDOMIZED CONTROLLED TRIALS

Randomized controlled trials can be broadly subdivided into explanatory and pragmatic. Explanatory RCTs are tightly controlled clinical experiments comparing an active treatment with either an inactive, placebo treatment or an equivalent treatment that has a previously determined treatment effect. The use of rigorous randomization and blinding can control the effects of bias and unwanted confounders in order to prove or disprove a causal connection between a specific intervention and a clearly measurable treatment effect.

Subjecting explanatory RCTs to a systematic review and meta-analysis aggregates the findings of different studies and further eliminates bias that may arise from an individual study in order to improve the estimate of how reliably these findings can be generalized to the whole population. However, despite the logic and intellectual appeal of this approach, we have already provided a critique of how vested interests that underpin this attempt to eliminate bias can in fact introduce a new bias that may provide a distorted and misleading notion of medical reality.

By contrast, pragmatic RCTs investigate usual care within a naturalistic clinical setting involving a heterogeneous sample population presenting with complex conditions and comorbidities that would normally be excluded from an explanatory RCT. Pragmatic trials are designed to evaluate the overall effect of more complex interventions, and as such have a particular relevance for many complementary therapies (MacPherson 2004) as well as conventional complex interventions such as psychiatry, physiotherapy, and many instances of primary care. Their weakness lies in their reduced ability to control for the effect of non-specific components of treatment, and this means that it is not possible using a pragmatic approach to identify a single specific causal factor that is the source of any reported therapeutic benefits.

OBSERVATIONAL STUDIES

Observational studies include research methods that compare groups but do not involve randomization. Examples include cohort and case–control studies, and cross-sectional studies that assess a group at a particular point in time.

A cohort study is a study in which subjects who currently have a certain condition, and/or receive a particular treatment or are exposed to a particular factor, are followed over time and compared with another group who are not affected by that condition, treatment or exposure. Conventionally, cohort studies are used when it would be unethical to allocate participants randomly to groups (e.g. smoking versus non-smoking); when large numbers of participants are required to identify relatively small treatment or exposure effects; when conditions are chronic and their natural course and prognosis are well known, so that the length of the study can incorporate fluxes in disease severity; or as a relatively inexpensive prelude to provide supportive data for a more rigorous RCT.

Cohort studies can either be prospective (where a group is followed over time) or retrospective (where data are collected for a group that was formed some time in the past).

Prospective cohort studies in East Asian medicines could be used, for example, to evaluate the long-term safety of herbal medicines (MacPherson & Liu 2005), or the effects of East Asian medical treatment in preventing certain age-related illnesses from developing. Retrospective studies could be used, for example, to consider any reduced financial burden on state-sponsored healthcare by those regularly using East Asian medicine.

The absence of randomization and blinding in cohort studies means that they are more susceptible to a number of potential confounders and biases. Observational cohort studies can describe an association between an intervention and an outcome, but they cannot ascribe a definite causal relationship between the two. Cohort studies are generally regarded as being prone to consistently overestimating the effects of a treatment (Ioannidis et al 2001). However, contrasting studies have revealed a more complex and ambivalent picture, with Kunz and Oxman (1998) demonstrating that non-randomization could lead to both increases in effect of 150% or more, and decreases of up to 90%, and other researchers finding no differences in estimates of treatment effects between RCTs and non-randomized observational studies (Concato et al 2000; Concato & Horwitz 2004; Benson & Hartz 2000; McKee et al 1999). Well-conducted observational studies that take into account known prognostic indicators during the evaluation of data and enrol participants using clear eligibility criteria can, according to one proponent, have the same internal validity as RCTs (Concato 2004), and (by virtue of the heterogeneous nature of trial subjects, more individually tailored treatments offered, and absence of some of the uncertainties and subsequent distorting effects of being part of a medical experiment) may also confer a greater external validity than the more artificial world of the RCT.

The relative value of observational studies versus RCTs continues to be debated in the research world. However, for the purposes of East Asian medical research, cohort studies offer a less expensive way of exploring possible health benefits resulting from an intervention that could be used to help build an evidence base that would add to the plausibility of East Asian medicines, facilitate their inclusion within mainstream healthcare, and encourage future research.

Case–control studies are used to help identify factors causing disease by comparing subjects that have a particular condition (cases) with an equal number of similar subjects (controls) who do not. These studies are generally retrospective and have been used, for example, to establish the convincing link between cigarette smoking and lung cancer (Doll & Peto 1976). In East Asian medicines case–controlled studies have been used to identify potential adverse reactions to Chinese herbal medicine (Melchart et al 1999). Case–control studies are relatively inexpensive, quick to provide data, and can be used to study relatively rare diseases, but they are highly susceptible to confounding factors and recall bias. For example, a case–control study indicated that use of hormone replacement therapy was associated with a reduced risk of coronary heart disease. However subsequent RCTs found the converse to be true (Rossouw et al 2002). This confusion occurred because the women using HRT were from a higher socioeconomic group than their controls and were more likely to eat healthier food and exercise regularly. It was these life-style factors that were mistakenly attributed to the HRT that caused a reduction in coronary heart disease.

Cross-sectional studies are surveys used to assess health issues relating to a sample of the population at a particular point in time. Conventionally they provide data on the prevalence of disease, or risk factors for disease such as obesity and alcohol use, or on the relationship between a number of variables occurring at the same time, such as income, obesity and diabetes. Their strength is that they are cheaper and provide data more quickly than prospective studies, but they are disadvantaged by being easily confounded by unsuspected or unknown variables and by being unable to distinguish a temporal sequence between variables. A cross-sectional study, for example assessing the relationship between marijuana use and unemployment, cannot determine which variable came first and could therefore be considered a causative factor. Cross-sectional studies would be useful to establish data such as the prevalence of East Asian medicines use among different populations, the different types of acupuncture used by East Asian medical practitioners, or the prevalence of herbal extract use compared to herbal decoctions.

Observational studies answer questions about the general effectiveness of a treatment package rather than the specific effects of a single therapeutic intervention. It is impossible using this approach to distinguish 'specific' from 'non-specific' effects, but if the purpose of the research is to prove effectiveness, evaluate potential side effects, or gain ideas about the cost-effectiveness of an intervention, then being able to attribute a single causative effect in treatment is not important. Observational studies are particularly relevant when the condition in question is chronic and its natural course and prognosis are well known, so that the length of the study can incorporate fluxes in disease severity (Walach et al 2002).

CASE STUDIES

Traditionally, East Asian medicines have relied heavily on individual case studies as a way of demonstrating theoretical principles in practice and exploring the subtleties and complexities of real-life case presentation and management. By illustrating both the 'rule' and exceptions to the 'rule', they offer a detailed insight into a clinical condition and into the mind of the practitioner involved in the process of diagnosis and treatment.

In EBM, case studies are typically regarded as anecdotal and useful only for providing advanced medical alerts, as in the case of thalidomide or AIDS, generating hypotheses to be explored in more rigorous trials, or to be used to explore the treatment of rare and unusual conditions (Bowling 2002). As such, they are frequently relegated to the bottom of the research hierarchy (Guyatt et al 1995).

However, proponents of 'real world' research challenge this. Robson (1997) defines a case study as 'a strategy for doing research which involves an empirical investigation of a particular contemporary phenomenon within its real life context using multiple sources of evidence' and continues to argue for the 'scientific' status of the case study as a process of enquiry governed by critical norms and standards of rationality. This ties in with the work of Forrester (1996), who argues that 'thinking in cases' represents not a flawed or inferior type of inductive thinking, but a distinctive 'style of reasoning' that belongs to science just as much as do other styles, such as deductive logic, experimental exploration, modeling based on analogies, or the statistical method. If, therefore, the Chinese, Japanese and Koreans have historically been attracted to such thinking and reasoning, this does not automatically signify a somewhat primitive way of thinking compared to that of the modern West. Rather, it can be seen as a cultural preference towards the concrete and experiential rather than the universal and abstract. There is value in both, but neither is intrinsically better than the other.

In addition, the application of qualitative methodologies to individual case histories can provide a way of systematically and deeply exploring the realities of clinical experience. Rather than creating research conditions where individual nuances are treated as confounding influences and hopefully excluded from the analysis, qualitative research sees that the value of the case study is its 'uniqueness', which can 'uncover the meaning of events in individuals' lives' (Janesick 2003). This emphasis on depth, uniqueness and exploring subjective meaning has often been seen in opposition to the kind of generalizable, objective data gathered by experimental trials (Pope & Mays 1995). Increasingly, though, both approaches are seen as distinct but complementary ways of investigating a particular question (Jones 1995), although among proponents of EBM there still exists a definite tendency to regard RCTs as the way of establishing a medical truth, and to use qualitative research to try and understand why patients are reluctant to comply with these proven benefits (Jones 1995; Donovan et al 2002).

n-of-1 STUDIES

n-of-1 studies are RCTs in individual patients. A patient can be randomized to either treatment A or treatment B, evaluated, and then given the treatment they did not initially receive. This is basically a crossover trial with a single subject. Both subject and researcher can be blinded, so there is a high level of internal rigor. n-of-1 trials are used conventionally to establish optimum drug dosages or to help clarify treatment responses in individual cases. Results can be pooled from several subjects, and the conclusions could be generalized beyond the individual patient to help characterize a subset of patients' responses to a specific treatment, or to characterize the heterogeneity of a disease (Madsen & Bytzer 2002).

n-of-1 trials are often cited as a way of bringing rigor into individual case histories. However, as with any crossover trial, treatments that have slow, long-lasting effects can seriously undermine the validity of the results because of an inadequate washout period. As this is the case in many complementary and alternative medical interventions, this is an important consideration to be taken into account.

CASE SERIES

Case series are a way of gathering data from different cases with the same presenting condition. Quantitative methods can be used to collate data through the use of validated questionnaires such as MYMOP (Paterson 1996;

Paterson et al 2010) or SF-36 (Jenkinson et al 1999) or other outcome measures. Although lacking the internal rigor of the RCT, large-scale long-term outcomes studies involving many practitioners is an affordable and practical way of generating significant data on effectiveness. This can then be used to help inform service providers and, with appropriate statistical methods such as predictive regression, data on prognostic characteristics or the contrasting benefits of different treatment regimens can also be assessed (Walach et al 2002).

QUALITATIVE RESEARCH

Qualitative research is concerned with describing and analyzing the qualities and meaning attributed to human experiences (Denzin & Lincoln 2003). Instead of attempting to quantify, statistically analyze and generalize reported data, qualitative research focuses primarily on the medium of the spoken and written word to elicit and evaluate the detailed life experiences of individuals and the social worlds they inhabit. There are diverse approaches and methodologies used in qualitative research. These may focus on exploring the subjective impressions or 'lived experience' of an individual (e.g. phenomenology) or take a broader social perspective by analyzing the way that a particular culture has developed, is maintained, and how it is changing (e.g. ethnography) (Grbich 1999).

Although qualitative research focuses on exploring the in-depth experience of individuals in a particular context, it also applies methodologies, such as grounded theory (Strauss & Corbin 1998), that can be used to identify common themes and processes that offer representative and explanatory models for human behavior. In a postmodernist world, where there is an acceptance of a multiplicity of truths, qualitative research can provide different but equally valuable insights as those provided by quantitative methods, into the nature of health, disease and medical intervention. Qualitative research will, hopefully, have an increasingly important role within the developing evidence mosaic of East Asian medicines and will contribute towards providing a more detailed understanding of how these practices affect human health and wellbeing.

DEFINING THE RESEARCH QUESTION

The selection of qualitative and quantitative methodologies depends entirely on the nature of the question that research is being used to address (Table 9.1). Different 'stakeholders' in the research process will require different types of information. For patients, the anecdotal accounts of case histories may be more relevant; individual practitioners might be more interested in a pragmatic comparison of different treatment regimens; health service providers may prioritize data relating to safety and economic impact; and scientists and clinical researchers might be seeking to identify a specific causal effect from an intervention. Each of these diverse stakeholders will have their own hierarchy of research methodologies according to the kind of data they need to address their particular area of inquiry.

Defining the research question, then, is the fundamental starting point from which the rest of the research design will follow. For example:

Table 9.1	Strengths, weaknesses and possible applications of different research methodologies	
Research method	Strengths	Weaknesses
Double-blind RCT	• Controls for bias and confounding factors • Proves a specific causal relation between an intervention and treatment effect	• Highly selective, homogeneous and unrealistic sample • Difficult to provide individualized treatments • Complex and expensive
In East Asian medicines a double-blind RCT could be used to establish the specific efficacy of a herbal intervention		
Pragmatic RCT	• Reflects 'real-world' practice in a heterogeneous sample population • Able to evaluate a treatment as whole system	• Unable to prove a specific causal effect • May be affected by unmeasured and unknown non-specific effects • Complex and expensive
Pragmatic trials could be used to evaluate the overall effect of East Asian medicines as they are routinely practiced in a real-world setting.		
Observational studies	• Affordable and relatively easy to organize • Reflects 'real-world' practice • Can be used to assess association between treatment and outcome	• May overestimate treatment effect • Subject to bias and confounding factors
Observational studies could be used to provide long-term data relating to safety and adverse effects from East Asian medicines.		
n-of-1; case history; case series	• Illustrates and evaluates individual strategy and clinical decision making • Rapid and inexpensive way to provide preliminary data on herb selection, dosage and safety	• Difficult to generalize data • Limited impact due to individual nature of cases • Subject to bias and confounding factors
n-of-1 trials could be used to establish optimum dosage of herbs prior to a larger clinical trial or case histories could be used in the process of establishing best practice guidelines		
Qualitative research	• Provides deep insights into the 'real-world' experience of receiving East Asian medicine • May be used to provide a model for how complex interventions work	• Does not provide quantitative data on effectiveness for statistical analysis and generalization to the wider population
Qualitative methods could be used to provide a detailed analysis of the impact of East Asian medicines on health and wellbeing		

- Questions relating to the specific efficacy of an East Asian medicine in treating a particular condition will require an explanatory RCT.
- Questions relating to the effectiveness of the whole system of East Asian medical intervention in normal practice will require a pragmatic RCT.
- Other questions may not require an RCT to provide the necessary data and could be better explored using other methods (Table 9.2).

Table 9.2   Matching research methodology to the research question

Research question	Methodology
What is the efficacy of East Asian medicine for a specific disease or condition?	Placebo-controlled, double-blind, randomized clinical trial
What is the effectiveness of an East Asian medical practice in 'real-world' practice?	Pragmatic randomized controlled trials
Are there long-term side effects from a specific East Asian medicine?	Observational study–longitudinal survey Case–control study
What is the patient's experience of taking a specific East Asian medicine?	Qualitative research
Which conditions seem to respond well to a specific East Asian medical practice?	Outcomes audit Cross-sectional survey of practitioners
What are the active ingredients of a particular herb?	Laboratory experimentation
What is the economic cost of a specific East Asian medical practice for treating a disease?	Health economic studies

Once the primary orientation of the research question has been decided and an appropriate methodology selected, the question needs to be further refined.

A RESEARCH STRATEGY FOR EAST ASIAN MEDICAL PRACTICES

A research strategy for East Asian medical practices should involve a progressive gathering of increasingly detailed data. As this grows into a convincing body of evidence, a balance between rigor (internal validity) and relevance (external validity) must be aimed for. Equal value should be accorded to the breadth of the objective generalizations that can be made, and the depths of the subjective experiences of people's real lives. Transparency within the research process should acknowledge that no single method can lay claim to the truth. All have their own distortions and at best, using a variety of methods, we can build up a complex, multidimensional map of the effects of an East Asian medical intervention. These effects may be physical, emotional, social, vocational, economic, intellectual, political and spiritual. Different researchers will use different methods to assess these effects of treatment, and each should be considered to be equally important and 'real.'

However, built into this framework are assumptions drawn from the research hierarchy (NICE 2004). Research strategies are frequently presented as a series of phases that provide a continuum of increasingly convincing evidence. Whereas it may not be the explicit intention of the writers, these phases tend to reproduce the levels of the conventional research hierarchy into a temporal sequence of research events. The RCT is considered definitive. Although the rigor of the RCT is widely accepted, we have seen there is a strong argument that observational studies may provide equivalent data. The conditions necessary for experimental research can create an artificial experience for both patients and service providers which can differ significantly from naturalistic clinical practice. Pragmatic studies have been presented as a viable alternative that can combine the rigor of the RCT with the relevance of observational studies, and as such may be a more appropriate method to be used in the evaluation of East Asian medical practices. However, we have also seen how qualitative studies offer a depth of insight that gives a different, but equally valid, truth to the generalizable averages of the RCT. Can East Asian medical research develop a new model which takes a more egalitarian approach to these diverse but equally important methods?

A PROPOSAL

Yin-Yang 阴 阳 is a philosophical concept that has had an important place in Chinese thought since the fourth century BC (Unschuld 1985). Yin (signified by a character which originally meant the 'shady side of a hill') and Yang (the 'sunny side of a hill') encapsulate a view of the world in which states, processes and relationships (such as night and day, or cold and hot) could be described as both opposing and complementary. Yin relates to that which is internal, unstructured, subjective and reflective, whereas Yang manifests as external, structured, objective and transformative. No one thing or activity is definitively Yin or Yang – its meaning is both relative and contextual. Thus a cold night is Yin in relation to the daytime sun but Yang in relation to absolute zero. Yin and Yang describe the natural dynamics of change from the ebb and flow of the tides to burnout from extended periods of stress. Also, and importantly, Yin and Yang can never be complete polar opposites: there is always an element of Yin within Yang and vice versa.

Can a seemingly esoteric 2000-year-old concept have any relevance to research questions in the 21st century? In practice there is much that can be incorporated from this ancient way of thinking. It is non-hierarchical: neither Yin nor Yang is considered 'better' than the other. It contains apparently opposing concepts and incorporates them within a complementary, mutually enhancing framework; and it allows for a dynamic interplay between the two polarities. If we attribute subjective experience, quiet listening and intuitive insights to Yin, then we can see how qualitative research, case studies and practitioner consensus have a more Yin aspect. By comparison, the objective, large-scale heavily controlled environment of the RCT belongs to Yang. Within the Yin–Yang symbol (Fig. 9.1) other research methods can be positioned. Now there is no hierarchy, just different stages in a research cycle that values the depth of the qualitative as much as the breadth of the quantitative, and encourages the development of one from the other.

Within each polarity these is an aspect of the opposite pole. Thus the Yin–Yang model encourages nested qualitative studies within the RCT process, and equally, qualitative work should utilize a more structuralist analysis of narrative to help develop key themes. Yin–Yang has the flexibility and comprehensiveness to be able to incorporate the spectrum of research methods and position them in a way that reflects both their particular strengths and their relationship to the whole cycle of research and investigation. This may be a fanciful

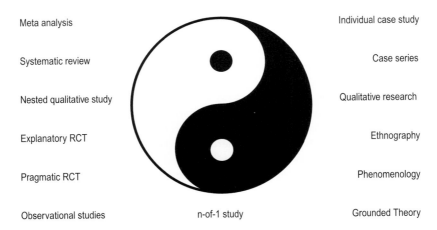

Meta analysis	Individual case study
Systematic review	Case series
Nested qualitative study	Qualitative research
Explanatory RCT	Ethnography
Pragmatic RCT	Phenomenology
Observational studies	n-of-1 study	Grounded Theory

FIG. 9.1 Example of a Yin–Yang research model.

attempt to fit new ideas into an old conceptual framework, but the interdependent movement of Yin–Yang is a simple but profound model that originated in early attempts to make sense of the world, and could perhaps still have a place in framing a research strategy for Chinese medicine some 2000 years later.

CONCLUSION

If East Asian medical practices are to move from the margins of healthcare to assume a more central and secure position in the Western world, it seems inevitable that they will have to generate a rigorous and convincing evidence base. To achieve this we have the option of two diverging paths. The first uses research methodologies developed to test the efficacy of pharmaceutical drugs and involves large-scale randomized controlled trials using standardized medical products. This may lead to the identification of reliable and efficacious herbal remedies or to the isolation of powerful active compounds that could progress down the long road to drug registration before being added to national formularies and then dispensed by conventional medics. This is one way to test East Asian medicines and disseminate any benefits to the broader population.

However, much may also be lost by this approach. The capacity of East Asian medical practices to offer individualized treatments that can be readily adjusted to meet changing clinical circumstances will not survive a movement towards standardized products. Nor will many of the adjunctive components of these treatments that emerge from the detailed and attentive questioning and observation that accompanies a traditional consultation – from descriptions of disease that use the richly metaphoric language of East Asian medical terminology; or from the dietary and lifestyle advice that frequently accompany herbal formulae or the needling of acupuncture points. Opting for research pathways that abandon these vital and precious aspects of these traditional medicines will undermine and diminish the very medical practices they are trying to investigate.

An alternative route is to use the rich assortment of available research methodologies to develop a deep and multifaceted understanding of the nature of

East Asian medical practices and to evaluate how they may affect individual and collective health. This approach embraces these practices as whole systems of medical care that otherwise might lose their potency and value if reduced into their component parts. Granting equal status but different values to qualitative and quantitative methods will enable East Asian medicines practices to be both explored and improved. Producing an evidence base using this approach will enhance rather than diminish these practices, and will also address the different needs of the various stakeholders in the process. Although there will doubtlessly be treatments that are shown to be archaic and ineffective, this will hopefully resemble the kind of pruning necessary to enable an old fruit tree to rejuvenate and produce a vigorous new crop.

REFERENCES

Bekelman, J.E., Li, Y., Gross, C.P., 2003. Scope and impact of financial conflicts of interest in biomedical research: a systematic review. JAMA 289 (4), 454–465.

Bensky, D., Gamble, A., 1986. Chinese Herbal Materia Medica. Eastland Press, Seattle.

Benson, K., Hartz, A.J., 2000. A comparison of observational studies and randomized, controlled trials. N. Engl. J. Med. 342 (25), 1878–1886.

Biagioli, M., 1999. The Science Studies Reader. Routledge, New York.

Bodenheimer, T., 2000. Uneasy alliance: clinical investigators and the pharmaceutical industry. N. Engl. J. Med. 342, 1539–1544.

Bowling, A., 2002. Research Methods in Health. Open University Press, Buckingham.

Cabana, M.D., Rand, C.S., Powe, N.R., et al., 1999. Why don't physicians follow clinical practice guidelines? A framework for improvement. JAMA 282, 1458–1465.

Campbell, R., Quilty, B., Dieppe, P., 2003. Discrepancies between patients' assessments of outcome: qualitative study nested within a randomised controlled trial. BMJ 326, 252–253.

Chalmers, I., 1990. Underreporting research is scientific misconduct. JAMA 263, 1405–1408.

Claridge, J., Fabian, T., 2005. History and development of evidence-based medicine. World J. Surg. 29, 547–553.

Colquhoun, D., 2009. DC's Improbable Science. http://www.dcscience.net.

Concato, J., 2004. Observational Versus Experimental Studies: What's the evidence for a Hierarchy? NeuroRx 1, 341–347.

Concato, J., Horwitz, R.I., 2004. Beyond randomised versus observational studies. Lancet 363, 1660–1661.

Concato, J., Shah, N., Horwitz, R.I, 2000. Randomized controlled trials, observational studies, and the hierarchy of research designs. NEJM 324, 1887–1892.

Daston, L., Galison, P., 2007. Objectivity. Zone Books. Distributed by the MIT Press, New York, Cambridge, MA.

Denzin, N.K., Lincoln, Y.S., 2003. Strategies of Qualitative Inquiry. second ed. Sage Publications.

De Vries, R.G., 2004. The warp of evidence-based medicine: lessons from Dutch maternity care. Int. J. Health Serv. 34, 595–623.

DiMasi, J.A., Hansen, R.W., Grabowsk, H.G., 2003. The price of innovation: new estimates of drug development costs. J. Health Econ. 22, 151–185.

Doll, R., Peto, R., 1976. Mortality in relation to smoking: 20 years' observations on male British doctors. BMJ 2 (6051), 1525–1536.

Donovan, J., Mills, N., Smith, M., et al., 2002. Improving design of randomised trials by embedding them in qualitative research: Protec T (prostate testing for cancer study). BMJ 325, 766–770.

Farquhar, J., 1994. Knowing Practice: The Clinical Encounter of Chinese Medicine. Westview Press, Boulder and Oxford.

Flanagin, A., Carey, L.A., Fontanarosa, P.B., et al., 1998. Prevalence of articles with honorary authors and ghost authors in peer-reviewed medical journals. JAMA 280 (3), 222–224.

Constructing an evidence base for East Asian medicines

Forrester, J., 1996. If p, then what? Thinking in cases. Hist. Hum. Sci. 9 (1), 1–25.

Giles, J., 2004. British drug company to put data online as criticism mounts. Nature 429, 793.

Goldenberg, M.J., 2006. Gift horse or Trojan horse? Social science perspectives on evidence-based health care. Soc. Sci. Med. 62, 2621–2632.

Grbich, C., 1999. Qualitative Research in Health. Sage Publications.

Guyatt, G.H., Sackett, D.L., Sinclair, J.C., et al., 1995. Users' guides to the medical literature. IX. A method for grading health care recommendations. JAMA 274, 1800–1804.

Hall, D.L., Ames, R.T., 1995. Anticipating China: Thinking Through the Narratives of Chinese and Western Culture. State University of New York Press, Albany.

Ioannidis, J.P.A., Haidich, A.B., Pappa, M., et al., 2001. Comparison of evidence of treatment effects in randomized and nonrandomized studies. JAMA 286, 821–830.

Janesick, V.J., 2003. The choreography of qualitative research design. In: Denzin, N.K., Lincoln, Y.S. (Eds.), Introduction. Strategies of Qualitative Inquiry, second ed. Sage publications, p. 70.

Jenkinson, C., Stewart-Brown, S., Petersen, S., Paice, C., 1999. Assessment of the SF-36 version 2 in the United Kingdom. J. Epidemiol. Community Health 53, 46–50.

Jones, R., 1995. Why do qualitative research? BMJ 311, 2.

Jørgensen, A.W., Jørgensen, K.J., Gøtzsche, P.C., 2010. Unbalanced reporting of benefits and harms in abstracts on rofecoxib. Eur. J. Clin. Pharmacol. 66, 341–347. Epub 2010 Feb 17.

Jullien, F., 1995. The Propensity of Things: Toward a History of Efficacy in China. Zone Books, New York.

Kunz, R., Oxman, A.D., 1998. The unpredictability paradox: review of empirical comparisons or randomised and non-randomised clinical trials. BMJ 317, 1185–1190.

McKee, M., Britton, A., Black, N., et al., 1999. Interpreting the evidence: choosing between randomised and non-randomised studies. BMJ 319, 312–315.

MacPherson, H., 2004. Pragmatic clinical trials. Complement. Ther. Med. 12, 134–140.

MacPherson, H., Liu, B., 2005. The safety of Chinese herbal medicine: a pilot for a national survey. J. Complement. Altern. Med. 11 (4), 617–626.

MacPherson, H., Peters, D., Zollman, C., 2009. Closing the evidence gap in integrative medicine. BMJ 339, b3335.

Madsen, L.G., Bytzer, P., 2002. Review article: single subject trials as a research instrument in gastrointestinal pharmacology. Aliment. Pharmacol. Ther. 16, 189–196.

Melchart, D., Linde, K., Weidenhammer, W., et al., 1999. Liver enzyme elevations in patients treated with traditional Chinese medicine. JAMA 282 (1), 28–29.

Montgomery, K., 2006. How Doctors Think: Clinical Judgment and the Practice of Medicine. Oxford University Press, Oxford, New York.

Munos, B., 2009. Lessons from 60 years of pharmaceutical innovation. Nat. Rev. Drug Discov. 8, 959–968.

NICE (National Institute of Clinical Excellence), 2004. Guideline Development Methods. NICE, London. (Chapter 7). http://www.nice.org.uk/pdf/GDM_Chapter7.pdf.

Paterson, C., 1996. Measuring outcome in primary care: a patient-generated measure, MYMOP, compared to the SF-36 health survey. BMJ 312, 1016–1020.

Paterson, C., Unwin, J., Joire, D., 2010. Outcomes of traditional Chinese medicine (traditional acupuncture) treatment for people with long-term conditions. Complement. Ther. Clin. Pract. 16, 3–9. Epub 2009 Sep 9.

Pickstone, J.V., 2001. Ways of Knowing: A New History of Science, Technology, and Medicine. University of Chicago Press, Chicago.

Pope, C., Mays, N., 1995. Qualitative Research: Reaching the parts other methods cannot reach: an introduction to qualitative methods in health and health services research. BMJ 311, 42–45.

Rawlins, M., 2008. De testimonio: on the evidence for decisions about the use of therapeutic interventions. Lancet 372, 2152–2161.

Robson, C., 1997. Real World Research. Blackwell, Oxford.

Rossouw, J.E., Anderson, G.L., Prentice, R.L., et al., 2002. Writing Group for the Women's Health Initiative Investigators. Risks and benefits of estrogen plus progestin in healthy postmenopausal women: principal results from the Women's Health Initiative randomized controlled trial. JAMA 288, 321–333.

Sackett, D.L., Rosenberg, W.M.C., Gray, J.A.M., et al., 1996. Evidence based medicine: what it is and what it isn't. BMJ 312, 71–72.

Strauss, A., Corbin, J., 1998. Basics of Qualitative Research: Techniques and Procedures for Developing Grounded Theory, second ed. Sage Publications.

Unschuld, P.U., 1985. Medicine in China. University of California Press, California.

Walach, H., Jonas, W.B., Lewith, G., 2002. The role of outcomes research in evaluating complementary and alternative medicine. In: Lewith, G., Jonas, W.B., Walach, H. (Eds.), Clinical Research in Complementary Therapies. Churchill Livingston, p. 38.

Constructing an evidence base for East Asian medicines

Treatment evaluation: an anthropologist's approach

Elisabeth Hsu

Treatment evaluation tends to be the domain of clinical scientists and statisticians. Their assessment is generally considered more 'objective' than the 'subjective' point of view of practitioners and their patients concerning the 'results of the treatment', in the terminology of their tradition of medical learning, or its 'quality', for which patients often lack words. The researcher who conducts randomized controlled trials (RCTs) and their meta-analyses, however, is also a sort of practitioner, just within a different playing field. Authors working within Science and Technology Studies have highlighted the subjectivities of science researchers, their social networks, and the technopolitics they participate in (ever since Latour & Woolgar 1979). With regard to an East Asian medical treatment, namely the Tibetan medical treatment for *Helicobacter pylori* infections, the same ultrasound results were differently evaluated by biomedical and Tibetan practitioners. This was due to many years of clinical training within different institutions of medical learning, resulting in different styles of appreciating what counts as evidence (Adams & Li 2008: 126).

In respect of currents within what would appear to most the same tradition of learning, namely 'modern Western science', historians of science have demonstrated that there is not just one sort of 'objectivity' but several different types, each suited to solving scientific problems particular to scientific fields in specific historical situations (e.g. Daston & Galison 2007; see Vignette 10.1). In other words, desirable as 'objective' assessments of treatment evaluation may be, it needs to be borne in mind that they are, in fact, the product of highly profession-specific, socially constructed and culturally accepted styles of knowing, ethics and aesthetics (e.g. Hacking 1991). The industry of knowledge production, however, in its very being and in its legitimation (i.e. the institutions housing health officers, administrators, statisticians and computers, who produce numbers on papers, which are recycled by media and electronic information devices), differs from the life worlds of patients and practitioners.

Health services research has come to acknowledge the importance of the patient's voice and funds large investigations into measuring patients' reported outcomes (e.g. http://phi.uhce.ox.ac.uk/home.php). However, these are operationalized and quantified in accordance with the rules of the above knowledge production industries. Medical anthropologists, by contrast, have emphasized that the subjectivities of the patients and practitioners matter, linking their personal transformation to societal change and newly emergent forms of political authority (Biehl et al 2007). Subjectivities matter also in treatment evaluation, as is argued here.

VIGNETTE 10.1 THREE STYLES OF OBJECTIVITY
ELISABETH HSU

Daston and Galison (2007) highlight three different epistemic virtues, each giving rise to a different research practice for obtaining 'objectivity' and each putting the researcher in a different role. The 19th-century botanist, for instance, who believed the species he described were 'universal' categories, would engage in a practice of 'selection' and 'synthesis' to draw an ideal-type specimen; the histologist, by contrast, who is convinced the defining characteristics of different kinds of human tissue are to be found in a 'particular sample', would engage in a scientific practice that would produce an 'automated transfer' of the specimen, such as photographs of his carefully colored preparations. The botanist is portrayed as a 'sage', whose 'reasoned' judgment allows him to produce the ideal-type specimen, the histologist as a 'worker', whose objective sample of tissue is obtained through 'mechanical' reproduction. A scientist who works like an astronomer, finally, is described as an 'expert', who recognizes and 'interprets' phenomena that are considered to have 'family resemblances' by engaging in the practice of 'pattern recognition.' All these modern Western scientists are considered to engage in a research practice that produces 'objective' scientific truths, although their epistemic virtues, their role as a scientist, their practices, and the ontologies of the categories they describe are very different.

'Subjectivity' is often understood, in somewhat contradictory ways, as (1) an aspect of individuality, (2) sometimes, tainted by feelings and personal concerns that are contrasted with objectivity, rational thought and clear judgment, and (3) more recently, as referring to all inner processes, regardless of whether they are emotional, moral or cognitive. Finally, the subjectivity of an artist, expressed in aesthetic form, is meant to strike a chord in other people, as well as those of other historical times and societies (Biehl et al 2007: p. 5–6). A focus on subjectivity need not result in a celebration of solipsism, individuality and cultural constructedness (see also the individual case histories discussed by Volker Scheid in Vignette 8.1). On the contrary, one can go a step further and focus one's research on subjective experiences that appear to transcend boundaries of class and culture. Individual patients' subjective experiences of betterment, which are constitutive of the highly specific medical practices that treatment evaluation is concerned with, sometimes show features that have striking cross-cultural commonalities.

RECENT MEDICAL ANTHROPOLOGICAL RESEARCH ON TREATMENT EVALUATION

Biomedical researchers have noted that randomizing and double-blinding is necessary to account for the 'placebo effect', which they treat as a sort of 'noise' that 'hinders' them from measuring the efficacy of the pharmacologically active substance (Sullivan 1993). However, medical anthropologists have pointed out that the efficacy these scientists are aiming to measure is a highly idealized entity. The late Cecil Helman, in a memorable introductory lecture (see also Helman 1990: 170), drew concentric lines around a dot in the middle of the blackboard that signified the active substance's pharmacological efficacy. The first circle depicted the efficacy of the color of the coating of the pill that contained the pharmacologically active substance, the second denoted the efficacy of the packaging within which the coated pill was presented, the third the efficacy of the general practitioner in a white coat in his consultation room handing over the packaging within which was the color-coated pill, and the fourth concentric line referred to the efficacy of the prestigious medical establishment, with its glorious history of medical success 'in the combat of disease' and its impressive technological equipment for future interventions, to which the general practitioner's practice belonged. For the patient the 'total drug effect' arose out of the totality of all these efficacies, which Helman had drawn on the blackboard in a Russian-doll-like fashion, while the RCT professional was interested only in the dot in the middle.

Didactically effective as it was to draw concentric lines around a dot, but it put the pharmacologically active substance centre-stage, when not necessarily always the material properties of the drug, but rather the sociopolitical dynamics of the assemblage of which it is part, may play a far more important role in how the patient experiences the efficacy (e.g. Waldram 2000) and how different scientific communities evaluate it (e.g. Barry 2006). Recently, the issue of treatment evaluation has become so central to medical anthropology that two monographs pertaining to it have been published, both with Cambridge University Press. Moerman (2002) proposed to do away with the concept of 'placebo' and emphasized that regardless of whether or not a drug had a pharmacologically active substance, people had a 'meaning response' to it; he highlighted symbolic aspects of its color, size, quantity, newness, mode of administration, and even reported on trials about innovative forms of heart surgery that highlighted how the meaning response affected treatment evaluation. Whyte and colleagues (2003), by contrast, emphasized the 'social efficacy' of medical treatment. Where Moerman reports on fascinating data from research trials, and therefore is easily comprehended and frequently cited by health professionals, Whyte et al. discuss findings arising out of long-term ethnographic research based on participant observation in the local language. A mother of a child with a cough in a shantytown of the Philippines, for instance, would not bother to know what the outcome of an RCT was. Her choice of treatment and purchase of the right brand of cough syrup would depend on habits within her life world, on whether her mother and grandmother used cough syrup too, on which brand the neighbors preferred, and on what was advertised on TV. Even if a mother was aware that cough syrup had no curative effects, it remained her first choice of treatment; by administering it, she would be seen as a good mother by neighbors and family, and upon his return from work in the evening her husband would not be irritated by constantly coughing children (which can become a liability for a marriage). So, although pharmacologically the cough syrup is not always curative, it was experienced as socially highly effective. In many ways that mattered more – all the more so if one could assume that a constitutionally strong child, who was meant to live, would eventually shake off the cough anyway.

THE PHENOMENOLOGICAL APPROACH TO TREATMENT EVALUATION

The above research has been conducted within the parameters of medical anthropology since its very beginnings, which owes its existence to researchers who started to carve out this field as one of worthy social scientific inquiry by emphasizing the difference between 'disease' and 'illness.' Disease was the biological dysfunction the biomedical practitioner attended to, whereas the anthropologist claimed competency in accounting for the social aspects of illness (Kleinman 1980) and sickness (Frankenberg 1980; Young 1982). With regard to treatment evaluation, this meant differentiating between the natural scientist's assessment of 'therapeutic efficacy' and the social scientist's of 'therapeutic success.' Research on 'therapeutic efficacy' was useful, but should not be overinflated, as it was merely one among many modes of treatment evaluation (Hsu 1996).[1] However, the differentiation between socially constructed illnesses and biological dysfunctions of disease, which once appeared a good first approximation to the problematic, has since been found to be derived from an epistemological fallacy.

With Margaret Lock's (1994) research into menopause in Japan and North America as 'local biologies', i.e. biological realities both to local scientists and to the local people they study, the Cartesian body affected by either disease or illness has been called into question, as has the split of legitimate scientific inquiry into either social or natural sciences. Social scientists have been made acutely aware of the 'thinginess' of the social processes they study, i.e. of the material, technological and natural scientific aspects of sociality (e.g. Latour 2000). Where structuralism and social constructivism provided anthropology with conceptual frameworks to reinforce the above Cartesian dichotomy intrinsic to medical anthropology, medical anthropologists today are searching for ways in which to account for the social in the biological and vice versa (e.g. Farquhar & Lock 2007). This should apply also to treatment evaluation. Some anthropologists have been inspired by phenomenology (e.g. Csordas 1994, 2002), fewer by ecological psychology (e.g. Ingold 2000; Hsu 2010). Others, particularly in the context of writing on ritual, have elaborated in terms of 'fractal scaling' on Mandelbrot's mathematics of self-similarity, which applies not merely to natural but also to the social and artistic phenomena (Mosko 2005).

Thomas Csordas gives the philosophy put forth in the *Phenomenology of Perception* (Merleau-Ponty [1945] 1962) a decisively anthropological twist. He meaningfully combines Merleau-Ponty's understanding of the body as the existential ground whence human beings experience the world with Bourdieu's practice theory, which posits that even the body that we may experience as primordial and natural is, in fact, 'history turned into nature' (and therefore, ultimately, derived from and informed by social practice). This approach, which posits that the social is intertwined with the natural in complex ways, explained partly by taking recourse to history, promises to provide a fertile theoretical framework for treatment evaluation. The phenomenologist's vantage point

---

[1] Furthermore, the practitioner's own assessment in terms of 'therapeutic results' mattered, as did the patient's assessment of the 'therapeutic quality.' The former are discussed in Vignettes 10.1–10.4, the latter is the theme on which this article expands.

overcomes the limitations of cultural constructivism as it allows for the theoretical possibility that some social practices are grounded in experiences common to human beings in different places and across historical periods.

How a patient feels after treatment depends ultimately on the way in which the treatment affects the patient's self and body, feelings and subjectivity, or rather as highlighted below, on intersubjectivities between patient and practitioner, patient and other patients, patients and their social and natural environment, patients and the material things they interact with. The crux is that feelings are often inchoate, i.e. difficult to pin down and define. They are experienced in response to the situation in its entirety, in which the treatment is administered, such that it is often impossible to disentangle which response the treatment itself triggered and which the social entourage and the institutional and ecological environment. Sometimes feelings are intense, but their intensity only occasionally lasts for a certain time, and some forms of medical treatment appear to achieve betterment in the patient through eliciting a sequence of different intense feelings, for example instigating intense fear followed by laughter and ridicule (Kapferer 1983). In general, however, feelings are fluid and difficult to pigeonhole; they are easily modulated by alterations in atmosphere and circumstance, social relation and institutional set-up. There is research to suggest that people do not have sensations and feelings as one possesses things, but that feelings are an aspect of interpersonal relationships (e.g. Chau 2008).

In what follows, an attempt is made to approximate how medical treatment in general, and Chinese medical treatment in particular, can affect the subjectivities of patients and their feelings. In contrast to the highly culture-specific, if not profession-specific, ways in which 'objectivity' has been defined in the modern Western sciences (see Vignette 10.1), it appears that, cross-culturally, certain aspects of medical treatment are directed at eliciting certain subjectivities in patients with surprisingly similar features.

FEELING LIGHTER

To be sure, what one feels after a treatment is often what one was told to expect before deciding to have the treatment. Indeed, this can be understood to imply that human beings are 'gullible.' Medical marketing strategies – including Asian and East Asian ones (e.g. Bode 2008; Banerjee 2009; Hsu 2009; Zhan 2009) – build on such 'gullibility.' However, rather than ridiculing the human capacity to be affected by another human and calling it 'gullibility', it can be viewed as fundamental to human sociality. As Moerman (2002: 36) noted, when it comes to delivering effective treatment, it is not so much the 'gullibility' of the patients that matters (as the notion 'placebo effect' implies, alluding to the psychology of the gullible patient), but that of the medical practitioners: their belief in themselves, in their methods and technologies, their knowledge and personal experience. Medical training, like any other form of learning, is possible only because of the human capacity for 'gullibility.'

What then are patients told to expect after treatment? "You will feel lighter", Ute Luig recounts in respect of a *ngoma* drumming session in Zambia, and Marina Roseman in regard of a trance dance among the Orang Asli in Malaysia (Oxford medical anthropology research seminars, Hilary Term 2005). The subjective experience of 'feeling lighter' generally is accompanied by a host of other more situation-bound and culturally specific transformations. Roseman pointed to the social relation between the young man who, upon awakening, assisted the young woman who had collapsed in trance, and Luig detailed the cosmology of different *jinn* and other spiritual beings that *ngoma* performances invoke. Yet, cross-culturally, the patient's subjective experience of effective treatment is frequently contained in the very same statement relating a bodily experience: you feel lighter.

Admittedly, trance dance is not actually considered medical treatment, although it is often considered therapeutic. In Europe, acupuncture is often taken as preventive care and experienced as 'relaxing.' When asked what 'relaxing' means, the answer is often 'I feel lighter.' Other complementary and alternative medicine forms of treatment, such as *qigong* meditation or zero-balancing, are also experienced as making one 'feel lighter.' In China, not only therapeutically applied *zhenjiu*(acupuncture) and *qigong* make patients say they feel more comfortable (*shufu*) after treatment – and 'not so heavy' (*buzhong*); also *zhongyi*, Chinese herbal medicine, embraces principles of treatment, which, patients say, makes them 'feel lighter' (*qing yidian*), including those herbal medications that are meant to evacuate the bowels, induce sweating or vomiting (*xia, han, tu*). In recent fieldwork, carried out in Shexian county in Huizhou, southern Anhui, between July 2009 and January 2010, a ninth-generation traditional medical doctor, who was known for his treatment of digestive problems, frequently heard among his patients the complaint of 'feeling heavy' (*zhong*). The herbs he prescribed affected their *qi* dynamics and thus regulated their stools. This, they said, made them 'feel lighter' (for an example of Korean medical treatment against constipation, see Vignette 10.2 by Seonsam Na).

VIGNETTE 10.2   KOREAN MEDICAL TREATMENT RESULTING IN THE SUBJECTIVE EXPERIENCE OF 'FEELING LIGHTER'
SEONSAM NA

In the Korean language the word for 'feeling lighter' is 'Gabyupda (가볍다)' or 'Gappunhada (가뿐하다)', which literally means 'light' or 'nimble.' The Korean word for 'feeling heavy' is 'Mugeopda (무겁다)' or 'Mujigeunhada (무지근하다)' which means 'heavy' or 'stuffy.' Patients mention these words when they are confronted with lack of strength or loss of agility. In modern biomedical categories, their closest equivalents are dysphoric states or the so-called chronic fatigue syndrome. In both conditions, patients commonly say 'Momi maleul an deuneunda (몸이 말을 안듣는다),' meaning their bodies (as they are so heavy) are not responding to their orders, and some even say, 'Momi chongeunmangeunida (몸이 천근만근),' meaning their bodies weigh thousands of pounds. It is generally observable that these patients are inactive, psychologically and behaviorally.

In East Asian medicine, including Korean medicine, the symptom of 'feeling heavy' has been typically related to dampness (濕). When one suffers from dampness, either directly through contact with fog, riverine environments or sudden rain (外濕), or through the decreased function of the alimentary organs which fail to successfully transform the ingested fluid into energy (氣化), leaving superfluous dampness running in the body

(內濕), one 'feels heavy (身重)' (Shin et al 2005, 538–543). Patients with this symptom have a propensity to lie down and sleep a lot (嗜臥) (Huh 1987, 115–118). Treatments target the obstructions (滯) and turbidity (濁) caused by dampness, by inducing light perspiration in the case of external dampness (微汗通經絡), or through diuresis and purgation (滲利) in the case of internal dampness that negatively affects the body's overall fluid metabolism (Hwang 1997, 53–54). The most frequently used formula for this condition is Oryungsan (五苓散), which consists of Taeksa (澤瀉), Jeokbokryung (赤茯苓), Baekchul (白朮), Jeoryung (猪苓) and Yukgye (肉桂), and it forms the basis of many dampness-treating prescriptions, such as Bungieum (分氣飲), Bunshimgieum (分心氣飲), Bojungchiseuptang (補中治濕湯) and Seungseuptang (勝濕湯). These formulas largely aim to rectify the body's fluid circulation by clearing up obstructions and refreshing turbidity (清而疎快)'(Hwang 1997, 198). Baekchul(白朮), in particular, is favored by practitioners treating dampness-related symptoms as it plays the double role of drying the dampness and replenishing decreased splenic function (Kim et al 1991, 536–537). As the 'feeling of heaviness' basically involves the condition of Defensive Ki depletion (衛氣虛), in that the depleted Ki causes the lack of the surface energy that propels agility and nimbleness (Huh 1987, 115–118), these formulas contain elements of replenishing agents such as Insam (人蔘) and Gamcho (甘草) along with such herbs with strong diuretic action as Jeoryung(猪苓) and Moktong (木通). In Bunshimgieum (分心氣飲), light purgation is designed to be achieved through agents such as Daebokpi (大腹皮) or Jigak (枳殼).

I remember, some five years ago, treating a middle-aged woman with constipation who suffered from prolonged fatigue and lack of strength, but without any clinical sign of depression. Her main complaint was that she felt too heavy. As she was troubled by reduced gastric activity, I used first a formula based on Pyungwisan (平胃散) to restore her basic alimentary function before proceeding with Bunshimgieum (分心氣飲) to tackle the dampness-induced obstructions in her body, with added ingredients to induce purgation and resolution of psychological tensions. Other than a brief conversation in my office about her current situation in the family, no other major psychological intervention was attempted. After a two-month-long treatment in which she took medicines without interruption, she reported 'feeling lighter', along with better bowel movements and a more positive outlook on her life in general.

It is surprising that cross-culturally in different languages people speak of 'feeling lighter' as a sign of betterment. If one assumes, as phenomenologists do, that people experience the world through their body and that the body is a generative principle (i.e. that the position of the self in space and its bodily projection into the surroundings is crucial for the ways in which a person knows the world), one may not be entirely surprised that people cherish a body that feels lighter, and that they do so cross-culturally. All bodies are affected by gravitation.

Treatment evaluation: an anthropologist's approach

TREATMENT EVALUATION FROM THE VIEWPOINT OF 'HOMO RITUALIS'

To recapitulate, the phenomenologist interested in patients' subjectivities and treatment evaluation notes that effective treatment makes them experience their body and self as 'feeling lighter.' This finding can be shrugged off as a 'so what?' From a biomedical viewpoint 'feeling lighter' is an unspecific effect. It is not classified as a therapeutic effect. Nor does the health literature depict it as a preventive medical measure, although it is often termed synonymous with 'relaxation.' 'Feeling lighter' is an unspecified agreeable state in a cross-cultural sample of patients' subjectivities about the effects of medical interventions. However, for the specialist interested in the complexities of treatment evaluation, it has not been an issue worth further consideration. Why?

Modern science and biomedicine is grounded upon the principle that the material world matters, even though a subfield 'psychosomatic medicine' was founded primarily to account for phenomena where the state of mind, the subjective bodily feeling and the psychology of the patient appear to be decisive for treatment outcomes. Without abandoning the basic principles of its science, biomedicine therefore admitted to certain so-called 'psychosomatic disorders.' Those appear to differ from others and, as anomalies, are dealt with in a separate department, that of psychosomatic medicine; or they are relegated to 'complementary' healthcare (which cannot deal with 'real' medical problems).

Along similar lines of argument, Chinese medical practitioners, who rightly emphasize that the effects of their treatment are those of a medical science, feel belittled by such an alignment of their sophisticated techniques of effectiveness with those cross-culturally observed unspecific effects of dance trance. No doubt, 'feeling lighter' is not the only effect of Chinese medical interventions. However, the seemingly unspecific 'feeling lighter' often is an important aspect of the patient's experience, also that of the Chinese medical doctor. It is not the mind affecting the body, as postulated by a psychosomatic rendering, nor is it a culturally constructed treatment outcome. Rather, it expresses a cross-culturally observed bodily experience.

Acupuncturists passing through Oxford (between 2001 and 2010) with whom I occasionally discussed this phenomenon have commented that 'feeling lighter' after effective treatment indicates a bodily awareness of a state of the mind–body where 'self-healing processes' can 'kick in' more effectively than otherwise. Convincing as their comment is for the patient, it does not provide a theoretically sound framework for an anthropologist wishing to account for the truth contained in these subjective experiences. These cross-culturally observed subjective experiences of 'feeling lighter' suggest that research on treatment evaluation that takes seriously the patient's voice requires us to revise our theoretical frameworks.

Let us recapitulate. Natural scientific research advocating ever more refined RCTs alludes to a *homo rationalis*, rational (wo-)man. Moerman's (2002) research does not question this scientific endeavor but emphasizes that the meanings relevant for treatment evaluation are generated by other means than rational argumentation only, such as color symbolism. Whyte et al (2003), however, put forth another paradigm to explain people's choices and evaluation of treatment: *homo sociologicus*, the social (wo-)man, who is also sometimes a *homo oeconomicus*, an economically astute (wo-)man. The phenomenologist's finding that patient subjectivities refer to bodily experiences that are cross-culturally surprisingly similar requires yet another framework. The one proposed here is that of *homo ritualis*, the (wo-)man who owes his/her achievements to ritual.[2] The aspect of ritual that is important to us here is that it alludes to a human being with a body that engages with other bodies in body techniques. Unlike the Cartesian body, which is central to RCTs and biomedicine, *homo ritualis* inhabits a body that is living, material, spatially positioned and concrete, and active, following a rhythm given by sociocultural temporalities.

THE PROCESSUAL ASPECTS OF RITUAL AND MEDICAL TREATMENT

When it comes to treatment evaluation, there is more to be learnt from what anthropologists say about ritual procedure and religious experience. Csordas (1983), for instance, emphasizes that internal, psychological preparation is necessary for treatment to be effective. In his discussion of charismatic healing among Pentecostals in the USA, Csordas differentiates three stages of a primarily psychic process, from 'predisposition' to 'empowerment' to 'transformation.' These, he says, are essential for making possible the all-compassing bodily, emotional and mental transformations that make treatment effective.

Csordas emphasizes that treatment can affect a patient only if he or she is predisposed to let a transformation happen. He identifies three stages in the ritual process, in line with the anthropologist of religion Victor Turner (e.g. 1967), who, in turn, draws on the folklorist Arnold van Gennep (1909) and his division of the rites of passage into 'rites of separation', 'rites of threshold' and 'rites of aggregation.' Important here is not that the patient's transformation takes place in *three* stages, but that the efficacy of medical treatment is a *process*. It does not arise from a single magic-bullet intervention to which the patient is passively exposed.

In *qigong* treatment delivered by a healer who worked in an urban area of the People's Republic of China, where petty private enterprise was thriving, effective treatment was found to depend not only on an individual's intrapsychic states but, importantly, on an interpersonal process that enhanced the social bonds of those participating in it (Hsu 1999, 58–67). One could identify five stages in this process. During the first, which concerned 'the choice of treatment', the patient would make the decision to either choose or reject *qigong* as a treatment suited to him- or herself; this stage was key to how the patient would evaluate the treatment in the end. The patient's choice of *qigong* as treatment was facilitated through the healer's 'forms of recruitment', which were subtle, multiple and situation specific.[3] Effective treatment was furthermore dependent on 'mutual commitment', which in

[2] Or, as James (2003) puts it, the 'ceremonial animal.' Accordingly, her opening chapter discusses dance. However, she does so from a structuralist viewpoint, rather than from the experiential one adopted here.
[3] If the patient were to choose Chinese medical treatment, the physician's calligraphy would belong among these forms of recruitment that affect the patient's choice and treatment outcome.

the case of this *qigong* healer involved treatment cycles of a minimum of ten sessions, and a 'reaching of consensus' on whether the results of the treatment were sufficient. The treatment was often terminated temporarily as the results of the treatment were not always very obvious and blatant. Since the *qigong* healer dealt mostly with chronic and recurrent conditions, and often delivered what a health professional would call palliative care to his many cancer patients, the treatment lasted, with intervals, sometimes for years. Often, the social bond between patient and healer would become stronger. Their families would undertake outings together, do errands for each other, or even start a joint business. Thus, friendship ensued in the fifth and final phase 'from patient to *pengyou* [friend].' In this *qigong* healer's case, medical treatment ideally resulted not only in the transformation of the patient's health status, but in a social transformation of patient and practitioner (which becoming friends is). Treatment evaluation in this case would have to attend not merely to processual aspects of *qigong* healing but also to interpersonal relations and their transformation in that setting, inclusive of those that affect the healer.

Let us take this a step further: ritual does not merely affect interpersonal relations, its effects are produced in the interstices between persons. In his ethnography of a Chinese temple festival in northern Shaanxi province, Adam Chau (2006: 156–159) first questions whether every ritual must have three stages. He notes that people converge to the temple grounds, mill around, enjoy the heat and noise they produce, until after some days, they disperse again. He draws on Durkheim's (1965: 246–247, 249–250) description of how scattered aboriginal groups in Australia would seasonally converge on one place, experience an intense sociality in togetherness, and disperse again. Where Durkheim points out the 'collective effervescence' that they produce, which impinges on the individuals' emotions and psychology, Chau emphasizes that the gathering produces *honghuo* (red fire) or *renao* (hot noise), a 'sociothermic affect' that arises from sensorial stimulation in interpersonal interaction. The sensorial in such a gathering, where thousands if not tens of thousands of people converge, resides in an interpersonal space of human interaction, Chau (2008) then maintains. It cannot be reduced to sensorial experiences in individual bodies. By reducing it to the physiological measurements or psychometric questionnaires of individuals, the point is missed. Evaluation of the temple festival's efficacy would have to attend to the sensorial dimension which is produced in the interstices between the individuals.

'GENERATING SYNCHRONICITY' AS A BODY TECHNIQUE IN MEDICORELIGIOUS PRACTICES

Just like a temple festival's ritual efficacy, medical efficacy may depend on 'generating synchronicity' and heightened intensity in the interstices of human interaction. Paying attention to how medical treatment can generate synchronicity emphasizes its processual aspects. Importantly, traditional medical cultures have developed sophisticated body techniques that induce synchronicity, which health scientists generally overlook, but practitioners and patients explicitly say is crucial for effective treatment.

The elicitation of *deqi* (得氣 obtaining the qi) is purported to be an important indicator for the effectiveness of an acupuncture treatment (Lai & Tong 2010). It is usually reported by the patient as a constellation of different sensations, or as a tightness or tenseness around the needle by the acupuncturist. Yet despite this perceived importance there remains confusion over *deqi*'s nature, role and exclusivity to the acupoint needling site. First mentioned in the *Huang Di Nei Jing* on six occasions (twice in the *Suwen* and four times in the *Lingshu*), the term was used in a different context on each occasion (Togo 2010). One of the earliest published English research studies on *deqi* involved the identification of the types of sensory fiber in humans that conduct the sensation (Hou 1979). Another important early study found that, contrary to popular opinion, *deqi* was not reported more frequently at classic acupoint sites than at non-acupoint sites (Vincent et al 1989). Since those early studies there has been a steady output of research publications concerning the types of sensation experienced (Park et al 2002; MacPherson & Asghar 2006; Mao et al 2007), the measurement of the sensations (White 2008; Kong 2007), and more recently the fMRI have correlated and anticorrelated brain networks associated with its presence (Asghar et al 2010; Hui et al 2010). Despite the increasing understanding of *deqi* there remain many questions. Is the dose or strength of *deqi* expression an important consideration? What is more relevant, the report of *deqi* by the patient or the sensation perceived by the practitioner? Do different regions of the body produce different *deqi* sensations when needled? And what about some styles of acupuncture that do not attempt to obtain *deqi* yet report therapeutic clinical outcomes? Even after three decades of study, clinicians and researchers still have many questions about the role of *deqi*, its importance, and the necessity of obtaining *deqi* to bring about a therapeutic clinical effect.

According to many practitioners and patients in China, *deqi* (attaining the *qi*) in acupuncture needling is thought to be the crucial event that decides whether treatment is efficacious or not (see Chris Zaslawski's summary of discussions about *deqi* in Vignette 10.3). The moment of *deqi* is one where patient and practitioner both attend to the same event, namely the needling of the patient such that the patient can feel it. In the moment of *deqi*, a patient may shiver slightly from the unusual sensation that the needle produces, or catch their breath or even exclaim 'dele dele', 'I got it' (the *qi*). Simultaneously, the practitioner may grunt with satisfaction or sigh with relief. The skilled needle prick generates a socially constructed time period of synchronicity between patient and practitioner, where both attend to the same event and to each other with heightened intensity (Hsu 2005). Only if the therapist can induce this momentary synchronicity is the needle prick thought to be effective. Accordingly, the efficacy of acupuncture can be interpreted to be ritually induced and bodily felt. Notably, it is located in the interstices between practitioner and patient. Contrary to what the medical canons proclaim, its effects may not be very specific but may induce an unspecific sort of vitality in a very direct and unmediated way. Some Chinese medical practitioners trace *deqi* to the concept of

Treatment evaluation: an anthropologist's approach

qizhi, which in the Han dynasty referred to sexual climaxing (Lo 2001): an eminently life-engendering form of generating synchronicity.

Likewise, ethnographers might find that the violent purging and vomiting that characterizes the opening phase of the Ayurvedic *panchakarma* treatment in Sanskrit texts, which is still practiced in parts of India today (Zimmermann 1992), is a body technique that generates a sense of synchronicity between the participants. Practitioners of Ayurveda regard these violent therapeutic interventions as purificatory. The anthropologist may want to go a step further. Because they are violent, they may have the intrapsychic effect of preparing the patient for an imminent therapeutic transformation, as Csordas (1983) outlines as being typical of the phase of predisposition. Pain causes presence (Scarry 1985), and therefore it may be intentionally inflicted in the opening phase of the *panchakarma* treatment, not merely to purify but also to awaken the patient and prepare themselves for the imminent transformation that the treatment should cause.

It would be wrong to assume that synchronicity can only be generated through socially recognized acute forms of pain infliction that cause presence. Touching, for instance, also causes presence. As a practice that heightens interpersonal communication through generating synchronicity, it has been used in pulse diagnostics and, as Gretchen de Soriano shows, also in *kampo*'s abdominal diagnostics (see Vignette 10.4). Dance and music generate synchronicity. So does song, with its rhythm and melody. Speech is in many societies thought to be a sense. Like song, it has rhythm and the power to bring people together into synchronous action. Odors can bring to mind long-forgotten memories, as can the taste of foods and medicines, thereby synchronizing participants partaking in the sensory experiences they generate. The Chinese medical treatment disciplines, from massage and acupuncture to herbal medicine, involve many body techniques that generate synchronicity through the activation of the senses. Practitioners and patients are often explicit about their importance, and this knowledge, which tends to be orally transmitted, if not tacitly assumed, deserves to be identified and described in detail.

Victor Turner emphasizes symbolic action, its interpretation, and in his later writings its effects on the brain, in particular the left hemisphere (e.g. Turner 1986). He thereby redefines Emil Durkheim's 'collective effervescence' that was thought to affect the psyche of the individual. Research on 'generating synchronicity' builds on Durkheim's and Turner's research that locates questions of ritual efficacy in the performers' brain and psyche, but goes a step further and highlights that there are medicoreligious traditions that have developed particular strategies of treatment. These rely on sophisticated body techniques that effect a synchronizing of the participants present. Needless to say, they are crucial for their evaluation of a treatment's effectiveness.

FUTURE RESEARCH

Research on treatment evaluation which relates to the human being as a *homo ritualis* with a living, active, material, spatially positioned body–mind, undergoing rhythmically distinctive processes of transformation, needs more refined methodologies. These should combine, in a non-myopic way, quantitative findings with the qualitative research based on long-term participant

In spring 2010 M sought treatment to 'complement' his biomedical treatments for Lyme disease. He was diagnosed in 2000 when episodic fevers began; in 2006 he was told he had been reinfected. The year 2010 brought a new series of fevers, further antibiotics, and an increase in the nervous system symptoms attributed to an autoimmune response to the insect bite. Through discussions with his NHS consultant and his general practitioner, and through his individual research, M learned he might never recover from arthritic joint pain, numbness in the face, loss of taste, pins and needles in his thigh, and an inability to stay awake. This he could not accept. M found published research on a herbal formula used in Lyme's disease, and came in search of it.

In *kampo*, the practice of Japanese herbal medicine, the initial encounter involves asking about the current symptoms and observing the patient, using the senses as a tool. Much of this examination is described in basic texts on Chinese traditional medicine; the categories are looking, listening/smelling, asking and palpating. The tactile examination is traditionally done last and includes the pulse and the abdomen. It was the *kampo* abdominal examination that provided the most significant information and it is described here. The initial touch is light, using the open hand to assess the overall strength and elasticity of the abdominal wall. The muscles here were tense and thin, as though stretched to the limit. Light pressure revealed rapid increasing pulsations along the aortic artery, and a movement of gas and air with gurgling noises inside the abdominal cavity; the surface was cold with sweat. This was interpreted as a *kyo* pattern (a frailty, emptiness) in the nervous system. According to the abdominal examination, M was drained of vitality and losing the struggle against the pathogen. As a result of this I felt guided to touch his hands below the pulse: they were cold, the knuckles white and shiny, and when squeezed the cold seemed to come from the bones themselves and not the flesh above. This kind of cold is called *kan*. It is associated with sensory numbness; the *kan* itself is a pathogen, and this very much dominated his body. I had a good understanding of his condition and believed that treatment would be successful. M followed my assessment with interest; he listened as I explained that there seemed to be a discrepancy between the biomedical fever and the Chinese traditional medical diagnosis. He agreed to take a herbal formula for two weeks, although it was not the formula his research had uncovered.

On his second visit M reported having experienced another of the episodic fevers, this one briefer than previous ones and with no resulting blisters inside the mouth. His joints were not aching; he wanted to continue with the same formula. The abdominal examination during this visit found the same muscular structures and pulsations as before, again a *kyo* pattern. The gas and air inside the abdominal cavity, the sweating and the gurgling noises were gone, indicating both an absence of *kan* and digestive functions normalizing. The tongue coat had changed, and was thicker and drier; this was also a sign of *kan* not dominating the body. A formula for this pattern was prescribed. Although the formula was changed during this and subsequent visits, the biomedical name and diagnosis did not vary.

There are two key messages from this vignette. First, a thorough and cooperative evaluative session between the practitioner and patient is the key to selecting an effective formula. And second, that touch is essential in order to create some kind of link between patient and practitioner that is important for effective practice.

Treatment evaluation: an anthropologist's approach

observation of patients and practitioners in their life worlds. Above, two techniques of generating synchronicity between all participants partaking in a medical treatment have been outlined (*deqi* in acupuncture and the therapeutic violence in the opening phase of the *panchakarma* treatment). Future research, it is hoped, will identify and focus on other body techniques in religiomedical traditions (as are the East Asian ones) that the patients and practitioners themselves explicitly identify as crucial for evaluating a treatment's effectiveness. It will account for their sequencing in several distinctive stages of treatment and record the ways in which they elicit the experience of different bodily, sensorial, emotional, spiritual and cognitive states in the interstices between patient, practitioner, and the social and natural environment. Health researchers are encouraged to stop being fixated on a decontextualized thing, such as a pharmacologically active substance of a medicine that acts like a magic bullet on the passive body of *homo rationalis*. Rather, they may find it more useful to take as starting point *homo ritualis*, the living, active, material, ecologically and spatially positioned web of persons and bodies undergoing multiple rhythmically distinctive processes of transformation.

ACKNOWLEDGEMENT

These ideas were developed in the context of the ESRC-project: Generating synchronicity as a medico-religious technique: vitality and relatedness in Southwest China, RES 000-23-1408, held between 2006–2010.

REFERENCES

Adams, V., Li, F.F., 2008. Integration of erasure? Modernizing medicine at Lhasa's Mensikhang. In: Pordié, L. (Ed.), Tibetan Medicine in the Contemporary World: Global Politics of Medical Knowledge and Practice. Routledge, London, pp. 105–131.

Asghar, A.U., Green, G., Lythgoe, M.F., et al., 2010. Acupuncture needling sensation: the neural correlates of deqi using fMRI. Brain Res. 22 (1315), 111–118.

Banerjee, M., 2009. Power, Knowledge, Medicine: Ayurvedic Pharmaceuticals at Home and in the World. Orient Blackswan, Hyderabad.

Barry, C.A., 2006. The role of evidence in alternative medicine: contrasting biomedical and anthropological approaches. Soc. Sci. Med. 62, 2646–2657.

Biehl, J., Good, B., Kleinman, A., 2007. Introduction: rethinking subjectivity. In: Subjectivity: Ethnographic Investigations. University of California Press, Berkeley, pp. 1–23.

Bode, M., 2008. Taking Traditional Knowledge to the Market: The Modern Image of the Ayurvedic and Unani Industry, 1980–2000. Orient Longman, Hyderabad.

Chau, A., 2006. Miraculous Response: Doing Popular Religion in Contemporary China. Stanford University Press, Stanford.

Chau, A.Y., 2008. The sensorial production of the social. Ethnos 73 (4), 485–504.

Csordas, T.J., 1983. The rhetoric of transformation in ritual healing. Cult. Med. Psychiatry 7, 333–375.

Csordas, T.J. (Ed.), 1994. Embodiment and Experience: The Existential Ground of Culture and Self. Cambridge University Press, Cambridge.

Csordas, T.J., 2002. Body/Meaning/Healing. Palgrave Macmillan, New York.

Daston, L., Galison, P., 2007. Objectivity. Zone Books, New York.

Durkheim, E., (1915) 1965. The Elementary Forms of Religious Life. Free Press, New York.

Farquhar, J., Lock, M., 2007. Introduction. In: Lock, M., Farquhar, J. (Eds.), Beyond the Body Proper: Reading in the Anthropology of Material Life. Duke University Press, Durham, pp. 1–16.

Frankenberg, R., 1980. Medical anthropology and development: a theoretical perspective. Soc. Sci. Med. 14B, 197–207.

Hacking, I., 1991. Two souls in one body. Crit. Inq. 17 (4), 838–867.

Helman, C.G., 1990. Culture, Health and Illness, second ed. Butterworth Heineman, Oxford.

Hou, Z., 1979. A study on the histologic structure of acupuncture points and types of fibers conveying needling sensation. Chin. Med. J. 92 (4), 223–232.

Hsu, E., 1996. The polyglot practitioner: towards acceptance of different approaches in treatment evaluation. In: Gosvig Olesen, S., Hoeg, E. (Eds.), Communication In and About Alternative Therapies. Studies in Alternative Therapy, vol. 3. Odense University Press, Odense, pp. 37–53.

Hsu, E., 1999. The Transmission of Chinese Medicine. Cambridge University Press, Cambridge.

Hsu, E., 2005. Acute pain infliction as therapy. Etnofoor 18 (1), 78–96.

Hsu, E., 2009. Wonders of the exotic: Chinese formula medicines on the East African Coast. In: Larsen, K. (Ed.), Knowledge, Renewal and Religion: Repositioning and Changing Ideological and Material Circumstances Among the Swahili on the East African Coast. Nordiska Afrikainstitutet, Uppsala, pp. 280–299.

Hsu, E., 2010. Introduction: plants in medical practice and common sense. In: Hsu, E., Harris, S. (Eds.), plants, Health and Healing: On the Interface of Ethnobotany and Medical Anthropology. Berghahn, Oxford, pp. 1–48.

Huh, J., 1987. Eastern Medical Compendium (東醫寶鑑). Reprinted Edition. Originally published in 1613. Namsandang, Seoul.

Hui, K.K.S., Marina, O., Liu, J., et al., 2010. Acupuncture, the limbic system, and the anticorrelated networks of the brain. Auton. Neurosci. doi.10.1016/j.autneu.2010.03.022.

Hwang, D., 1997. The Combined Handbook of Formulars and Medicines (方藥合編). Reprinted and translated by Namsandang (Eds.). Originally published in 1887. Namsandang, Seoul.

Ingold, T., 2000. Perception of the Environment: Essays in Livelihood, Dwelling and Skill. Routledge, London.

James, W., 2003. The Ceremonial Animal: A New Portrait of Anthropology. Oxford University Press, Oxford.

Kapferer, B., 1983. A Celebration of Demons: Exorcism and the Aesthetics of Healing in Sri Lanka. Indiana University Press, Bloomington.

Kim, et al., 1991. The Textbook of Herbeology (本草學). Yeonglimsa, Seoul.

Kleinman, A., 1980. Patients and Healers in the Context of Culture: An Exploration of the Borderland Between Anthropology, Medicine, and Psychiatry. University of California Press, Berkeley.

Kong, J., Gollub, R., Huang, T., Polich, G., Napadow, V., Hui K., et al., 2007. Acupuncture de qi, from qualitative history to quantitative measurement. J. Altern. Complement. Med. 13 (10), 1059–1070.

Lai, T.X., Tong, Z., 2010. A study on the classification and the catching of the 'arrived qi' in acupuncture. J. Tradit. Chin. Med. 30 (1), 3–8.

Latour, B., Woolgar, S., 1986 (1979). Laboratory Life: The Construction of Scientific Facts, second ed. Princeton University Press, Princeton.

Latour, B., 2000. When things strike back: a possible contribution of 'science studies' to the social sciences. Br. J. Sociol. 51 (1), 107–123.

Lo, V., 2001. The influence of nurturing life culture on the development of Western Han Acumoxa therapy. In: Hsu, E. (Ed.), Innovation in Chinese Medicine. Cambridge University Press, Cambridge, pp. 19–50.

Lock, M., 1994. The politics of mid-life and menopause. In: Lindenbaum, S., Lock, M. (Eds.), Knowledge, Power and Practice: The Anthropology of Medicine and Everyday Life. University of California Press, Berkeley, pp. 330–363.

MacPherson, H., Asghar, A., 2006. Acupuncture needle sensation associated with deqi: a classification based on experts' ratings. J. Altern. Complement. Med. 12 (7), 633–637.

Mao, J.J., Farrar, J.T., Armstrong, K., et al., 2007. Deqi: Chinese acupuncture patients' experience and beliefs regarding acupuncture needling sensation: an exploratory study. Acupunct. Med. 25 (4), 158–165.

Treatment evaluation: an anthropologist's approach

Merleau-Ponty, M., 1962 (1945). Phenomenology of Perception. Routledge, London.

Moerman, D., 2002. Meaning, Medicine and the 'Placebo Effect'. Cambridge University Press, Cambridge.

Mosko, M., 2005. Introduction: a (Re)turn to chaos: chaos theory, the sciences, and social anthropological theory. In: Mosko, M., Damon, F.H. (Eds.), On the Order of Chaos: Social Anthropology and the Science of Chaos. Berghahn, Oxford, pp. 1–46.

Park, H.J., Park, J.B., Lee, H.S., et al., 2002. Does deqi (needle sensation) exist? Am. J. Chin. Med. 30 (1), 45–50.

Scarry, E., 1985. The Body in Pain. The Making and Unmaking of the World. Oxford University Press, Oxford.

Shin, et al., 2005. Eastern Medical Compendium at a Glance (Korean). Deulnyok, Seoul.

Sullivan, M.D., 1993. Placebo Controls and Epistemic Control in Orthodox Medicine. J. Med. Philos. 18, 213–231.

Togo, T., 2010. Historical background of deqi. Presented at the 10th International Congress of Oriental Medicine, Chiba, Japan.

Turner, V., 1967. The Forest of Symbols: Aspects of Ndembu Ritual. Cornell University Press, Ithaka.

Turner, V., 1986. Body, brain, culture. Performing Arts Journal 10 (2), 26–34.

Van Gennep, A., 1909. Le rites de passage. Nourry, Paris.

Vincent, C.A., Richardson, P.H., Black, J.J., et al., 1989. The significance of needle placement site in acupuncture. J. Psychosom. Res. 33 (4), 489–496.

Waldram, J.B., 2000. The efficacy of traditional medicine: current theoretical and methodological issues. Med. Anthropol. Q. 14 (4), 603–625.

White, P., Bishop, F., Hardy, H., et al., 2008. Southampton needle sensation questionnaire: development and validation of a measure to gauge acupuncture needle sensation. J. Altern. Complement. Med. 14 (4), 373–379.

Whyte, S., van der Geest, S., Hardon, A., 2003. The Social Lives of Medicines. Cambridge University Press, Cambridge.

Young, A., 1982. The anthropologies of illness and sickness. Annu. Rev. Anthropol. 11, 257–285.

Zhan, M., 2009. A doctor of the highest caliber treats an illness before it happens. Med. Anthropol. 28 (2), 166–188.

Zimmermann, F., 1992. Gentle purge: flower power of ayurveda. In: Leslie, C., Young, A. (Eds.), Paths to Asian Medical Knowledge. University of California Press, Berkeley, pp. 209–223.

Endangered practices: challenging the discourse of healthcare integration

Paul Kadetz

INTRODUCTION

The policy discourse on the integration of heterodox or non-biomedical healthcare practices and practitioners into contemporary biomedically domi-nated healthcare systems (henceforth 'healthcare integration') is replete with assumptions. These assumptions primarily concern the beneficent outcomes of this integration in terms of improvements to healthcare access, safety and efficacy, as well as the overall health of the population. Although this dis-course can be located historically in both colonial and missionary healthcare interventions, the modern movement to promote healthcare integration has been most visibly led at the global level by the World Health Organization (WHO).

The WHO has promoted healthcare integration as a means to achieve 'health for all' since its formal introduction in the 1978 Declaration of Alma Ata (WHO 1978a). Although this goal has not been achieved, healthcare inte-gration has remained a primary focus of the WHO's Traditional Medicine Unit in Geneva and in its regional divisions. The Western Pacific Region Office of the WHO has been especially committed to healthcare integration. The Philippines, a member state of the Western Pacific Region, approved the legislation of a national adaptation of the WHO's policy for healthcare integra-tion via the Traditional and Alternative Medicine Act in 1997 (PITAHC 2009). By virtue of this law, a corporation affiliated with the Department of Health of the Philippines, the Philippine Institute for Traditional and Alternative Healthcare, was established to help promote and integrate traditional medi-cine in the Philippines (Mendoza 2009).

As a result of its varied geography, marked economic disparity, decen-tralized healthcare system and cultural diversity, the Philippines provides a unique context for understanding the impact and challenges of health-care integration. Furthermore, the literature on healthcare integration has focused predominantly on the integration and globalization of established het-erodox healthcare systems, such as traditional Chinese medicine, Ayurveda and Tibetan medicine. The unique and mostly local heterodox healthcare practices of the Philippines offer a contrast to these established and more stan-dardized healthcare systems and thus can challenge the normative integra-tion discourse supported by them.

Considering the extensive research and funding appropriated to study het-erodox healthcare practices for purposes of integration, it is curious that no research to date has assessed the actual effects of implementing healthcare integration on local populations and local healthcare systems.[1] With an estimated 80% of populations in low-income countries using heterodox healthcare practices, such assessments are clearly warranted (Bodeker & Burford 2007). This chapter will therefore examine the intended and unintended outcomes of healthcare integration, as well as assess the assumptions of beneficence embedded in the healthcare integration discourse. An analysis of the concepts of 'traditional medicine', 'integration' and 'standardization' will serve as a basis for this discussion. This analysis will be further supported with a presentation of the author's own research assessing healthcare integration at the local level in communities of the Philippines, where the practitioners of heterodox healthcare include albularyos who treat with local herbs, hilots who perform 'spiritually guided' massage and bone-setting, and traditional birth attendants.

'TRADITIONAL MEDICINE'

A HISTORICALLY INCONSISTENT TERM

The concept of 'traditional medicine' is central to the discourse of healthcare integration. The term has been used in WHO documents and the general literature to refer to healthcare practices that are specific to a particular geographic location and indigenous group; healthcare practices that are specific to particular ethnic groups, regardless of geographic location; and/or all non-biomedical healthcare practices, regardless of geographic, temporal or cultural origin. These different understandings have often appeared simultaneously in any given WHO document (WHO 2002a, 2002b).

Traditional medicine is often poorly distinguished from complementary and alternative medicine, which is widely identified as standardized heterodox practices that have been exported to other countries, regardless of their country of origin (e.g. acupuncture, Ayurveda and reflexology). However, conflicting understandings of complementary and alternative medicine have appeared in both WHO documents and the general literature (WHO 2002a, 2003, 2009).

The Traditional and Alternative Medicine Act of the Philippines clearly distinguishes between traditional medicine (i.e. those healthcare practices local to the Philippines) and alternative healthcare modalities (i.e. imported heterodox healthcare practices). Yet, in printed literature and communications from the Philippine Institute for Traditional and Alternative Healthcare, the two categories are merged. This has resulted in acupuncture, acupressure and chiropractic now being typically identified as constituting traditional medicine or 'Trad Med' (PITAHC 2009). This particular use of the term traditional medicine can present challenges concerning whether imported or local traditional medicines are subsequently standardized and integrated. Therefore, in this chapter, the term 'heterodox' will be used as an alternative to 'traditional.'

---

[1] The term local healthcare, as used in this chapter, comprises both a formal healthcare system (usually a predominantely biomedical system that is administered and regulated at the national, regional and/or local levels and is part of the formal economy) and an informal healthcare system (usually comprised of local heterodox practitioners who are often unregulated by the state, act independently, contribute to the informal economy, and are employed by individuals independent of the formal healthcare system).

'TRADITIONAL' AS A REPRESENTATION OF INVENTED TRADITIONS

Hobsbawm & Ranger (1983) proposed that traditions are often invented for the functional ends of social cohesion and the legitimizing of social action and institutions in the creation of modern nation states. 'Invented tradition' is defined as 'a set of practices of a ritual or symbolic nature, which seeks to inculcate certain values and norms of behaviour which automatically implies continuity with the past' (1983, 1). Hence, invented traditions can serve as a means by which to justify desired social changes by linking them to a (real or invented) past, thereby granting them validity, honor and automatic obligatory veneration. Tradition can also be an invented conception of the traditional 'other.' In relation to non-European culture, this may be understood as a Western invention of a romanticized, mysticized and orientalized parallel world that can then be compared to modern European beliefs. The attached evaluations maintain ethnocentric standards of Western intellectual and scientific superiority along with continued justification for modernization of, and paternalism toward, lower-income and non-European countries (Said 1978). In terms of traditional medicine, these purported links with the past can imply that healthcare practices are the same as are indigenous to a given locale, and that they have somehow never changed since first used.

Therefore, if what is labeled traditional medicine is actually an invented tradition, and if medical systems are normatively represented as a pluralism of traditional medicines and biomedicine, then this representation of medical pluralism must also be questioned.

BEYOND MEDICAL PLURALISM: UNBINDING THE CONCEPTUALLY BOUND

In the literature, medical pluralism characterizes healthcare as a grouping of multiple, discrete, bounded heterodox health practices with biomedicine (Hsu 2008). Thereby, all components of a healthcare system are depicted as equal, automatically thwarting any inquiry into power relationships (Baer 2004). Furthermore, unstructured combinations of healthcare practices that are dynamic and altered according to cultural, environmental and social (particularly political and economic) pressures are similarly unaccounted for in this conceptualization. For example, Adams (2008, 2003) demonstrates how the integration of heterodox health practices in Tibet can result in pressures for economic competition of Tibetan medicine with biomedicine, as these practices enter into the formal economy.

To be bounded, a practice must by definition be separate from others and maintain structural integrity when transmitted. However, if, as observed in the Philippines, practitioners often receive their training primarily through dreams and visions, and do not practice what a given practitioner category designates, but rather arbitrarily engage in practices reserved for other practitioner categories or simply create their own version of a practice, then the conception of bounded healthcare systems is seriously challenged.

Yet this issue is not only true of unbounded healthcare practices, but can be identified in seemingly bounded systems as well. Farquhar (1994) and Scheid

(2002) demonstrate that the apparent boundedness of traditional Chinese medicine (TCM) disintegrates when the plurality of individual practitioners is considered. Similarly, the circuitous logic that being a bioscience renders biomedicine beyond the influence of social construction, is based upon the false proposition that science is not socially constructed. Hence, the same argument has been made with respect to the cultural and individual interpretations – or 'art' of biomedicine, which more accurately would be labeled biomedicines, challenging the conception of a global uniformly interpreted practice (Berg & Mol 1998). Therefore, the concept of medical pluralism may not be appropriate for depicting *any* healthcare system, regardless of the presumed boundedness of the practices found therein.

West and Luedke (2006) attempt to remedy these shortcomings of medical pluralism with a model of medical landscapes. This model facilitates both the influence of social processes on local healthcare, as well as movement across purported epistemological and practice boundaries. But even medical landscapes may be too bounded in its representation of practices. Although it facilitates a reflexivity in perception of local healthcare, it simultaneously suggests mutually regulating, albeit separate, practices.

A far more fluid conceptualization of local healthcare is therefore needed. The term 'healthcare currents' may provide a more representative metaphor for the actual formal and informal healthcare used and created by local populations. This metaphor can be depicted as countless tributaries of local and national, formal and informal healthcare practices all flowing into four separate, but frequently intersecting, rivers of unequal sizes. These four rivers represent the use of local heterodox practices, imported heterodox practices, local biomedicine and global biomedicine that all empty into a local sea filled with the overall formal and informal local healthcare system. Thereby, a dynamic current of local healthcare is perpetually recreated. For these reasons, it is problematic to employ the concept of 'traditional medicine', which will merely render all local heterodox healthcare practices an undifferentiated swamp.

THAT SWAMP CALLED 'TRAD MED':

The problem with the concept of 'traditional medicine' in the Philippine context

Structure and power are embedded in concepts that become normative. Conceptually, biomedicine established a hegemonic status with regard to other healthcare practices by segregating itself from all that was not biomedicine. This process can be identified in the resulting labels of traditional, indigenous, complementary and alternative – all defined by what they are not, namely biomedical or bioscientific. Not surprisingly, then, 'integrative medicine' frequently becomes a strategy for legitimizing unscientific healthcare practices through the establishment of their biomedical evidence base.

The question then arises, for whom is this process of legitimization? In research conducted by this author in the Philippines (see Vignette 11.1), 95% of community informants reported no concern with scientific proof of safety

A mixed methods study of qualitative and quantitative data collection was conducted over a period of 16 months to determine the effects of, and test the assumptions of, healthcare integration on local healthcare systems in the Philippines.[i] Communities of two municipalities that implemented healthcare integration policy top-down (via physicians and nurses practicing acupuncture through the Municipal Health Office) in Bagabag[ii] versus bottom-up (via volunteer community health workers trained in the use of local herbs) in Murcia were assessed.[iii] These were contrasted with communities of two socioeconomically similar municipalities that did not implement integration (Bontoc and Siquijor).

Improvements to physical and financial access to healthcare were not demonstrated during the period before and after integration (2005–2010). In fact, top-down integration demonstrated the least improvement in distance to one's primary practitioner. The cost of a primary care visit either remained the same or was markedly increased with integration. For example, some traditional birth attendants that previously accepted donations requested payment after receiving training. Nor does integration appear to foster the use of local heterodox practices. Any increase in the use of local heterodox practitioners was predominantly correlated with financial necessity.

According to Birn (2005), to whom practitioners refer their patients can indicate the extent of integration. Heterodox practitioners demonstrated a consistently high level of patient referrals to biomedical practitioners, irrespective of healthcare integration. However, patient referral from physicians to heterodox practitioners appears to be more a function of community accessibility to biomedicine than of integration, as a majority of biomedical practitioners were opposed to healthcare integration.

The one criterion that demonstrated a significant difference between integrated and non-integrated communities was the number of heterodox practitioners who reported they would participate in standardized training: significantly higher in integrated Murcia (90%) and Bagabag (80%) than in Bontoc (50%) and Siquijor (44%). Hence, integration may be correlated with a willingness for standardized training among heterodox practitioners where integration has already occurred.[iv]

Although marked differences between top-down and bottom-up integration are not illustrated along the criteria assessed, important differences were identified in interviews and participant observation, especially in terms of individual healthcare choice, control and self-determination. Top-down healthcare integration, as implemented in Bagabag, was reported to *not* engender plurality of healthcare choice, but maintained a locus of control with the physician. No local heterodox practitioners are being integrated in these communities. Furthermore, local heterodox practitioners in Bagabag reported a reduction in their patients from 2005 to 2010, as well as a feeling of deliberately being marginalized via this process. Whereas bottom-up healthcare integration, as implemented in Murcia, sought to encourage plurality and self-determination in both awareness of choice of available practices and in terms of self-managed healthcare options. This was particularly evident in the community health workers' focus on the use of herbs available in one's backyard.[v]

i Semi-structured interviews were employed individually and in focus groups of convenience and snowball samples (N = 500) of community residents, heterodox practitioners, biomedical practitioners, council members, and key policy actors. Since healthcare integration in the two municipalities assessed occurred from 2006, questions were asked regarding changes that may have occurred for informants from before the time integration started (or 2005) to 2010 in order to determine if any changes occurred during this five-year period that could be correlated with integration.

ii Bagabag (in the Province of Neuva Vizcaya) has been implementing the policy of integration top-down via Trad Med trainings and practice (mainly acupuncture and tui-na) through the regional Department of Health hospital, Veteran's Regional Hospital, and through the municipal health office.

iii Murcia (in the province of Negros Occidental) conducted bottom-up implementation of the imported heterodox healthcare practices of acupressure and tui-na, the local heterodox healthcare practice of herbal use, and the biomedical practice of sanitary and hygienic education via the trainings (by physicians of the NGO, *INAM*) of lay volunteer community health workers working in their own communities at approximately the same time (three years ago) that Bagabag instituted top-down integration

iv However, it should be clarified that compliance with attendance at standardized training is not to be confused with a willingness to replace one's heterodox practice with standardized practices. In fact, no traditional healer interviewed would agree to replace what they traditionally practiced with the standardized training they might learn.

v However, this is not to suggest that top-down integration is always about control and bottom-up integration always generates autonomy. Walt (1994) notes that decentralization to the local level may merely mean that power is now in the hands of local landowners and the local power elite. This is particularly germane in the decentralized Philippine context, where landowners generally comprise the elite and control politics and healthcare decisions at even the lowest of administrative levels (Bello 2009).

or efficacy for their local heterodox healthcare practices.[2] Furthermore, what are being labeled 'Trad Med' by the Philippine Institute for Traditional and Alternative Healthcare, are predominantly imported heterodox practices, such as acupuncture, that have already earned a modicum of approval via biomedical legitimization. However, no national plans exist for legitimizing, and thereby designating as Trad Med, the majority of heterodox practices local to the Philippines beyond the use of a few local herbs.

In blurring the distinction between local and imported healthcare practices, the term Trad Med challenges an accurate understanding of what is actually being integrated, and can thereby potentially affect community accessibility to both formal and informal heterodox healthcare practices. Furthermore, as a result of the overtly vague and unspecific language of the WHO integration guidelines, who and what are integrated can be a highly political process often left entirely to the discretion of local authorities and key stakeholders (Pillsbury 1982). Accordingly, if the concept of traditional medicine is the primary component of integration, and if traditional medicines are generally

[2] Safety and efficacy, though a primary concern identified in almost every WHO healthcare integration document, was a concept that was so foreign to community members queried, that many did not understand the concept. The predominant sentiment was that unless a local practitioner gives one reason for concern, there is no conception of risk with local practices. Hence, safety and efficacy may be culturally relative concepts that cannot be assumed to be universally interpreted in the same manner, but may change from one local context to another.

invented traditions, then the concept of integration – built on the premise of traditional medicines as bounded separate medical systems – may be similarly ill-conceived.

INTEGRATION

DEFINING INTEGRATION AS AN HISTORICAL AND POLITICAL PROCESS

Integration is a broad category in the literature that generally describes the extent of a nation's acceptance of non-biomedical practices and practitioners into the formal (predominantly biomedical) healthcare system. However, Hyma and Ramesh (1994, 66) identify that 'The WHO's review of national experiences in the 1980s indicates that there is no single universally accepted concept of integration.' In order to understand the process of healthcare integration, it is therefore necessary to examine the historical development of this concept.

It is significant that the WHO chose to base their model of healthcare integration on Mao Zedong's call to unify TCM and biomedicine from the 1950s to the 1970s. However, this choice appears to have been based upon several misinterpretations of historical events.

TCM IS NOT CHINESE MEDICINE: A BASIC MISUNDERSTANDING IN THE WHO MODEL OF INTEGRATION

On closer analysis it becomes apparent that the WHO's concept of integration was based on a historically misinterpreted model of integration, exemplified by such statements from the WHO as: 'The decision to combine Chinese medicine and modern Western medicine at all levels of health services in medical research has led to the evolution of a new form of "integrated medicine" which seeks to apply the best of both systems, and to offset the weakness of each. In this way, the two systems are being gradually fused together' (Bannerman et al 1983, 34). This statement confused Chinese medicine, i.e. the numerous currents of local healthcare practiced in China prior to the formation of TCM from the mid-1950s, with the nationalized traditional Chinese medicine; thereby implying that TCM was a completely separate system from biomedicine.

In this chapter, traditional Chinese medicine is to be understood as an 'invented tradition', which is already an integrated system. During Mao Zedong's administration from the mid-1950s to the mid-1970s, biomedical physicians who graduated from short Chinese medicine training programmes, Chinese medicine practitioners, Chinese Communist Party leaders such as Zhou Enlai, and Ministry of Health bureaucrats were chosen to study and assemble the parts of the local healthcare practices of China that they deemed relevant to biomedicine, and standardize that which was not formally standardized along a biomedical model through a lens of Marxist dialectical materialism and disseminated in the manner of Western medical schools, textbooks, research centres and hospitals (Taylor 2005). The remainder of the traditional medicine of China, which did not correlate with a biomedical understanding, such as spiritual elements, was discarded (Lucas 1982). However, this markedly simplifies what was 'an undetermined and piecemeal process' over many years (Taylor 2005, 151).

CHAIRMAN MAO AND THE ROCKEFELLER FOUNDATION

The structure of the healthcare system through which Mao and the Chinese Communist Party operated was developed and implemented in the 1920s by the League of Nations Health Organization and supported privately by the Rockefeller Foundation (Loughlin & Berridge 2002). The Rockefeller Foundation also funded the Peking Union Medical College, the International Health Board and the China Medical Board, all of which were extremely influential in building the modern Chinese healthcare system from the 1920s through the 1940s. According to Johnson (2008), it is difficult to separate Chinese government health policy from the policy of the Rockefeller Foundation and its China Medical Board, which funded healthcare programmes in China from 1913 to 1949. As a result, there was little dispute in China that the Ministry of Health, established after the foundation of the People's Republic of China in 1949, was to function entirely on the basis of biomedicine (Taylor 2005, 6). Lucas (1982, 1) also maintains that the various political upheavals from the 1949 revolution to the Cultural Revolution did not alter the basic policies of national medicine first diffused to China in the late 1920s through the League of Nations Health Organization. Hence, when Mao Zedong chose biomedical physicians – trained predominantly in American and European biomedical schools (Lucas 1982) – to lead the integration of the various local systems of Chinese medicine into TCM, it is questionable whether he was acting completely autonomously and was not, to some degree, influenced by the healthcare paradigm established by the China Medical Board, the International Health Board, the League of Nations Health Organization, the standardization of US medical school education, and ultimately the Rockefeller Foundation.

In the mid-1960s, Mao began a program to train community health workers, or 'barefoot doctors', in a combination of TCM and biomedicine to serve as a first line of healthcare in the rural areas of China (Lucas 1982). After China joined the World Health Organization in 1973, their purported success with both the barefoot doctors program and the integration between TCM and biomedicine in the formal healthcare system was adopted by the WHO as *the* model by which to address health disparity in many developing countries (Sindiqi 1995). At the urging of Russian WHO delegates, and possibly influenced by the Chinese nationals in positions of power at the WHO at the time, China's model of healthcare integration became an integral component of the Declaration of Alma Ata (Sindiqi 1995). Thereby, the erratic and sometimes violent political process that resulted in the invention of TCM and the formation of the plural Chinese healthcare system has remained the primary model for healthcare integration as advocated by the WHO.

The relevance of the WHO using TCM as a model for healthcare integration, albeit not acknowledging that TCM was already an integrated system, is that it (a) falsely projects that any heterodox practice can be integrated, while disregarding that few may be as systematized and standardized as TCM;

(b) may thereby be facilitating the integration of only those heterodox practices that have been systematized, standardized and legitimated by biomedicine; and (c) makes it appear as if integration can be achieved by any nation at any point in time, regardless of political and socioeconomic contexts, as comprehensively as the People's Republic of China (PRC) *appeared* to do. This last point is particularly problematic.

HOW TCM WAS WON: A MODEL FOR FORCED HEALTHCARE INTEGRATION

Basing all healthcare integration on the integration of TCM and biomedicine in Maoist China poses important challenges when applied to other countries, or even to China today. First, it is imperative to acknowledge that healthcare functions within a given political economy. The formation of TCM and the barefoot doctors' program were conceived and implemented within an egalitarian–authoritarian economic and social system, which may not be transferable into liberal–democratic or other economic and social systems (Walt 1994).

Second, although Mao believed that the integration of Chinese medicine could provide an opportunity to redress rural health inequities with the practitioner resources already available, he had to overcome opposition from biomedical physicians, the Ministry of Health, and the modernization movement of the early Chinese Communist Party; who originally sought to extinguish Chinese medicine (Lucas 1982). Therefore, since healthcare integration in China could not be achieved by complete consensus, force and coercion were employed (Rosenthal 1981). This was accomplished on several fronts: (1) Mao's rhetoric of Chinese medicine as a 'national treasure' to serve alongside biomedicine, was influential amongst the populace, but was more the result of a nationalist movement that included a revival in many of the arts of China, than of any consideration for its therapeutic value (Taylor 2005). (2) Physicians were forced to engage in TCM studies. Those who resisted integration were labeled bourgeois, criticized, and/or exiled to distant areas (Taylor 2005). (3) At the onset of the Cultural Revolution, the Ministry of Health was blamed for ignoring rural health and the Chinese Communist Party took over complete administration of healthcare in order to facilitate integration, insisting that practitioners of Chinese medicine be placed in biomedical hospitals and clinics (Rosenthal 1981; Birn 2005). However, this centralization, which was necessary for full integration in China, would be challenged in a decentralized healthcare system such as the Philippines.' (4) During the Cultural Revolution, the same social pressures that had previously been directed toward biomedical physicians were now directed with even greater ferocity towards those Chinese medicine practitioners who sought to maintain autonomy and ideological separation from biomedicine. Classic medical texts were burned, Chinese medicine schools were closed, and classic Chinese medicine practitioners were the object of ridicule or physical attack and their practices and pharmacies destroyed (Scheid 2002).

Third, although presented as a complete process, integration was merely intended as an early stage of Mao's original goal of complete unification of TCM and biomedicine in order to form a unique new medical system. According to Taylor (2005), Mao believed that Chinese medicine – the reputation of which had been in decline since the early 19th century – had to be 'raised' to a certain scientific level before it could be unified with bio-medicine. However, owing to the extensive opposition from both party and practitioners, among other factors, integration and the formation of TCM became part of Mao's unfinished project.

Finally, it is questionable whether the outcome of Mao's attempt at integra-tion even qualifies as full healthcare integration. For actual practice may be the most significant indicator of full integration. As Croizier (1975, 30) notes, 'In the decade from 1955 to 1965 it was clear that, although integration of Chinese and Western medicine was the official policy, in practice, the administration of med-ical policy still gave [Chinese medicine] a secondary position.' Furthermore, the extent to which heterodox practices are integrated in the minds of the public may reveal the most about the actual extent of integration. In modern China, TCM has been employed primarily according to perceived best interventions for particular ailments (Scheid 2002). Hence, Rosenthal suggests, Mao's attempt at integration may be more accurately classified as a *selective* form of integra-tion, as was demonstrated in the selective development of TCM, for institutional arrangements left the biomedical physicians 'utilizing combined treatment extensively, but on their own terms' (Rosenthal 1981, 610).

Clearly, as illustrated here, the policy and process of healthcare integra-tion is not shaped solely by a biomedical agenda, but is very much a prod-uct of specific political, economic, philosophical and cultural forces that may not be replicable from one context to another. For example, the success of Cuba's formal healthcare integration programme of the 1990s may be attrib-utable not only to a specific climate created out of economic necessity (due to the US embargoes, particularly of biomedical supplies), but also to an egalitarian–authoritarian economic and social system that was sufficiently similar to China's in the 1950s (Kadetz & Perdomo 2010).

According to Birn (2005, 7), 'In many developing countries that subse-quently tried implementing primary healthcare loosely based on the Chinese model, there was never enough commitment from the political system, and it ended up being a semi-autonomous system outside of the regular medical hierarchy, underfunded and with low status.'

The unique circumstances of China's healthcare integration under Mao is made even more obvious when contemplating the possibility of its transfer to the China of today, where subsequent healthcare reforms have resulted in reduced accessibility to both biomedicine and TCM, especially in rural areas (Liu et al 1999). Hence, it is doubtful whether TCM would even have emerged in China's current political and economic climate (Birn 2005). This context specificity of healthcare integration is likewise required for any model that attempts to define the extent of healthcare integration in any country.

A PROBLEMATIC CLASSIFICATORY SYSTEM OF INTEGRATION

Several overlapping classificatory systems have been proposed that struc-ture the extent of healthcare integration in any country into between four and seven categories, representing a nation's acceptance or rejection of local heterodox healthcare practices and practitioners into the formal healthcare system (Singer & Baer 2007; Bodeker 1994; Hyma & Ramesh 1994; Young 1994; Pillsbury 1982; Green 1980). Thus, at one end of this continuum is complete official sanction and total incorporation of non-biomedical healthcare practices and practitioners into a nation's healthcare system. This is most often classified as *integration* and has been identified in the healthcare systems of Cuba and China (Bodeker et al 2005). At the other end of this continuum is complete prohibition of all non-biomedical practices via restrictive legislation. Such suppression was prevalent in many colonial healthcare systems, with Zaire serving as a well-documented example (Dauskardt 1990). In between these extremes are gradations of acceptability of local non-biomedical practices considered worthy by regulators, and leading to an informal coexistence with biomedicine known as *parallelism* (Bodeker 1994; 2001; Leslie 1992). This has been identified in Ayurveda's coexistence with biomedicine in India as well as in the recent regulation of practitioners of Chinese medicine in Australia (see Jon Wardle's discussion in Vignette 11.2).

This unidimensional classificatory system of healthcare integration depicts heterodox healthcare practices as a uniform, undifferentiated, aggregate national-level category. Hence, such a model cannot distinguish the degree to which all of the possible heterodox practices and practitioners of any country may be individually integrated. In a country such as the Philippines, where some heterodox practices are actively integrated whereas others are ignored, such a general model is bound to misrepresent the extent of integration of all practices and practitioners.

VIGNETTE 11.2   REGULATION OF CHINESE MEDICINE PRACTITIONERS IN AUSTRALIA
JON WARDLE

The practice of Chinese medicine has a longer history in Australia than in many other Western countries. The arrival of Chinese immigrants during the Victorian gold rushes helped establish the medical system, extending beyond the immigrant community by 1911; Chinese herbal formulations were readily available, with English labels and directions. By 1925 Chinese herbalists were organized enough to defeat the introduction of the *Pharmaceutical Chemists Act*, which would have restricted the dispensing of Chinese herbal medicines to pharmacists (Loh 1985). At the height of herbal medicine in Victoria in 1925, over one-fifth of all herbalists were Asian (Martyr 2002). This base was expanded, as in many other countries, by the renewed interest in alternative forms of medicine from the 1960s, with the proliferation of Chinese medicine colleges from this time (Baer 2007). In the 1990s Chinese medicine use had become significant enough – with over 2.8 million consultations annually – for the Victorian, Queensland and New South Wales governments to explore regulatory options (Bensoussan & Myers 1996). In 2005 Australian use had increased to over 12.3 million consultations with acupuncturists or Chinese herbalists (Xue et al 2007). The Victorian government followed the recommendations of the 1996 report by implementing the *Chinese Medicine Registration Act* 2000, the only state to do so.

Regulation of health practitioners in Australia is based on the *Australian Health Minister's Advisory Council Criteria*, and is focused primarily on potential risk to the public. Although potential benefits of regulation to a profession are acknowledged, they are generally not taken into consideration under these criteria. Legislation surrounding regulation makes it explicitly clear that the intention is to protect the public rather than promote the interests of the profession, and offers several protections against 'aspiring' professions that aim to use regulation as a professional development tool. Regulation of Chinese medicine practitioners has proved a worthwhile move for patients. Complaints against practitioners rose fivefold once a centralized reporting mechanism had been enacted, and the legislative power to act on these complaints enabled them to be corrected (Lin et al 2005). Advertising violations, record keeping, professional ethics issues (such as fraud or restricted title use) and treatment issues (dangerous practices or financial exploitation) have been the major areas of complaints (Lin & Gillick 2006), though there have also been enforceable protections in other areas – such as the inappropriate or unsustainable use of endangered herbs.

Currently a transition is taking place from state-based regulation of health practitioners to the centralized *National Registration and Accreditation Scheme*. This has delayed the expansion of Chinese medical practitioner regulation. However, from 2012 Chinese medicine will be part of this national process, which aims to reduce the regulatory costs to government by standardizing and sharing regulatory infrastructure amongst all health professions' Boards, while retaining individual Board autonomy to develop accreditation, registration and practice standards for their respective professions. Implementation of regulation has not been without problems: heterogeneity in qualifications – particularly unrecognized foreign qualifications – meant that grandparenting existing practitioners was difficult, with 10% of initial applications being refused – though these were primarily for 'character' reasons (Lin & Gillick 2006). The increased standards of education have also resulted in a significant consolidation of education providers. There has been a shift to the university sector, which has been associated with access to a broader range of opportunities and resources to promote the profession and integrate further within the broader health sector. This integration has been driven largely by Chinese medicine practitioners and, in turn, has supported development of academic and research capacity in the field. Regulation has also had clear benefits for the practice of Chinese medicine in Australia. Fears of loss of professional autonomy have been largely unfounded: the inclusion of minimum levels of clinical experience and traditional philosophy in the Chinese Medicine Registration Board of Victoria course accreditation guidelines has in fact saved Chinese medicine from the loss of control of input in practitioner education experienced by Australia's largest unregulated health profession, naturopathy (Lin et al 2005). The assurance of minimum standards among practitioners has also led to the return of previously restricted therapeutic tools, with the Victorian health minister announcing in 2010 that the Chinese herbal medicines *ban bian lian*, *zhi fu zhi* and *ma huang* would be inserted into Schedule 1 of the Poisons List, making them available for prescription for qualified Chinese medicine practitioners, a first for a Western nation.

POOR THEORETICAL MODELS DON'T EASILY DIE: THE WHO ADAPTATION OF THIS CLASSIFICATORY SYSTEM

The WHO Western Pacific Region Office's *Regional Strategy for Traditional Medicine in the Western Pacific 2002–2010* encourages member states to use a particular adaptation of this classificatory model to assess their country's integration: 'Countries are encouraged to conduct assessments to identify how far TM/CAM has been recognized and integrated into mainstream health services. The extent of the integration of TM/CAM can be graded according to a typology of: Integrated, Supported, Recognized, Neglected' (WHO 2002a, 11).

As this is essentially the same classificatory scheme as previously presented, the same shortcomings are illustrated in the WHO-WPRO typology. Particularly problematic is the dependence on one designation to apply to all of the heterodox practices in a given country. Using this typology to determine the extent of healthcare integration in the Philippines, *Supported* would best describe the classification of certain imported heterodox practices (specifically acupuncture). The only local healthcare practice that could be designated as *Integrated* are ten indigenous herbs approved and regulated by the Bureau of Food and Drugs. However, almost all local Filipino heterodox practices, such as hilot-bonesetting, hilot-massage, and albularyos, would be best classified as *Neglected*, given that they have neither been included nor acknowledged in any healthcare integration planning.[3] Therefore, simply by virtue of using this model, practices that are unaccounted for will be rendered invisible and thereby further *Neglected*.

Furthermore, this classificatory system presumes that a national healthcare integration policy is somehow uniformly implemented across all levels of a nation or, alternatively, that one local level assessment can be generalized to the entire nation. This is pertinent to a context such as the Philippines, a diverse archipelago of 7107 islands, in which only a few municipalities have implemented healthcare integration. Hence, a far more nuanced classificatory system is needed in order to generate a more accurate understanding of the extent of all heterodox practice and practitioner integration.

INTEGRATION AS A DISCOURSE OF ASSUMED BENEFICENCE

As previously stated, there is a marked assumption in the literature on healthcare integration that this process is inherently beneficent to a population's health and to a healthcare system in general (WHO 1978a,b, 1984, 2002a,b, 2003). It is also assumed that healthcare integration will promote the use of local heterodox healthcare practices (Republic of the Philippines 1997). Yet, if a practice is not included in the agenda for integration, it may be restricted by a newly regulated medical pluralism, that

---

[3] Few heterodox practices are regulated by The Department of Health of the Philippines (specifically massage and traditional birth attendants) or the Bureau of Food and Drugs of the Philippines (i.e. herbal regulation). Though the Philippine Institute for Traditional and Alternative Healthcare (PITAHC) is planning to certify acupuncture, acupuncture is already being offered at several hospitals on an outpatient basis.

is, if it becomes officially recognized at all. Vignette 11.1 critically evaluates several of these assumptions in the context of an empirical research study situated in the Philippines.

STANDARDIZATION: THE HEART OF INTEGRATION

CONTEXTUALIZING MEDICAL STANDARDIZATION

The issues identified in the way in which the concepts of traditional medicine and integration have been employed, highlight the inherent problems in the normative concept of standardization. The modern standardization of healthcare can be traced to the early standardization of biomedicine. The Carnegie Foundation commissioned Abraham Flexner to assess the curriculum of American medical schools at the turn of the 20th century (Hewa 2002). By 1910, Flexner had provided a report complete with recommendations for the need to standardize medical schools and a curriculum by which this could be realized. The Rockefeller Foundation hired Flexner to implement this standardization, resulting in the closure of over half of the medical schools in the United States between 1910 and 1935. In those schools that remained, a unified curriculum purportedly assured the public that any US physician from any US medical school had successfully completed training to a certain standard and thereby was qualified to practice medicine. Most importantly, this process defined who and what should be standardized, thereby creating a narrowly constrained paradigm of what denotes safe, efficacious and appropriate healthcare practices and practitioners.

This standardization process, embedded in the curriculum of the Rockefeller-funded Peking Union Medical College, is likely to have influenced the subsequent standardization of TCM, and thereby the future standardization of other heterodox healthcare practices and practitioners via WHO integration policy. This example also demonstrates that even as its proponents present standardization as a scientific process, it, like integration, is simultaneously a political, economic and social process, whereby all four of these factors influence one another.

THE ISSUES OF STANDARDIZING HEALTHCARE PRACTICES IN THE PHILIPPINES

Standardization assumes bounded healthcare practices or practices that can be systematized. If, as in the Philippines, a majority of local heterodox practitioners are self-taught, then possibly no member of a given labeled practitioner category will practice in the same manner, nor might a standard for this practitioner category ever be even theoretically identified. Although local healthcare practices may conform to the dominant Filipino cosmology, it is doubtful that such a cultural standard could be translated into an acceptable biomedical understanding of standardization.

Furthermore, there is no single universal system of classification of local heterodox healthcare practice across the Philippine islands (Tan 1987). Attempts to organize local practices and practitioners have been incomplete, containing

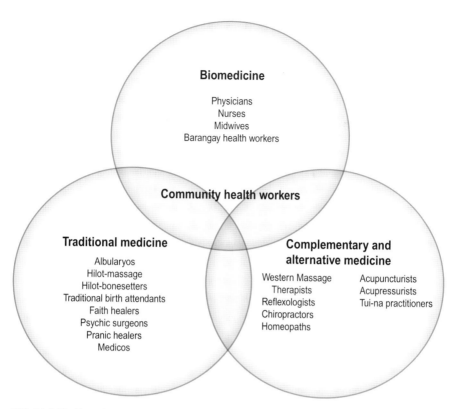

FIG. 11.1 The Formal and Informal Health Care System of the Philippines Depicted as a Representation of Bounded Medical Pluralism.

only certain practice and practitioner labels specific to the particular community studied.[4] Additionally, overlapping categories of local healthcare practices and practitioners are commonly identified. For, even when practice categories are representative of a given local level, practitioners rarely strictly practice as per their given title. Hence, 'herbalists' may primarily be performing massage and 'bone setters' may only prescribe herbs (Kadetz 2008a, 2008b). These challenges to the conceptualization of basic practice/practitioner categories would present

---

[4] Some general categories that have been found in the literature include the *albularyo* (usually referring to a practitioner whose primary treatment is herbal. However, other practitioner categories identified use herbs, and *albularyos* use prayer and other diagnostic and treatment modalities); the *hilot* (*hilots* are comprised of the *manghihilot* – usually using some form of physical manipulation, massage or touch, but they can also use *ventosa*, a form of cupping – and the *magpapaanak* or *commadrona* or TBA primarily treating prenatal, delivery, and postnatal care involving touch, herbs, prayer, and any combination thereof); *medicos* (a category reserved for local practitioners that incorporate training in imported heterodox practices and/or biomedicine into their practices) and *diviners* and *faith healers* (whose practices any of these local healers can and do incorporate). However, it should be noted that these general designations, and the practices that fall under them, change from province to province and even community to community within a municipality and that practitioners can be far more specialized, for example there are practitioners who only treat dog bites or remove fish bones (Kadetz 2008b). For more in-depth discussions see Jocano 2004; Turner 1999; and Tan 1987.

insurmountable problems for a Western conception of standardization dependent upon such discrete categories. Figure 11.1 illustrates the shortcomings of a bounded, and hence false, representation of the formal and informal healthcare system of the Philippines that would be necessary for standardization.

Lastly, and possibly most problematic for standardization, is the fact that many local practitioner informants found the concept of standardization inherently ignorant, for they believed that what was given to them as a gift from God could neither be taught nor standardized, nor should it be shared. However, the dominant conceptualization of standardization leaves little room for such variations in cultural and belief systems.

Yet, on a more fundamental level standardization may be a misdirected and naïve goal, in assuming that all heterodox healthcare practices, and the systems of knowledge from which they were conceived, can and should be reducible to a biomedical paradigm or else risk being discarded. The potential for unintended negative outcomes embedded in this goal is illustrated in the case study of traditional birth attendants (see Vignette 11.3).

INTEGRATING EAST ASIAN MEDICINE

VIGNETTE 11.3   A CASE STUDY OF STANDARDIZATION: THE 'REINTEGRATION' OF TRADITIONAL BIRTH ATTENDANTS IN THE PHILIPPINES

PAUL KADETZ

From 2004 to 2008, the World Bank, USAID (2004), the European Commission (2008) and the Asian Development Bank issued reports concerning the funding of a project to reduce infant and maternal mortality in the Philippines via 'skilled' deliveries within in-birthing facilities. The Asian Development Bank's (2007) independent evaluation was the only report to *not* recommend funding the project, finding it both infeasible, unsustainable, and substantiated by unreliable aggregated Department of Health data.[i] However, with substantial loans from the remaining funders, the Department of Health of the Philippines issued an Administrative Order in 2008 stating that all women in the Philippines are to be considered 'at risk' during pregnancy and must only deliver in-facility by 'skilled professionals' (Department of Health of The Republic of The Philippines 2008). Traditional birth attendants, having received UNICEF training in delivery since 1952, are to be *integrated* into the maternal child health team only if they agree to not perform deliveries again.

Interviewing community members from the same municipalities previously investigated (see Vignette 11.1), the feasibility and sustainability of implementing this policy were found to be challenged along numerous criteria. First, 80% of Filipino women in rural or isolated areas prefer to deliver at home, usually with the assistance of traditional birth attendants (ADB 2007).

To replace at-home delivery by traditional birth attendants, indigent women will be covered by the national insurance, Philhealth, for up to US$130 for a maximum of four deliveries. However, this does not fully cover the cost of a hospital delivery, and women must still pay for medications (before reimbursement by Philhealth), transportation to the facility, and any costs beyond the allocated coverage – all of which may be beyond a family's budget.

The locations of in-birthing facilities are chosen by a municipal health officer with possible input from a provincial governor. However, facilities were not always planned for those communities furthest from hospitals; where women were least likely to be able to access emergency care. But regardless of their location, several municipal health officers reported very infrequent use of in-birthing facilities.

The feasibility of increased hospital deliveries is also challenged. Several hospital chiefs reported that their numbers of admissions for normal spontaneous deliveries was overtaxing an already overtaxed hospital system, and that hospital obstetric staff have had to encourage women deemed not to be at risk to deliver at home.

No provisions have been offered for increasing the number of 'skilled' birthing professionals to replace traditional birth attendants. This imbalance may prove difficult to overcome in a country with well-documented mass migration of medical professionals.

If the reality of this situation is that Filipino women will continue to have at-home births with traditional birth attendants – who are now no longer being trained or supplied with sterile birthing kits – then there is a potential for increased maternal and infant morbidity and mortality, especially in remote, poor and inaccessible areas where the implementation of this policy is least feasible. Hence, the main objectives behind healthcare integration – to reduce health inequity and improve healthcare access – are negated by this particular form of 'integration.'

---

[i] Furthermore, Hogan, Foreman, Naghavi, et.al. (2010) and Rajaratnam, Marcus, Flaxman et.al. (2010) challenge the accuracy of the WHO's global maternal and infant mortality measurements respectively.

CONCLUSION: THE CONTEXT-DEPENDENCE OF INTEGRATION

INTEGRATION BY AND FOR WHOM?

In discussing how healthcare integration was implemented in the Philippines, one municipal health official noted, that 'the goal is to completely retrain them to our standard of safety.' The official then outlined an explicit plan to render all local heterodox practitioners 'safe' by retraining chosen practitioners in those practices that have been approved as safe and effective by the Philippine Institute for Traditional and Alternative Healthcare, the Bureau of Food and Drugs, and the Department of Health of the Philippines. Thereby, albularyos that would normally use an abundance of local herbs for treatment will be retrained to only treat with the ten herbs approved by the Bureau of Food and Drugs; Hilots employing 'spiritually guided' massage will be retrained in the Department of Health of the Philippines' approved massage; and traditional birth attendants will assist midwives, but no longer deliver. If the practitioner was unwilling to be retrained or was found to not comply with training, they would not be allowed to continue practicing. Hence, standardization and integration are being used in this context to narrow the practices that heterodox practitioners can use, or even to completely eradicate them.

The fact that local heterodox practitioners may help communities by serving important social and cultural functions, and that their practices may be altered to the point of being no longer socially meaningful, or specifically able to address culture-bound illnesses and thereby of questionable utility for the local context, are valid concerns that are neglected by the current discourse on integration.

GLOBAL INTEGRATION POLICY: ONE SIZE DOES NOT FIT ALL

The unintended negative consequences of healthcare integration presented in this chapter can be understood as a microcosm of the larger problems embedded in the domains of global health policy and global health governance. Feasibility, sustainability, and outcomes for a given local context are often not assessed to the degree that they are assumed in healthcare integration policies (Oxman et al 2007). This may be a reflection of the hegemony of biomedicine in global health policy, wherein local contexts are universalized according to the needs and agendas of higher-income countries. It may also reflect the WHO policy making process, whose transparency and structure is brought into question. Oxman and colleagues' 2007 assessment of the WHO's systematic and transparent approaches to policy making identified an over-reliance on experts; lack of attention to Member State adaptation of global recommendations; lack of attention to local needs, conditions, resources, costs, and values; lack of attention to effective dissemination and implementation strategies and their rigorous evaluation; and a failure to develop recommendations that address existing health systems.

The fact that different local contexts have different needs presents challenges to the entire universal paradigm of global governance and global health policy. However, this is not to denigrate local policies and interventions that have most certainly benefited from global and international coordination. One is immediately reminded of the successes of numerous vertical disease eradication programs, with the eradication of smallpox marking one of the triumphs of global healthcare policy and coordination through multilateral institutions. But it is important to note that these programmes are addressing specific healthcare issues that best fit within a medical model of intervention.

According to Cunningham and Andrews (1997, 4), 'The subject of Western scientific medicine is power.' It has been argued in this chapter that the subject of integration is also power disseminating from the global, national and local levels. Although it is beyond the scope of this chapter, it is imperative to explore the effects of the WHO's choice to define and champion integration in terms of a model that is historically tied to the top-down assertion of governmental force and control (TCM in China), rather than a model of integration achieved by more equitable political power and agency, as demonstrated by the powerful political lobby of Ayurvedic practitioners in India (Bala 2007; Leslie 1992). Whether such political and social capital is necessary for heterodox practitioners to achieve the 'separate but equal' status of parallelism is not clear, but may be one element that effects the type of integration a given heterodox practitioner group seeks and achieves. One may further question whether the WHO's choice of the Chinese model has engendered an inequity of power between key actors and stakeholders in healthcare by virtue of its historical use and structure.

All of the executions of power presented in this chapter can combine in complex and unpredictable ways that must be considered along with other political, economic,[5] social, and cultural forces in order to understand the potential unintended consequences of healthcare integration. One such combination of these forces joining in the legal arena concerns the ownership of local medical knowledge (see Gerard Bodeker's discussion in Vignette 11.4).

This chapter has argued for more rigorous and context-dependent conceptual models of healthcare that will facilitate accurate representations of all formal and informal healthcare practices. In order to achieve this, the models employed by policy makers must be able to differentiate between intention and actuality, for the healthcare structures intended by policy makers do not always describe how healthcare is actually used and structured by individuals and communities. To put it simply, one representation cannot fit all.

THE THIRD DIMENSION: 'EXTERNAL' VERSUS 'INTERNAL' INTEGRATION

In this chapter, integration is presented as occurring in two dimensions, namely, a dimension of top-down/bottom-up (presented in the research findings in Bagabag and Murcia, see Vignette 11.1) and a dimension within the individual practitioner (as discussed in Farquhar (1994) and Scheid's (2002) findings of individual plurality in TCM practitioners). However, a third dimension can be identified that occurs organically within communities, as opposed to being externally imposed. This was illustrated in Murcia (see Vignette 11.1), where healthcare disparity generated an increase in biomedical referrals to heterodox practitioners, resulting in an integration based more upon local or internal needs, rather than external needs or external perceptions of local needs.

Another example of internal integration is illustrated in the Philippine municipality of Sadanga, where poor access to biomedical healthcare has required the local heterodox practitioners to be the primary care givers for the majority of the population. These practitioners will refer to physicians as needed. This integration of biomedicine into a predominantly heterodox healthcare system has reportedly worked well for this municipality.

That integration should require experts who often know little about local heterodox healthcare practices, and that communities are often considered by

---

[5] The economic benefits of standardization and integration must be considered a potent force in shaping the particular way in which healthcare integration unfolds. China has led the way for the global exportation of heterodox practices, as demonstrated in the Philippines among many other countries (Hsu 2002; Kadetz 2008a). But more so, PITAHC's corporate status forces it to prioritize those practices that are the most profitable. The four herbs processed at PITAHC's manufacturing plants are sold in abundant supply in local and municipal health units and generate a substantial source of income. Also, the Chamber of Herbal Industries in the Philippines Inc., accounting for 70% of the local herbal market, estimated sales in excess of US$600 million in 2007 (CHIPI 2010).

Patenting of traditional medicine products is an increasing global trend. Japan, for example, has a strong culture of patenting and holds multiple patents on the processing and use of the important traditional Chinese medicine *Ganoderma lucidum* (known as *Ling Zhi* in China and *Reishi* in Japan).

The growth of the herbal sector, and the constant demand for new and marketable products, has led the herbal industry worldwide to assume that traditional medical knowledge is available for all to commercialize, generally without sharing benefits with customary owners.

Yet there has been increasing international debate and legal challenge over the patenting of traditional knowledge and its products, following two broad positions.

The first, by non-indigenous individuals and organizations, claims ownership of indigenous knowledge for commercial gain. The second is by indigenous representatives and developing countries to prevent this from happening, and either to take ownership of such products themselves or to engage in partnerships with fair sharing of benefits for the commercial development of their knowledge, products or processes (Bodeker 2007).

This has taken place against the backdrop of two international legal frameworks that contradict each other: the Convention on Biological Diversity, and the World Trade Organization's Trade-Related Aspects of Intellectual Property Systems.

The Convention on Biological Diversity (1993), through Article 8(j), assigns ownership of biodiversity to indigenous communities and individuals, thereby giving them the right to protect this knowledge. The more powerful Trade-Related Aspects of Intellectual Property Systems, however, makes no reference to the protection of traditional knowledge and holds that if knowledge is not patented it is not owned. The long-running Doha Round of the World Trade Organization negotiations has called for harmonization between the Convention on Biological Diversity and the Trade-Related Aspects of Intellectual Property Systems. This focuses on benefit sharing, based on prior informed consent of traditional holders who share their knowledge with companies (a provision of the Convention on Biological Diversity, and a counter to so-called 'biopiracy') and whether the Trade-Related Aspects of Intellectual Property Systems should be amended to take this into account. At the time of writing, this review is still in progress.

Meanwhile, the 2007 United Nations Declaration on the Rights of Indigenous Peoples recognizes the right to maintain, control, protect and develop traditional knowledge, including medicines, and to maintain traditional health practices. Several countries have reorganized their traditional knowledge into systems that Western patent offices can reference for 'prior art', i.e. existing inventions already in the public domain. India's Traditional Knowledge Digital Library, with details of 4500 Ayurvedic medicinal plants and thousands of yoga postures, is one of the most sophisticated protective responses to biopiracy (Patwardhan et al 2010). And the United Nations University has documented examples where communities are developing their local and unique systems of benefit sharing, independent of patent regimes (Suneetha & Pisupathi 2009).

For integrated healthcare to succeed, it needs to draw on a full range of traditional treatments, including yoga, tai chi, acupuncture, detoxification therapies and diet. While these are largely absent from existing intellectual property rights debates, they play an increasing role in global public health. Intellectual property rights regimes need to catch up.

these experts to be incapable of making the best healthcare choices on their own, is another significant unchallenged assumption of this healthcare policy domain. This particular assumption is especially contradictory for communities that have been entrusted with the stewardship of their local healthcare, by virtue of a decentralized healthcare system such as in the Philippines, yet are rendered incapable of making decisions concerning preferred healthcare use.

THE QUESTION OF HOW TO 'DO' INTEGRATION: 'DONE TO', 'DONE WITH', OR NOT DONE?

In conclusion, there is an unchallenged conception of inherent beneficence to health and wellbeing in the discourse of healthcare integration that is not substantiated by the data presented in this chapter. This is not to imply that these findings are generalizable beyond the communities studied, or that the potential value in the concept of healthcare integration – with its agenda of decreasing healthcare disparity – is being challenged. What is questioned, however, is precisely how healthcare integration is being implemented, and whether the best practices specific to each local context are being considered in the policy making process.

The cases presented here ask whether healthcare integration is something that really needs to be 'done to' a population, 'done with' a population, or whether it is something a population will organically arrive at if left to its own devices? Is external intervention really necessary, or could local, state, non-governmental organizations and multilateral resources be better directed toward other healthcare needs? Do communities and individuals really need to be protected from themselves and from making their own healthcare decisions? And ultimately, can informal local healthcare systems be externally controlled? Although the model for integration chosen by WHO emphasizes a normative conception of integration as something that needs to be 'done to' a population,[6] it is suggested here that there is no one way to 'do' integration, which may be best determined by the local context itself. For in reality, population preferences, ruled by changing sociocultural factors, may be most central in generating the demand for the supply of particular local healthcare practices and thereby create the ensuing local network of practitioners. Hence, I would argue that context is everything,

[6] According to Zhang (2000:140), the primary function of the traditional medicine division at WHO is to 'encourage and support member states in integrating traditional medicine into the national healthcare system and in the proper use of traditional medicine by supporting national programs of research and training, technical guidelines and international standards.'

regardless of the geographic or political designation to which healthcare integration is applied.

Although this analysis was not intended to advocate either for or against healthcare integration, the research findings do suggest that integration policy implemented in a manner that ignores the specific needs of local contexts may negatively affect informal local healthcare systems, access to healthcare, and ultimately the health of communities. Clearly, the field of healthcare integration demands more local research in order to provide an evidence base for healthcare policy that benefits population health in practice, as opposed to doing so only in theory. But this would only be useful if policy makers were interested in the outcomes of their policies, and then use the derived evidence as a feedback mechanism to establish best practices.[7]

Finally, this research suggests that what may be gained by adhering to a beneficent concept of healthcare integration must be considered in terms of what may be lost in local level healthcare and how this may ultimately alter the social fabric of communities and the delicate mechanisms that function to maintain the health of vulnerable populations.

ACKNOWLEDGMENTS

My sincere gratitude to Dr. Jessica De Leon, Sister Dulce Corazon Velasco, Dr. Jenny Madamba, Dr. Penny Domogo, Eva Javier, Emilda Villacin, Rhiza Escote and Professor Ruben Caragay for their assistance in the Philippines. Ms. Charlotte Strum for her valuable assistance in the use of the *Rockefeller Foundation Archives*. Dr. Kim Small and Dr. Gerard Finin of the *East-West Center* for support in archival research as an affiliate scholar. Dr. Beth Sommers, Theresia Hofer, Sheila Bibb and Rachel Irwin for their helpful critiques. Professor Gerard Bodeker, Dr. Dawn Chatty, and Dr. Proochista Ariana for their valuable guidance. Dr. Volker Scheid and Dr. Hugh MacPherson for their thoughtful suggestions. And Dr. Vivienne Lo, Penny Rogers, and Sara Boynton for their valued support.

[7] According to Oxman et al (2007), in their study of the WHO policy process, WHO directors interviewed 'singled out the use of evidence more commonly than any other area for improvement. Evidence is generally not retrieved, appraised, synthesized, and interpreted using systematic and transparent methods. Few directors reported using data about potential harms or explicitly considering values—i.e., the relative importance or worth of the consequences (benefits, harms, and costs) of a decision. Using data about potential harms was not considered for public health or policy interventions' (1885–1886).

REFERENCES

Adams, V., 2003. Integrating abstraction: modernising medicine at Lhasa'a Metsikhang. In: Schrempf, M. (Ed.), Soundings in Tibetan Medicine: Anthropological and Historical Perspectives. Brill, Leiden.

Adams, V., 2008. Integration or erasure? Modernising medicine at Lhasa'a Metsikhang. In: Pordie, L. (Ed.), Tibetan Medicine in the Contemporary World. Global Politics of Medical Knowledge and Practice. Routledge, London.

Asian Development Bank, 2007. Philippines: Women's Health and Safe Motherhood Project. Performance Evaluation Report. Retrieved on 1/5/10 from: http://www.adb.org/Documents/PPERs/PHI/27010/27010-PHI-PPER.pdf.

Baer, H., 2004. Medical pluralism. In: Ember, C., Ember, M. (Eds.), Encyclopedia of Medical Anthropology. Kluwer, New York.

Baer, H., 2007. The drive for legitimation in Chinese medicine and acupuncture in Australia: successes and dilemmas. Complement. Health Pract. Rev. 12, 87–98.

Bala, P., 2007. Medicine and Medical Policies in India: Social and Historical Perspectives. Lanham, Lexington.

Bannerman, R.H., Burton, J., Wen-Chieh, C., 1983. Traditional medicine and healthcare coverage: a reader for health administrators and practitioners. WHO, Geneva.

Bello, W., 2009. The Anti-Development State: The Political Economy of Permanent Crisis in the Philippines. Anvil, Pasig City.

Bensoussan, A., Myers, S., 1996. Towards a Safer Choice: The Practice of Chinese Medicine in Australia. University of Western Sydney, Sydney.

Berg, M., Mol, A. (Eds.), 1998. Differences in Medicine: Unraveling Practices, Techniques and Bodies. Duke University Press, Durham.

Birn, A., 2005. Chinese barefoot doctors, a viable model today? Working Paper. IDSC 11. Stian Haklev.

Bodeker, G., 1994. Traditional healthcare and public policy. In: Islam, A., Wiltshire, R. (Eds.), Traditional Health Systems and Public Policy. IDRC, Ottawa, pp. 96–109.

Bodeker, G., 2001. Lessons on integration from the developing world's experience. BMJ 322, 164–167.

Bodeker, G., 2007. Intellectual Property Rights and traditional medical knowledge. In: Bodeker, G., Burford, G. (Eds.), 2007. Traditional Complementary and Alternative Medicine: Policy and Public Health Perspectives. Imperial College Press, London.

Bodeker, G., Burford, G., 2007. Traditional Complementary and Alternative Medicine: Policy and Public Health Perspectives. Imperial College Press, London.

Bodeker, G., Ong, C.K., Grundy, C., Burford, G., Shein, K., 2005. WHO Global Atlas of Traditional, Complementary, and Alternative Medicine. World Health Organization, Kobe. http://www.pchrd.dost.gov.ph/submitted-news/1-press-releases/295.html.

Chamber of Herbal Industries of the Philippines, Inc 2010. About Us. Retrieved on 1/2/10 from: http://new.chipi.org.ph/about-us/.

Croizier, R., 1975. Medicine and modernization in China: an historical overview. In: Kleinman, A., Kunstadter, P., Alexander, E.R., et al. (Eds.), Medicine in Chinese Cultures: Comparative Studies of Healthcare in Chinese and Other Societies. Geographic Health Studies, Washington, D.C.

Cunningham, A., Andrews, B. (Eds.), 1997. Western Medicine as Contested Knowledge. Manchester University Press, Manchester.

Dauskardt, R.P.A., 1990. Traditional medicine: Perspectives and policies in healthcare development. Development Southern Africa 7 (3), 351–358.

Department of Health of the Republic of the Philippines, 2008. Administrative Order 2008–0029 Implementing Health Reforms for Rapid Reduction of Maternal and Neonatal Mortality.

European Commission, 2008. Mid-term review of the health sector policy support programme (ASIE/2005/017638) in the Philippines. Commission of the European Communities.

Farquhar, J., 1994. Knowing Practice. The Clinical Encounter of Chinese Medicine. Westview Press, Boulder.

Green, E.C., 1980. Roles for African traditional healers in mental healthcare. Med. Anthropol. 4 (4), 489–522. http://www.socresonline.org.uk/6/4/han.html.

Hewa, S., 2002. Rockefeller Philanthropy and the 'Flexner Report' on medical education in the United States. Int. J. Social. Soc. Policy 22 (11), 1–47.

Hobsbawm, E., Ranger, T. (Eds.), 1983. The Invention of Tradition. Cambridge University Press, Cambridge.

Hogan, M., Foreman, K., Naghavi, M., et al., 2010. Maternal Mortality for 181 countries, 1980–2008: a systematic analysis of progress towards Millennium Development Goal 5. Lancet (375),1609–1623.

Hsu, E., 2002. 'The medicine from China has rapid effects'; Chinese medicine patients in Tanzania. Anthropol. Med. 9 (3), 291–313.

Hsu, E., 2008. Medical pluralism. In: Heggenhougen, K., Quah, S. (Eds.), International Encyclopaedia of Public Health, vol. 1(4). Elsevier, Oxford, pp. 316–321.

Hyma, B., Ramesh, A., 1994. Traditional medicine: its extent and potential for incorporation into modern national health systems. In: Phillips, D., Verhasselt, Y. (Eds.), Health and Development. Routledge, London.

Jocano, L., 2004. Folk Medicine in a Philippine Municipality: An Analysis of the System of Folk Healing in Bay, Laguna, and Its Implications for the Introduction of Modern Medicine. Tamarind, Manila.

Johnson, T.P., 2008. Yang Chongrui and the First National Midwifery School: childbirth reform in early twentieth-century China. Asian Med. (4), 280–302.

Kadetz, P., 2008a. A model for understanding Change in an indigenous medical system. Unpublished Dissertation, University of Oxford.

Kadetz, P., 2008b. A Pilot Study of Medical Pluralism in Batac, Philippines. Unpublished Research.

Kadetz, P., Perdomo, J., 2010. The integration of Traditional Chinese Medicine in the Cuban Healthcare System. In: Asian Medicine: Tradition and Modernity. Brill Publications, Boston (forthcoming).

Leslie, C., 1992. Interpretations of illness: syncretism in modern ayurveda. In: Leslie, C., Young, A. (Eds.), Paths to Asian Medical Knowledge. University of California Press, Berkeley.

Lin, V., Bensoussan, A., Myers, S., et al., 2005. The Practice and Regulatory Requirements of Naturopathy and Western Herbal Medicine. Department of Human Services, Melbourne.

Lin, V., Gillick, D., 2006. Is registration of Chinese medicine protecting public health and safety? Health Issues 88, 20–24.

Liu, Y., Hsiao, W., Eggleston, K., 1999. Equity in health and healthcare: the Chinese experience. Soc. Sci. Med. 49, 1349–1356.

Loh, M., 1985. Victoria as a catalyst for western and Chinese medicine. J. R. Hist. Soc. Vic. 39–46.

Loughlin, K., Berridge, V., 2002. Global health governance: historical dimensions of global governance. Centre on Global Change & Health, London School of Hygiene & Tropical Medicine, London.

Lucas, A., 1982. Chinese Medical Modernization: Comparative Policy Continuities 1930s–1980s. Praeger, NY.

Martyr, P., 2002. Paradise of Quacks: An Alternative History of Medicine in Australia. Macleay Press, Sydney.

Mendoza, R.L., 2009. Is It Really Medicine? The Traditional and Alternative Medicine Act and Informal Health Economy in the Philippines. Asia Pac. J. Public Health 20 (10), 1–13.

Oxman, A., Lavis, J., Fretheim, A., 2007. Use of evidence in WHO recommendations. Lancet 369 (9576), 1883–1889.

Patwardhan, B., Bodeker, G., Shankar, D., 2010. Ending medical dominance over the developing world. SciDev 30 June. http://www.scidev.net/en/opinions/ending-medical-dominance-over-the-developing-world.html (accessed 23.08.10).

Pillsbury, B., 1982. Policy and evaluation perspectives on traditional health practitioners in national healthcare systems. Soc. Sci. Med. 16, 1825–1834.

PITAHC, 2009. Retrieved on 10/10/09 from: http://www.doh.gov.ph/pitahc/Index.html.

Rajaratnam, J.K., Marcus, J.R., Flaxman, A.D., et al., 2010. Neonatal, postneonatal, childhood, and under-5 mortality for 187 countries, 1970–2010: a systematic analysis of progress towards Millennium Development Goal 4. Lancet 375, 1988–2008.

Republic of the Philippines, 1997. Republic Act no. 8423; The Traditional and Alternative Medicine Act.

Rosenthal, M., 1981. Political process and the integration of traditional and western medicine in the People's Republic of China. Soc. Sci. Med. 15(5), 599–613.

Said, E., 1978. Orientalism. Vintage Books, NY.

Scheid, V., 2002. Chinese Medicine in Contemporary China. Plurality and Synthesis. Duke University Press, Durham.

Sindiqi, J., 1995. World Health and World Politics: The World Health Organization and the UN System. Hurst & Co, London.

Singer, M., Baer, H., 2007. Introducing Medical Anthropology: A Discipline in Action. Alta Mira Press, New York.

Suneetha, M., Pisupathi, B., 2009. Learning from the Practitioners: Benefit Sharing Perspectives from Enterprising Communities. United Nations Environment Programme (UNEP) and United Nations University Institute of Advanced Studies (UNU-IAS).

Tan, M., 1987. Usug, Kulam, Pasma. Traditional Concepts of Health and Illness in the Philippines. AKAP, Quezon City.

Taylor, K., 2005. Medicine of Revolution. Chinese Medicine in Early Communist China. Routledge, London.

Turner, J., 1999. Formalizing 'traditional' healing: experience and practice on Samar Island. Unpublished MA Thesis.

USAID, 2004. Newborn Health in the Philippines: A Situation Analysis. Basics Support for Institutionalizing Child Survival Project (BASICS II). United States Agency for International Development, Arlington, Virginia.

Walt, G., 1994. Health Policy: An Introduction to Process and Power. Zed Books, London.

West, H.G., Luedke, T.J., 2006. Introduction: healing divides: therapeutic border work in Southeast Africa. In: Brokers and Healers: Brokering Therapeutic Resources in Southeast Africa. Indiana University Press, Bloomington.

World Health Organization, 1978a. Declaration of Alma Ata. WHO, Geneva. Retrieved on 22/06/10 from http://www.paho.org/English/DD/PIN/alma-ata_declaration.htm.

World Health Organization, 1978b. Primary healthcare, the Chinese experience. Report of an inter-regional seminar. World Health Organization, Geneva.

World Health Organization, 1984. Report of the Working Group on the Integration of Traditional Medicine in Primary Healthcare. WHO Regional Office for the Western Pacific, Manila.

World Health Organization, 2002a. Regional Strategy for Traditional Medicine in the Western Pacific 2002–2010. WHO Regional Office for the Western Pacific, Manila.

World Health Organization, 2002b. WHO Traditional Medicine Strategy 2002–2005. WHO, Geneva.

World Health Organization, 2003. Second Consultation Meeting on Traditional and Modern Medicine: Harmonizing the Two Approaches. WHO Regional Office for the Western Pacific, Manila.

World Health Organization, 2009. Traditional Medicine Definitions. Retrieved on 3 May 2009 from: http://www.who.int/medicines/areas/traditional/definitions/en/index.html.

Xue, C., Zhang, A., Lin, V., et al., 2007. Complementary and alternative medicine use in Australia: a national population-based survey. J. Altern. Complement. Med. 13, 643–650.

Young, D., 1994. Models of healthcare pluralism. In: Islam, A., Wiltshire, R. (Eds.), Traditional Health Systems and Public Policy. IDRC, Ottawa, pp. 62–70.

Zhang, X., 2000. Integration of traditional and complementary medicine Into national healthcare systems. J. Manipulative Physiol. Ther. 23 (2), 139–140.

Endangered practices: challenging the discourse of healthcare integration

Branding Indian aromatherapy: differentiation through transnational networks

Laurent Pordié

Branding is about differentiation. In the wellness industry,[1] it generally refers to the creation of original products, techniques or services, or to the conferring of value on exceptional locations and landscapes. A brand rests on the abilities of its creators to build a unique identity in this fast-growing and competitive sector. A health and wellness centre located in the Bordeaux region in France may thus differentiate itself from its competitors by offering vinotherapy products based on the antioxidant properties of wine. Other firms may market wellness cruises in the Caribbean, or relaxing outdoor mud baths in scenic Arizona. The possibilities are infinite.

Most spas offer signature treatments that are usually created to encapsulate their brand. A paradox arises, however, when these treatments are at the same time contemporary innovations and presented as very ancient therapeutic traditions. This paradox is only obvious when viewed from a certain angle. For the creators or the managers of the brand, there exists no contradiction. The 'tradition' legitimates new practices, which eloquently represent and identify the brand, its underlying concept and ethos – and sometimes its geographical location. The process is circular. The identity of the brand rests on a given therapeutic tradition, which is revisited and adapted to modern circumstances and consumers. This revisiting and adaptation are important conditions to differentiate the brand from its close competitors.

Such is the case for the Indian aromatherapy treatments found at Mango Spa,[2] a successful chain in India of about 20 high-class, standardized centres prominent in the wellness tourism industry and spread across the country and abroad. The identity of these treatments is claimed to be Indian, implicitly

---

[1] The wellness industry embraces a wide range of activities, including recreational tourism, treatments in health resorts, 'pancha karma' retreats, thalassotherapy, yoga, meditation, etc. (see Smith & Puczkó 2009, 83–104). One of the most widespread wellness structures is the spa. In the wellness industry, the use of this term involves a semantic shift: from the age-old water treatments (balneotherapy and hydrotherapy) located in places renowned for the medicinal properties of their springs, such as the town of Spa in Belgium, known since the Roman times for its baths, the term 'spa' in today's world tends to increasingly designate a healing and wellness center where virtually all kinds of practices, invented or stemming from any place on the planet, can be found. Although these centers do not limit their offers to water treatments, for commercial purposes the word 'spa' is often presented as the acronym (a 'chronologically reversed acronym', in fact) of the Latin *salus/sanitas per aquam* or 'health through water.' However, no clear origins of the term 'spa' have yet been established.

[2] I have changed the name of the spa company, its lead manager and the staff.

Ayurvedic, but a careful study of their genealogy shows that they were, and still are, largely inspired by the global wellness industry, and further shaped by the needs and desires of managers, therapists and clients together. This tension between claims of authenticity and the innovation processes involved in the making of these 'Indian therapies' is rendered all the more apparent by the fact that the chain won a prominent National Innovation Award for 'reviving the ancient knowledge of India.' Clearly, the logic here is that of branding.

However, combining novelty with the Old World does not reveal much about the processes by which a brand is created. While it is acknowledged that a strong brand creates a relationship between the brand itself and the consumers, this chapter will show that a brand like Mango Spa is primarily produced *through* relationships. In the case of Indian aromatherapy – the brand flagship – these relationships are established across extended transnational networks. They offer a grid from which to read 'the cultural specificities of global processes' (Ong 1999). The insertion of the company into these networks is not only a necessary condition for its healthy functioning, but it also engages Mango Spa in a relational universe fundamental to its dynamism and its creativity.

To study this phenomenon therefore entails the use of various lenses, focusing on small local units of activity, but taking into account 'the worlds that pass through them, that encompass them, constitute and reconstitute them' (Augé 1994: 178). The unpredictable encounters of distant worlds are rendered possible, even normalized, in the wellness tourism industry. I will argue that the imagined or factual encounters that occur within a space such as Mango Spa bring creative invention into existence, and appear as a fundamental condition in the branding of Indian aromatherapy.

A BUSINESS FOR THE 'METROSPIRITUALS'

Mango Spa's managing director, Leena, is a woman in her 40s formally trained as a lawyer and based in a wealthy locality of Mumbai. Leena and her husband, who is also in the 'health, fitness and wellness' business,[3] spent a part of their life in the US and came back to India, where they remained involved for many years in the life of a Siddha Yoga ashram in Maharashtra. There, they put into practice their entrepreneurial and project-management skills for the ashram's foundation in a variety of domains, including wellness and the healing arts for both Indians and foreigners. Leena attempts to bridge her thriving business with humanism and higher, spiritual preoccupations. This blending, she says, is the key to her success and that of Mango Spa. The services offered to the clients or guests — the terms used in preference to 'patients' — are embedded in a larger moral frame personally inculcated by Leena to her staff, which gives considerable attention to the subjects' needs and, according to her, remains focused on their spiritual elevation. This woman explicitly targets those whom she calls 'the metrospirituals.' These are urban individuals in search of a meaningful

---

[3] The husband was at the head of the company in the very first years before resigning to take up an executive position with an international spa firm.

existence and willing to satisfy their consumerist appetite with the expensive services offered by Mango Spa.[4] Indeed, her clientele consists exclusively of wealthy Indians and Westerners spending luxury holidays.

Leena insists on creating new forms of transactions in which the social and spiritual dimensions of exchange help to produce a harmonious physical and ethereal environment for her clients. She therefore distinguishes two levels in the relationship of her brand to the guests: an immediate exchange in the domain of the individuals and a long-term exchange that transcends worldly affairs. In this way, she not only sells a service or a product but, most importantly, she also makes a gift to others and to herself by working at bettering the world. Her economics of practice therefore challenges the distinction between gift and monetary transaction, and reveals – to paraphrase Bloch and Parry (1989) – a pattern of two related but separate transactional orders: a transaction concerned with the social or cosmic order and a 'sphere' of short-term transactions concerned with the arena of the individual.

When one of the senior executives of a prominent luxury hotel chain in India came to see Leena and her husband in the early 2000s and offered to initiate a new spa line, she could not have foreseen the phenomenal success that was in store for their enterprise after its creation in 2004. This successful business-woman affirms that she was guided by 'something in her.' She sees the success of Mango Spa as resulting from the wishes of higher powers that intervened through her. In just a few years of its existence, Mango became a prominent spa brand that resulted in a remarkable development in India and managed to export itself overseas.[5] Mango Spa acquired "good 'brand equity'", a management and marketing term which in Leena's words means that the brand adds value to the spa's activities and products. She systematically emphasizes the competitiveness and quality of her company's services by such statements as "while [Mango Spa] is the only Indian spa brand that operates worldwide, and while our methods are deeply rooted in ancient teachings, our aim is certainly not to convert our clients to the principles of ayurveda, for instance, but simply to provide a superior spa experience." Among the impressive numbers of awards won every year – sometimes two or three – nationally and internationally since the inception of the company, Mango Spa received in 2008 the renowned Innovation Award I mentioned earlier.

The brand has certainly benefited from the image of India as the source of numerous therapies and spiritual practices, among which Ayurveda and yoga, respectively, enjoy worldwide repute. Ayurveda enjoys a very noticeable success in India. It is promoted for national and international tourists by both private and governmental agencies, and even elevated in Kerala as a unique selling proposition of state tourism.[6] However, the success of Ayurvedic tourism has largely been a byproduct of the widespread availability of

---

[4] See Langford (2002) for an elaboration on this kind of articulation between indigenous remedies, spiritual quest and consumption.
[5] Although the achievements of Mango Spa are certainly uncommon, its development has to be understood in the larger context of the phenomenal growth of the spa industry in Asia, which only made its debut in the mid-1990s.
[6] The quantitative research conducted by Robinet Jecob (2008) shows that over 80% of international tourists in India experience Ayurveda and spas at least once during their stay in Kerala, which indicates if not an exact figure, a certain trend.

treatments in hotels and popular holiday resorts. To a large extent, Ayurveda is an additional offering provided by the tourism industry, rather than an independent, self-sustaining industry, which medical tourism perhaps is. The same is true of the services offered at Mango Spa. Ravichandran and Suresh (2010, 211) question in this context the relatively poor placement of India in terms of inbound tourism, and suggest creating 'brand India as a provider of wellness services.' This reflects the current perception that wellness elements are important for destination branding (Gelbman 2009).

Going beyond a wish to merge material and spiritual dimensions in her business, Leena thinks of herself as a visionary who also possesses knowledge of and experience in 'implementation and team building in multinational and multicultural arenas.' This was reflected in her ambition to revive and adapt 'the ancient healing science and wisdom of India.' Such a project required her to combine numerous therapeutic and material cultural horizons so as to produce Indian healing methods agreeable to a cosmopolitan clientele.

The ethos of the brand is summarized in the following extract taken from one of the documents produced by the company:

> [Mango Spa] offers a spectrum of authentic, traditional Indian wellness treatments and experiences in a stylish and soothing setting. Drawing from ancient Indian healing wisdom and Ayurveda, [Mango Spa] believes that a spa unfolds a way of life within which the life force is the bedrock of wellness. [Mango Spa] embraces a deep understanding of mind, body and spirit[7]; their individual needs and their interdependences. The [Mango Spa] programs are thoughtfully designed to luxuriously pamper and indulge, heal and nourish, restore and rejuvenate. [Mango Spa] offers a new lifestyle awareness that is both internal and external.

The idea of 'experience' is central to the brand and to others in the industry. Spas offer a particular type of experience to their guests and guidance for their lifestyle. "Otherwise," adds a spa manager, "a spa would just be a luxury massage parlour." The healing modalities offered at Mango Spa are presented as part of a larger approach to life. They are designed to guide people toward positive self-transformation – an emphasis also found among students of Chinese medicine in the US (as described by Sonya Pritzker in Vignette 12.1). The menu and the spa management and general direction are emphatic that their brand is distinct from all others in India, owing to its 'Indian character' and its strict use of what they call Indian wellness practices – which include Ayurveda.[8] Everything in the spa is made to emphasize its Indian identity: the treatments have Sanskrit names, the patients are greeted by a reverential namaste and offered garlands of jasmine on their departure, statues of Hindu deities decorate the rooms, etc. Leena notes that 'the Eastern influence continues to be strong, influencing products, services and spa design', and she hopes to benefit from it. The menu indicates different categories: Indian therapies, Indian aromatherapy, scrubs and wraps, beauty, Ayurveda

INTEGRATING EAST ASIAN MEDICINE

---

[7] This is a common theme in the wellness industry. See for example Laing and Weiler (2008), and Smith and Kelly (2006).
[8] While all spa brands in India also make use of treatments of Indian origin, most, if not all, indeed include 'international wellness experiences', 'cranial osteopathy', 'Tibetan', 'Balinese', 'Swedish' or 'Thai' massages, etc.

VIGNETTE 12.1 TRANSFORMING SELF, WORLD, MEDICINE: THE TREND TOWARDS SPIRITUALIZATION IN US CHINESE MEDICINE
SONYA PRITZKER

12

For Katie Cohen, the decision to study Chinese medicine emerged out of a desire to contribute to the world in a meaningful way. Working as a model in New York City, she always had a sense that she wanted to do 'something deeper' with her life. Until marital crisis forced her to face her innermost fears and desires, however, she did not know what that looked like. She desperately wanted to participate in the improvement of society, either through environmental action or some form of healthcare. After coming to California and hearing about Chinese medicine, and experiencing a visceral sense of recognition when she went to a talk emphasizing the spiritual–emotional components of the medicine, she decided to take up the study of acupuncture and herbal medicine. From her perspective, this medicine, with its connection to ancient Daoist and Buddhist notions of personal and spiritual harmony, was a perfect match for her personal, spiritual and moral mission. She promptly began the four-year endeavor to become a practitioner, and from the beginning of her program engaged with the medicine in a very personal way, taking guidance from her teachers on how to incorporate meditation and self-reflection into her studies. By her second year, Katie felt completely transformed by this work, and was more committed than ever to establishing a practice that emphasized spiritual growth and self-realization.

Katie is like many others studying Chinese medicine in the US, motivated to change themselves and the world through healing. Like Katie, many of the students see Chinese medicine as an ideal avenue for the personal and spiritual development that will allow them to create a career based on helping themselves and others find harmony in their lives and ultimately change the world. By emphasizing the spiritual roots of the medicine, many schools, teachers and practitioners market themselves directly to these transformation-seeking students. Some scholars have argued that such marketing practices distort the medicine, misrepresenting it as the holistic, spiritual opposite of biomedicine (Unschuld 2009). Admittedly, the strong emphasis on spirituality in US Chinese medicine circles does tend to highlight certain aspects of the medicine, such as its relationship to Daoism and Buddhism, and downplay others, such as its historical privileging of the male gender. In the worst-case scenario, this is seen as distorting the medicine. From another vantage point, it is seen as leading to the formation of hybrid practices that simply evolve the medicine. From still an other perspective, it is a positive transformation that fully aligns with the needs of society and person, and represents the most authentic interpretation of Chinese medicine for our time.

No matter which perspective one chooses, it is important to get to know people like Katie and her classmates. Her struggles with divorce and self-definition, along with her strong connection with Chinese medicine and its practices, reveal the deeply personal, embodied nature of her experience. Seeing her classmates also struggling with the desire to transform themselves and the world through healing, it is clear that Katie is linked to a cultural context in which there is a strongly felt need for something profoundly different. The reality and authenticity of these needs is unquestionable at the level of experience, and recognizing how Chinese medicine fits into this experience is an important step towards appreciating the 'authentic' Chinese medical practice in the West.

and yoga. Among these, the local brand of aromatherapy holds a central place. It is an innovative practice that is said to stem from the Ayurvedic tradition, despite the overarching creative influence of the spa direction.

MOLECULES, HOLISM AND THE GLOBAL

This influence is acknowledged by Leena herself, who is very aware of what makes for a good brand in the spa industry: "What's cutting edge in spas is really Old World, transported from the past into this millennium on a carpet of imagination," she remarks. And imagination she has in plenty! Her loud proclamations of the Indian traditional identity of the spa have not come in the way of her interest in all kinds of healing forms, her life experience and the meaning she tries to give to it – all of which have introduced novelty into the spa. She projects her self and infuses her ideas into her brand.

For example, Leena subscribes to the 'message from water' theory of the Japanese Masaru Emoto. Relatively famous in New Age circles, this man has attempted to prove with factual evidence that human vibrational energy, thoughts, words, ideas and music affect the molecular structure of water, an essential element of the human body and of the earth itself. Emoto has documented these molecular changes by taking microscopic photographs of frozen water. His results show various molecular shapes for water collected in many environments and conditions, such as the Arctic, Lourdes, pristine Japanese streams or polluted rivers in industrialized regions, or before and after exposure to prayers, Tibetan mantras or classical music. This study allowed him to develop a theory according to which the environment of a person has a profound impact on his or her own molecular structure, which in turn may improve or harm his or her life.

This is the reason why, in front of each massage table in the spa, there rests on the floor just below the head of the client a clay pot filled with water in which nine stones are placed. Each of these stones is inscribed with one of the nine virtues claimed for Mango Spa, such as Love, Joy, Honesty and Integrity, and Respect and Responsibility. This is meant to positively affect the clients, the therapists and the rest of the staff, by changing their own 'water structure.' However, this molecular approach to wellbeing is not revealed to either the staff or the clients. The reason for this secrecy can be traced to the unhappy experience Leena had earlier with crystal therapy. It was considered too esoteric – and perhaps not really Indian – by the spa's guests, who were therefore reluctant to choose this type of treatment. "The clientele is not yet ready to receive this kind of New Age therapy," she says. She conceals the most esoteric aspects of her approach to healing, but she sees them as important assets of her brand. Emoto's theoretical concerns are blended with the Ayurvedic humoral theory and some explanatory frame corresponding to the therapeutic effects of the aroma of oils – all without the spa management perceiving any contradictions. The sum of the individual effects of each of these therapeutic methods is expected to act synergistically, according to Leena's own epistemological heterodoxy.

One could cite more examples of how the approaches, techniques and epistemologies at Mango Spa bear Leena's personal imprint, whether apparent or hidden, and shape the spa's brand and treatments. But it is expedient at this stage to revisit what I said earlier. While Leena presents the implementation of these ideas as hers, she acknowledges that her many years in the US in the Indian diaspora (a transnational community *par excellence*) and her numerous visits to different spas in that country prior to setting up Mango, have affected those ideas, and that her frequent and close contacts with foreigners during her ashram life have influenced her a great deal. However, these influences are both concrete and abstract, and their impact is not readily measurable: she finds it hard at this point in time to clearly say how much of her success she owes to her own thinking and how much to other influences. It would be a bit like trying to divide the total corpus of her knowledge into clearly defined segments – the knowledge she gained while a law student, the knowledge she acquired during her practice as a lawyer, and the knowledge that has grown as a result of her own reflection. The boundaries become blurred, and more so as time passes. What becomes evident here is that her transnational journey, in India and abroad, has exposed her to a variety of people, things, ideas, methods and techniques through specific encounters which have played a significant role in the mechanisms of both knowledge and brand production at Mango Spa.

We could press this further: Leena has attended international meetings, such as the Global Spa Summit, an event that brings together a considerable number of delegates and executives. Such meetings are certainly useful in promoting brands and in gaining credentials within this network, and they also provide a learning experience on a variety of topics ranging from management, marketing and design to the current trends in the international market of complementary and alternative therapies. While such collective events of the global spa industry – and the encounters therein – do tend to have a certain homogenizing effect on both the knowledge and the practices of the spa industry executives, they also provide matters for comparison and ideas for differentiation – in other words, potential for branding. These gatherings not only carry the label 'global', but they actually embody the global. Some authors thus speak of 'spa culture' (Frost 2004) or 'global spa culture' (Cohen 2008, 12–13). Clearly, local therapeutic knowledge at Mango Spa is not solely a product of Indian individuals, firms or institutions, but is in fact a product of wider influences and market operations (see Trina Ward's description of cosmetic acupuncture, Vignette 12.2). Global processes, in turn, are at *all* times local processes embedded in communities, households and individuals. They are therefore not uniform, nor are they elements of a context, which determine local practices from outside. As can be seen in the case of Leena, 'global patterns' are deeply inserted within local practices. The global appears to be small and diversified (Law 2005) rather than big and homogeneous. These considerations must be taken into account in any attempt to understand the way in which a spa business is shaped and its brand created or reinforced.

THE INDIAN-NESS OF AROMAS

The Mango Spa brand has been built by very rigorous management techniques, which comprise internal and external audits, weekly and monthly reports (revenues, cleanliness, performance of the therapists, etc.), and most importantly a system of feedback involving the clients. These techniques are aimed

The recent rise of cosmetic acupuncture in the UK can be seen as a creative reinterpretation of the role of acupuncture. Moving acupuncture out of the sphere of medicine, into the domain of beauty under the banner of wellbeing, further reinforces rather than challenges the hegemony of biomedicine.

Some disparagingly view the practice of cosmetic acupuncture as 'purely commercial, so that it is not so much about medicine anymore, as wellbeing' (Deadman et al. 2009). Similarly, feminists have argued that women engage with cosmetic acupuncture treatments as a response to sexism and agism (Hurd et al 2008). Thus acupuncture, dispensed to fulfill beauty consumption patterns, entrenches such stereotypes. The implication is that this is not the route to wellness, let alone health.

The discourse of wellbeing is, however, readily adopted in a positive light by many practitioners. It is one that marks practitioners out as different, but from what? The familiar terms that are used, such as revitalize, enhance, holistic, natural, are found throughout the Western acupuncture world. The meaning of such language has subtly engaged with a social reference based on a culture of youth. Cosmetic acupuncture is also known as facial enhancement, facial revitalization or facial rejuvenation acupuncture – discourse that successfully differentiates the practice from violent surgery and poisonous Botox. However, such terms fail to differentiate it from that of other beauty treatments, which also feed off the wellness culture.

This creates a problem: the shifting of domain, from medicine to beauty, requires further differentiation (Zhan 2009b). That is, a need arises to redefine boundaries between the industries. What is more, as the local treatment, of basically sticking needles into and around wrinkles, is not surprisingly a technology that can be applied with little training, cosmetic acupuncture is now being taught in beauty colleges. The angry response of those wanting to control this market is to accuse those providing cosmetic acupuncture with little training as being unprofessional, of diluting acupuncture, and their approach as an unacceptable and untrustworthy practice (Adkins 2009).

But who has done the diluting? The quote in the title of this vignette is from a leading bioethicist calling for medicine to declare its independence from cosmetic procedures (Dreger 2009). There are some acupuncturists who feel the same way about the medicine they practice: they would rather see Chinese medicine questioning the authority of biomedicine and thereby offering a genuine alternative to modern healthcare, rather than entrenching stereotypical concepts of beauty.

Chinese medicine in the UK is clearly bound up with the commodification and marketization of healthcare which inevitably results in a defining of Chinese medicine's aims and clientele that is at odds with those at the basis of the National Health Service: available free at the point of use based on need, thus allowing biomedicine in the UK to retain its hegemony unchallenged.

at ensuring an improvement of the brand. The spa managers I met told me that this style of functioning put them under extreme pressure. The clients have the possibility of commenting on all aspects of their experience in the spa: disturbing sounds in the corridors, the appearance of the linen and the staff, types of massage, perceived quality and pressure of strokes, oils, decoration, etc. Many of the guests do fill out the relevant forms, whereas others opt to convey their opinions directly to the staff. This has led to several innovations. One important concern that emerged from the feedback, for example, related to the smell of the oils used. As one of the spa managers remarked, "We do not call what we do Ayurvedic aromatherapy, because the guests thought it was Ayurveda. It is Ayurveda in fact, but we branded it as Indian aromatherapy to make clear that we do not provide any stinking oils." Indeed, most traditionally manufactured Ayurvedic oils have peculiar odors, which penetrate the skin and hair and may persist for long periods. Aromatherapy was thought to be more appealing to the clients owing to its perceived popularity in the West. Mango Spa wished to modify the scent and hence the composition of the oils.

So as to obtain international standards quality for its oils, which in a sense would reflect the standard of the guests themselves, Mango Spa took a decision to outsource their manufacture. All started incidentally, when Leena came across a book entitled *Magic of Ayurveda Aromatherapy*, written by Farida Irani (2001). Irani is an Indian woman formally trained in Ayurveda in Pune, and today established in Australia, who claims to have pioneered Ayurveda Aromatherapy. Her book states that she combined the 'ancient science of Ayurveda' with the 'science of Aromatherapy', and that she has been successful in reviving the use of essential oils in Ayurveda.[9] The book and its author became important inspirations for Leena. She chose to deal with Subtle Energies, Irani's natural products manufacturing company established in Sydney in 1993, to create and produce the exclusive oils of the brand. Four main oils, which correspond to the main Indian aromatherapy massage treatment categories, are currently in use under the names of Relaxation Blend, Energizing Blend, Deep Tissue Muscular Blend and Facial Blend. These (essential) oils, needless to say, are not traditional, but are nevertheless claimed to be Indian, as the plants themselves are collected and processed in India before they are sent for oil extraction and production to Australia.[10] A therapist told me that it was fundamental that the plants grow in India, so that the 'feel of Indian-ness was experienced even in the aromas.'

This rather onerous creative process is explicitly intended to satisfy the clients' desires, to pamper their skin, and to avoid offending their sensitivity to smell.[11] The massage itself is therefore softened and adapted to the

[9] There is, however, an older book, written in 1995 and titled *Ayurveda & Aromatherapy* (Miller & Miller 1995). Interestingly, this book, co-authored with the writer's husband, adopts exactly the same approach as Irani's, and was the work of a woman of Indian origin living abroad, in the US. Born as Jyoti, she calls herself Light. She and her husband are the owners of Earth Essentials, a company producing essential oils.

[10] The same applies to the products used for facial and bath salts and scrubs and wraps, which are manufactured by Arcania Apothecary, a company based in the UK.

[11] While the brand managers are aware of the differences existing among their clients, whom they do not consider homogeneous, one may argue that once the market niche is defined – here wealthy 'metrospirituals' – the practice of branding tends to overlook social and individual asperities.

guests.[12] The guests are now systematically offered the opportunity 'to fra-grance[13] the oils', so that they can experience the sensuous smell of the new 'traditional' products before the massage. These kinds of phrase abound and concern virtually each and every aspect of the guest experience in the spa. They are taught to the staff during their training and are included in their manual. This forms an integral part of the branding process, which aims to achieve standardization and consistency. Clients from various ori-gins 'fragrance the oils', 'drink a detoxifying herbal tea', or 'use towels in organic cotton' while listening to the meditation music played to enhance the peacefulness of the place. Such practices are generally called 'rituals' in the spa management industry at large. They purport to 'communicate care and attention to details, and contribute to the brand with minimal impact on the time or cost of treatment' (Foster 2008, 200). The therapists then fol-low through by profiling the constituents of the oils and by explaining 'their effect on the body and the mind', according, they solemnly affirm, to the Ayurvedic pharmacopeia. The massage then takes place, after the washing of the feet of the guest with medicated water and essential oils, a ceremony presented as an 'old Indian ritual.' Positioning the clients at the centre of the brand development is fundamental to the company's philosophy. The core value at Mango Spa has been shaped by an old Sanskrit adage, *atithi devo bhavaḥ*, 'the guest is God.'[14]

The Mango Spa brand draws its sustenance from its transnational relation-ships. These operate at two levels: at one level, a long-term arrangement with foreign companies ensures the supply of 'Indian products', and, at the other, the meetings between Mango Spa's clients and its personnel generate incen-tives for the adaptation of the Mango Spa brand to its steadily growing client list, Indian and foreign.

THE THERAPISTS' APPEARANCE AND BEHAVIOR

Playing a key role in the success of the Mango Spa brand have been the spa's therapists. Most of them, however, have never received any formal medical training, only 12 weeks of intensive massage training at Mango Spa. Over 70% of these therapists are female. In its early stages, the firm appointed therapists with a massage background. Since 2007, however, most have been recruited from catering schools and hospitality colleges, and this for three reasons. First, the knowledge they have gained in the hospitality industry is seen as being of primary importance in the wellness industry. Second, lack-ing professional experience, they are hired on a lower salary scale. And third, as they do not have prior experience, they are thought to be more amenable to the new teaching they will receive on the brand standards and the treat-ment techniques at the spa. 'The Mango Spa senior management feels that it

[12] On the transformation of Ayurveda along similar lines, see the seminal work by Francis Zimmermann (1992).
[13] The phrase is meant to suggest smelling the oils.
[14] The Indian Ministry of Tourism claims to have pioneered the use of this maxim in the tourism sector in order 'to help tap into the full potential of tourism in India' (http://www.incredibleindia.org/newsite/atithidevobhava.htm).

is difficult for experienced therapists to unlearn what they already know, and they tend to adulterate the treatments with their own strokes', confided a spa manager. This kind of adulteration is seen by the spa management as potentially undermining the brand image.

Despite this standardizing process at work, however, each therapist develops her or his own style. What really unites them is their provenance. In earlier times, most massage therapists came from the southern states of India – Kerala, for instance, which today is considered the heart of Ayurveda – but over the years the northeastern Indians of Tibeto-Burmese origin have come to compose 90% of the number employed. Most of these people come from the states of Manipur, Mizoram, Assam or Nagaland, and a small group from among the exiled Tibetans in India. They usually belong to impoverished families and are ready to travel across India for job opportunities. Always willing to relocate, they do not resist internal transfers within the Mango Spa group. Most of them are educated and speak a good level of English.

But the massage therapists are primarily recruited on the basis of predefined cultural stereotypes. One important reason northeastern Indians are favored is their physical appearance.

"They look like Thai or Japanese people," says a Keralite member of the staff, "and they are always polite and well mannered. The Hindus [meaning the South Indians, despite the fact that there are Hindus in the northeastern states also] are rough, often very traditionalist and badly educated." A spa manager from Tamil Nadu adds, "It takes less time to groom them to the hospitality industry [than the South Indians]. They are hard working, but they show a herd mentality. They join in groups and leave in groups. Loyalty is less. They would happily jump to another spa company for a couple of thousands extra. Since [Mango Spa] started hiring northeast Indians, the attrition rate has been very high. But I would still prefer to have them if I were to run my own spa. I find them more professional and much easier to work with than South Indians."

This poses a set of problems as far as attrition and identification are concerned. A high turnover of personnel is seen as potentially undermining a spa's brand value through its effect on its quality of service. What is more, spa management specialists emphasize the fact that it is preferable to engage people who are easily identifiable with the brand, so as to 'send a strong message about the authenticity' (Foster 2008, 199–200): Thais in Thai massage spas, for example. Indeed, a large majority of the therapists at Mango Spa do not evoke India for most of the international guests, who for the most part associate them with South-East Asia at first glance. This cannot but create a conflict with the desirable perception of the Indian identity of the Mango Spa brand. This contretemps becomes even more explicit for the treatments presented as Ayurvedic. As notes a spa manager, "The message that only Keralites can perform Ayurveda treatments properly is so deeply instilled in the minds of people that I have had guests who refused to take treatments from therapists from other states." The question therefore arises: why are northeasterners preferred by the direction? The salary difference between them and the others could not be a factor. The willingness of northeastern masseuses to carry out massages on men is a very central reason behind the overwhelming choice of these women in the spa. Traditionally, male masseurs only work on male clients, and masseuses on female clients. However, responding to market demand, most spas in India have allowed the pattern to reverse itself, and Mango Spa is no exception to the trend. Coming from a cultural milieu that they present as having little or no concern about caste and purity, the northeastern masseuses see nothing wrong with falling in line with the new attitudes to the business. They view it as a sign of openness and emancipation. In contrast, most south Indian women would shrink from touching men, even in the context of therapy.

The inclination of northeastern masseuses towards cross-gender massage should be understood as liberating, holding new possibilities for individual achievement and self-realization. Bodies become sites for the production of values against the background of a traditional society.

CONCLUSION

This chapter has shown that the imagination involved in the creative process of making and sustaining a brand is not only affected by the desires of those at great social, cultural and geographic distance, as globalization theory would have it, but also by linkages in the form of contacts, discussions and interactions between individuals that cross the borders of nation-states. That is to say, transnationalism plays an instrumental role in shaping the brand. Transnationalism is here conceived as the sum of intermittent connections and bodily co-presence among distinct individuals across the borders of nation-states. This approach follows the criticism expressed by some authors about the relative disengagement of the social sciences – and of transnational studies for that matter – regarding the role of 'distance contacts' such as travel and occasional encounters in holding social life together (Urry 2004). This involves temporality. The cross-border linkages do not need to last very long to fall under the purview of transnationalism as long as they are repeated and maintained across time. It is here the space that is transnational, and not necessarily the individuals on holiday. In these transnational spaces, people from various cultural backgrounds contribute to the creation of new therapies.

The encounters brought about by Mango Spa play a major role in the making of therapeutic practices. This configuration emphasizes the many networks and ramifications involved in the creation of healing practices, which make irrelevant many of the common assumptions about single-sited and one-dimensional origins of 'ancient therapies' (see, for example, Mei Zhan's description of Chinese medicine in this context in Vignette 12.3). These encounters bring creative invention into existence, a fundamental condition for the successful branding of Indian aromatherapy. Training programs, body techniques, gender or caste restrictions, or again the fragrances of oils have all been meticulously revisited in order to meet the needs of the market of wellness tourism. The brand therefore rests at the same time on claims of Indian-ness and authenticity, and adaptive creativity. The first two qualify the brand and the last differentiates it.

The branding of Indian aromatherapy thus conciliates otherwise contradictory situations, pertaining to the innovation processes involved in the creation and differentiation of objects and techniques that are claimed to be local but inevitably placed under strong and decisive global influences. These objects and techniques do gain legitimacy through tradition, but also need at the same time to challenge those traditions to become visible on their own terms.

'Where did traditional Chinese medicine come from? How did you become interested? Is it scientific?' New acquaintances at informal gatherings sometimes ask me these questions as a conversation starter. Yet, having conducted more than a decade of ethnographic research at clinics, hospitals and other organizations of traditional Chinese medicine in the San Francisco Bay Area and Shanghai, I find it impossible to answer with a simple origin story befitting such social occasions. As argued by the anthropologists Sylvia Yanagisako and Carol Delaney (1994), origin stories are particular narratives that construct the order of things in the world, as well as relations among things and people. As such, conventional origin stories can obscure more complex relations and processes of encounter, entwinement and displacement in social formation. It is precisely these relations and processes that are at the heart of my ethnography of the 'worlding' of traditional Chinese medicine – how dynamic forms of Chinese medicine are constituted through translocal encounters and entanglements from which particular visions and practices of what makes up the world and our places in it also take shape (2009 Zhan; 2009a).

Although I was born and raised in China, my entry as an ethnographer into the worlds of Chinese medicine did not start there. Nor did it originate in a traditional clinic or herbal shop in an American Chinatown. When studying at Scripps College I trained with Dr David Sadava, a biologist working on gene therapies for small cell lung cancer. In encouraging my studies in biology, Dr Sadava enlisted me for a research project to test the effect of Chinese herbs – the ones practitioners often prescribe for cancer patients today – by applying their extracts to lung cancer cell cultures. It was in the laboratory that I developed a fascination with anthropological studies of science, especially how knowledges are produced and contested in everyday practice, as well as an interest in the mutual shaping and simultaneous production of biomedicine, bioscience and traditional Chinese medicine that extend beyond the confines of the laboratory and are embedded in translocal politics of difference. This fraught experience of 'culture' and 'science' was soon to find resonance in my fieldwork encounters. I had initially planned to work in the Bay Area only. Yet the fact that practitioners and advocates – as well as ideas, techniques and practices – traveled constantly between both sides of the Pacific, meant that my project inevitably became multisited. When introducing myself to practitioners in Shanghai, I had to explain why I 'came back' for Chinese medicine. 'What is anthropology? What does it have to do with Chinese medicine?' they would ask. My answer that as a medical anthropologist I was interested in 'cultural' practices of healing was usually recognized as adequate. After all, many proponents of Chinese medicine in China often highlight it as a matter of cultural legacy rather than emphasize its scienticity, which has come under increasing attacks as China 'gets on track with the world.' Yet for those practitioners who aspire to a future that is on par with their biomedical counterparts, culture only serves to accentuate the marginality of Chinese medicine. At an interview with a practitioner known for publicly voicing such aspirations, my usual speech about culture was greeted with silence. Finally, when I told him that I also studied biology, his eyes lit up: "Ah, *now* we have something in common!"

No exotic tales of ancient origins. No simple out-of-China narratives to describe the 'globalization' of traditional Chinese medicine. The worlding of Chinese medicine involves multiple and sometimes unexpected origins, trajectories and associations through which both knowledges and worlds are made.

These practices stand in their own right as important forms of innovation. This type of consideration differs from the numerous works concerned with the transformation of learned indigenous knowledge through their contact with the West and its people,[15] where their current globalized forms holding strong commercial potential are often disparagingly presented as diluted or corrupted versions of a greater tradition.

---

[15] In the case of Ayurveda, this specific kind of encounter has led to what some authors have termed 'New Age Ayurveda' (Reddy 2002; Zysk 2001).

REFERENCES

Adkins, P., 2009. http://www.cosmeticacupunctureuk.com.

Augé, M., 1994. Pour une anthropologie des mondes contemporains. Flammarion, Paris.

Bloch, M., Parry, J., 1989. Introduction. Money and the morality of exchange. In: Bloch, M., Parry, J. (Eds.), Money and the Morality of Exchange. Cambridge University Press, Cambridge.

Cohen, M., 2008. Spas, wellness and the human evolution. In: Cohen, M., Bodeker, G. (Eds.), Understanding the Global Spa Industry. Spa Management. Elsevier, Amsterdam.

Deadman, P., MacPherson, H., Maxwell, D., et al., 2009. Chinese medicine in the west 2009. J. chin. Med. (90, 6–18).

Dreger, A., 2009. Medicine needs a declaration of independence from cosmetic procedures. Hastings Cent. Rep. 39 (5).

Foster, S., 2008. Branding and spas. In: Cohen, M., Bodeker, G. (Eds.), Understanding the Global Spa Industry. Spa Management. Elsevier, Amsterdam.

Frost, G., 2004. The spa as a model of an optimal healing environment. J. Altern. Complement. Med. 10 (1), 85–92.

Gelbman, A., 2009. Using wellness elements for branding an exclusive image of tourism sites in the north of Israel. In: Smith, M., Puczkó, L. (Eds.), Health and Wellness Tourism. Elsevier, Amsterdam.

Hurd Clarke, L., Griffin, M., 2008. Visible and invisible ageing: beauty work as a response to agesim. Ageing Soc. 28 (5), 653–674.

Irani, F., 2001. Magic of Ayurveda Aromatherapy: Discover the Magic & Rare and Unique Ayurveda Aromatherapy Oils in Harmony with Universal Healing Success. Subtle Energies, Sydney.

Jecob, R., 2008. Health Tourism and Ayurveda. Abhijeet Publications, Delhi.

Laing, J., Weiler, B., 2008. Mind, body and spirit. Health and wellness tourism in Asia. In: Cochrane, J. (Ed.), Asian Tourism: Growth and Change. Elsevier, Amsterdam.

Langford, J., 2002. Fluent Bodies. Ayurvedic Remedies for Post-Colonial Imbalance. Duke University Press, Durham and London.

Law, J., 2005. And if the global were small and noncoherent? Method, complexity, and the baroque. Soc. Space 22, 13–26.

Miller, L., Miller, B., 1995. Ayurveda and Aromatherapy. The Earth Essential Guide to Ancient Wisdom and Modern Healing. Lotus Press, Twin Lakes.

Ong, A., 1999. Flexible Citizenship. The Cultural Logic of Transnationality. Duke University Press, Durham, NC.

Ravichandran, S., Suresh, S., 2010. Using wellness services to position and promote brand India. International Journal of Hospitality & Tourism Administration 11 (2), 200–217.

Reddy, S., 2002. Asian medicine in America: the Ayurvedic case. Ann. Am. Acad. Pol. Soc. Sci. 583 (1), 97–121.

Smith, M.K., Kelly, C., 2006. Holistic tourism: journeys of the self? Journal of Tourism Recreation Research 31 (1), 15–24.

Smith, M., Puczkó, L., 2009. Health and Wellness Tourism. Elsevier, Amsterdam.

Unschuld, P.U., 2009. What Is Medicine?: Western and Eastern Approaches to Healing. University of California Press, Berkley.

Urry, J., 2004. Connections. Soc. Space 22, 27–37.

Yanagisako, S., Delaney, C., 1994. Introduction. In: Yanagisako, S., Delaney, C. (Eds.),

Naturalizing Power: Essays in Feminist Cultural Analysis. Routledge, New York.

Zhan, M., 2009a. Other-Worldly: Making Chinese Medicine Through Transnational Frames. Duke University Press, Durham, NC.

Zhan, M., 2009b. A Doctor of the Highest Caliber Treats an Illness Before It Happens. Med. Anthropol. 28 (2), 166–188.

Zimmermann, F., 1992. Gentle Purge: The Flower Power of Ayurveda. In: Leslie, C., Young, A. (Eds.), Paths to Asian Medical Knowledge. University of California Press, Berkeley.

Zysk, K.G., 2001. New Age Ayurveda or what happens to Indian medicine when it comes to America. Traditional South Asian Medicine 6, 10–26.

The Cuban Chinese medical revolution

Vivienne Lo (羅維前), Adrian Renton

> **"**....*es sentido del momento histórico; es cambiar todo lo que debe ser cambiado*...
> Fidel Castro, 1 May 2000, Plaza de Revolucion[1]

In Chinese medicine, as in other traditional medicines, practitioners commonly try to align their practice with a single 'authentic' lineage. Different schools or teachers claim the right to represent a timeless tradition dating to an eminent Chinese ancestor, or even the revelations of the mythical Yellow Emperor. This quasi-religious impulse to be the latest living proponent of the 'Real Thing' obscures the complex interplay that exists between the faithful transmission of knowledge and practice across millennia, and the ways in which old medicines are often reinterpreted for new contexts. The historical development of Chinese medicine in late 20th-century Cuba provides a unique case study where the mutability of Chinese medicine is seen as a positive quality in the service of revolution. In this chapter we describe the Cuban Chinese Revolution, which provides an opportunity to reflect on the overall themes of this book, with its focus on authenticity, best practice and the evidence mosaic.

Reflective commentators on the globalization of Chinese medicine tend to acknowledge that 'living traditions', successful by definition, constantly transform themselves in order to remain meaningful outside the social and cultural context of their origins (Lo 2009; Zhan 2009). In interpreting and adapting traditional ideas to fit modern clinical and educational settings, European and American practitioners of Chinese medicine and their patients have changed Chinese medicine, often out of all recognition to Chinese practitioners (Barnes 2009). This is so much the case that to protect their traditions against the tide of foreign appropriation and 'misconception' about traditional Chinese medicine, contemporary Chinese government initiatives are pouring money into standardized teaching abroad, and authorized translations of Chinese medical terminology as discussed in several chapters of this book. Such are the anomalies of the nationalization and globalization of Chinese medicine. But because the very survival of a tradition demands change, scientists and researchers looking for a Chinese medicine to study are faced with the need to still this ceaselessly emerging practice. By taking a random snapshot of an art in progress, it can be imagined that it will constitute a sufficient slice of the tradition to represent the whole. How that modern image is linked to what Scheid (2007) has styled the 'currents of tradition' that fed it in the past raises complex questions

---

[1] 'It is the feeling of the historical moment; it is changing all that must be changed.'

for historians and clinical researchers alike. Those scientists involved in clinical research looking for reproducible results or to debunk tradition, for example, have to be challenged with the question, Does the Chinese medicine that you are studying have any claim to historical authenticity?

Could there be some core stability to Chinese medicine, something common in the diagnostic systems, the myriad acupuncture techniques and manual therapies such as massage and bone adjustments, the 'simples', the polypharmacy, the ritual and calendrical medicine, that we can identify as distinctively Chinese and to which scientists can address themselves – an historically authentic Chinese medicine that will provide a foundation for generating relevant research questions and formulating appropriate research protocols? Or are we limited to isolating and testing the techniques and substances as they present themselves today without identifying them as Chinese or traditional, without recourse to history – just as medicine in the broader universal sense?

The issue pertains not only to Chinese medicine outside China, where transformations of meaning are more easily seen in practice. Late 20th century modernization, nationalization and professionalization of Chinese medicine in China have standardized traditional medicine according to criteria that have contributed to the success of so-called Western medicine (a term that ignores all the non-European and American contributions to modern medicine). Tradition was rooted in a newly constructed empiricism, claims were made for being able to treat modern diseases, teaching was transformed from an art transmitted through scholarly or family lineages into a university discipline (Taylor 2005). In the process Chinese medicine became a very different phenomenon, no longer the work of artisans and scholar physicians but a formally approved part of China's National Health Service (Lei 2002).

Precisely because of its disregard for authenticity, as we shall see, the Cuban case provides a unique opportunity to chase what matters in defining Chinese medicine, that elusive object of academic and scientific research, and to reflect upon the wider issue of the appropriate design of research protocols for medical techniques and ideas that claim an origin in China. Another reason to choose Cuba as research context is that 20–30 million patients are treated with Medicina Traditional y Natural there each year, much of it identified as Chinese (Ministerio de Salud Pública 2003, 2008; Dirección Provincial de Salud-Matanzas 2008). In 2008 the authors visited Cuba in order to see for ourselves how Chinese medicine has been blended into the Cuban health service and to make a preliminary assessment of the kind of research undertaken there. To this end we were accompanied by Marcos Diaz, an Honorary Member of the Centre for Medicina Traditional y Natural of the Ministry of Public Health of Cuba.

SKETCHING THE CONTEXT

In 1959, Castro inherited a country that by Caribbean and South American standards had very positive health indices and more doctors per capita than Britain, France, Holland and Japan. Clearly, not all the conspicuous contemporary successes of the Cuban healthcare system are the products of socialist revolution (Chomsky 2000). However, with this head start Cuba went on to better even those countries within their own socialist networks. By 1984,

Cuba's life expectancy was higher than in any other Warsaw Pact country and its infant mortality rate lower than all but one (Feinsilver 1995). So how do Cubans continue to enjoy First World health in a Third World economy – in particular after the catastrophic collapse of Soviet support in 1989? Cynics will say that Cubans, while making distinct improvements in their diet in the last ten years, do not yet have First World diseases of wealth and, of course, they dance (Feinsilver 1995). Stereotypes aside, with the loss of the Soviet preferential prices for sugar, Cuba lost some 85% of its foreign trade and was faced with severe economic challenges in the delivery of food, let alone medicine. There are many theories about its ability to survive. Chomsky (2000) argues, for example, that real impact comes from the proper distribution of resources. Certainly, Cuban state policies have ensured better access to healthcare for all, as well as massive improvements in education, food, employment, sanitation and vaccination programmes.

Sketching the context, Diaz points to the links between poverty, landlessness and health that were highlighted in Castro's speech in his defence after the attack on the Moncada fortress, *History will Absolve Me* (1953). The health of the population became a key indicator of revolutionary success, with the Cuban patient cast as a 'biopsychosocial being within the community and environment' (Feinsilver 1995). Together with their investment in supporting local communities in the creative use of local resources, Cuban health programmes anticipated the principles of plural medicine enshrined in the Alma-Ata declaration on Primary Care by 20 years.[2]

Did this concentration on 'locality', especially as expressed through the 1964 establishment of the polyclinics as medicine's door to the community, make the Cuban authorities more sensitive to indigenous traditions, including the exogenous practice of its Chinese communities? At this stage in our research, we do not know the shape and location of these communities and to what extent they were targeted in the campaign. In the 18th century, hundreds of thousands of Chinese were imported on exploitative work contracts to supplement the African slave workforce on the sugar plantations, particularly during the long period of 'emancipation.' Stories of medical prowess in those early Chinese communities name legendary figures: Kan Shi Kom, Domingo Morales, Liborio Wong (aka Wong Seng) and Juan Chang Bom Bia. The latter is well known to have practised traditional medicine in the late 1800s in Matanzas province, so there is no doubt that the Chinese indentured labor brought their healing traditions with them (Roig de Leuchsenring 1965).

To someone of mixed Chinese–British blood (Vivienne Lo) there is something familiar about the wide, high set of the cheekbones, the shape of the eyes and one particular shade of the myriad Cuban skin colors that suggests

---

[2] The Declaration of Alma Ata, International Conference on Primary Health Care, USSR, 6–12 September 1978, adopted a concept of health as a state of complete physical, mental and social wellbeing, and not merely the absence of disease or infirmity; and affirmed health as a fundamental human right. It asserted that health inequalities between countries were unacceptable and recognized that improving health requires the action of many other social and economic sectors in addition to the health sector. It affirmed that health was a key element in the foundation of economic prosperity and identified primary care as a key feature in the development of all public health systems and asserted the right and duty of people to participate individually and collectively in the planning and implementation of their healthcare.

the absorption of those migrant Chinese, and as we shall see, some of their healing techniques as well. The four blocks of Chinatown and the ostentatious Chinese cemetery testify to the survival of an ethnically distinct Chinese community. The Chinese restaurant in Havana's old-town tourist precinct displays the usual miscellany of heat rubs, cold tonics and virility aids found in Chinatowns around the world. In 2008, reflecting the growing global prestige and economic power of their traditional medicine, the annual gathering of the Chinese elders of the *Casino* (a peculiarly Cuban Chinese term for the Havana meeting house, no longer a gambling den) was celebrated with a conference dedicated to Chinese medicine. Chinese medicine exists in the Chinese community outside of the hospitals and polyclinics as an exotic alternative to modern standard medicine, as it does in all overseas Chinese neighborhoods (Feinsilver 1995). There is also no doubt that the importance of the Chinese community has been a consideration in government support of acupuncture (Delgado Garcia 1995). However, what has happened with Chinese medicine in the Cuban public health service is quite different from other stories of the Chinese medical diaspora around the world.

CHINESE MEDICINE IN CUBA

The gradual absorption of the healing practices of old Cuban and South American Chinese communities into the ethnically Hispanic/local medical environment is not substantially different from that in Chinese communities worldwide. But the seeds of the acupuncture that we see in the Cuban public health system today were first planted by visitors from the West. In 1963, a prominent Argentinian acupuncturist, Floreal Carballo, held the first acupuncture seminar in Havana. Although this initiative was followed by some provision of acupuncture in the Cuban Public Health System, notably the modern practice of acupuncture analgesia, it was limited in range and impact (Acosta Martínez 2000). During the 1980s and early 1990s various American practitioners held short courses teaching their idiosyncratic interpretations of Chinese medicine. They gathered a core group of medical intellectuals interested in Chinese philosophy. One of these was Marcos Diaz.

Diaz's book *La Medicina China Tradicional y la Medicina del Futuro: qué, por qué, cómo y dónde* (Traditional Chinese Medicine and the Medicine of the Future: what, why, how and where) slips seamlessly between quotations from the revolutionary father of modern Cuba, José Martí, and citations from the Canon of Change (*Yi jing* 易經). In evoking the *Canon of Change,* the Chinese divinatory oracle that explains the nature of transformations in the universe, Diaz appropriates classical Chinese authority to highlight the revolutionary pedigree of ancient Chinese philosophy. But the roots of the kind of Chinese medicine that we see flourishing today in Cuba can be traced to a specific historical moment at the end of the 1980s, part of the late 20th century program of socialist science and technology exchange. This was more than a decade after China had sent cohorts of doctors to Africa, following the teams detailed to build railways in places such as Tanzania in the early 1970s (Hsu 2002). At the time, there was a growing realization of the power of medicine as a peculiarly effective ambassador for nation states. It was a significant moment for Chinese medicine when, with the visit of President Nixon in 1972, the televising of a brain operation using acupuncture anesthesia alone and without chemical analgesia, had demonstrated the spectacular benefits of traditional practice. Acupuncture became effective political propaganda, synonymous with national cultural genius – and we can add to this catalogue of indigenous pride all the other technological innovations that we saw China boasting in the opening ceremony of the Beijing Olympics (on 8 August 2008): printing, the magnetic compass, kites and paper.

Reflecting on the shared ideals of national cultural genius in a socialist context, it is not coincidental, then, that the development of Cuba's Chinese medicine has been led by its military medical service – a fact which somehow emphasizes its role in the country's struggle to survive. With his basic training in Chinese medicine, in 1988 and 1989, just before the loss of Soviet subsidies that underwrote so much of the Cuban economy, Diaz was busy setting up the specialty of traditional military medicine. Three consultants from military medical academies in North Korea, North Vietnam and China were invited by the Ministry of Military Affairs, then under Raul Castro. They linked up with those medical intellectuals such as Diaz who, until then, had trained in idiosyncratic American interpretations of Chinese medicine and were eager for teachers bringing the traditions fresh from the East. Dr Dong, with his translator, Kim, and a masseur named Jun from the Institute of Traditional Medicine of the North Korean Army, were assigned to a hospital in Havana. Together with Chinese and Vietnamese specialists, they looked at local herbs and started a process which is still ongoing to establish similarities and categorize Cuban substances, hitherto unknown in the Chinese materia medica, according to the system of Chinese medical potencies.

The timing was right: as the economic effects of the loss of Soviet subsidy started to bite, the Cuban health economy could no longer purchase basic food or drugs to support the health of its population and, critically, its military personnel. This crisis in supply was further intensified by the Toricelli (1992) and Helms-Burton (1996) Acts in the United States, which aimed to bring unprecedented pressure on suppliers of medicines and food to Cuba. Resolutely self-sufficient, Cuba's move away from Soviet-type reliance on high levels of chemical fertilizer towards organic farming was accompanied by nationalizing the cultivation of medicinal herbs and substituting herbal treatments for imported pharmaceuticals. Their choice to sponsor traditional medicine mirrors that of Mao Zedong in the 1950s after the breakdown of Soviet relations and the withdrawal of Soviet medical aid. By the mid-1990s, the eclectically titled Medicina Traditional y Natural became a formal branch of Cuban public health, with a new office in the Ministry of Public Health, alongside surgery, cardiology and all the other disciplines more familiar to readers. In 1997 the National Program set standards which dictated, for example, that 20% of all patients to be seen, for example by the hospital at Matanzas, should receive traditional and natural medicines. In 2002 the *Acuerdo del Comite Ejecutivo del Consejo de Ministrio* (Agreement of the Executive Committee of the Council) 42.82 put in place the regulatory framework for practice.

The integration of Chinese medicine into the Cuban health system has been driven by the economic need to fall back on local and national resources, the aid programs of historical socialist military alliances and influential enthusiasts.

Intrinsically the polysemous nature of Chinese medicine itself, its ability to embrace all the meanings that different audiences have invested in it, is also a perfect fit with the principles of continuing revolution that are at the core of the Cuban Revolution. Cuban Chinese medicine has created distinctive and unique opportunities for research and practice that do not sidestep the paradox that, to survive, a tradition must be intrinsically dynamic and be made relevant within changing cultures and societies.

CASE HISTORY: A VISIT TO FAUSTINO PEREZ HOSPITAL, MATANZAS

Next to the warning not to touch the broken blue window frame on the staircase, slogans affirm the ideal of continuing revolution and the fragile survival of Fidel's Cuba. Through a doorway a group of women sway gently through their *Taiji quan* 太極拳 steps. The well-scrubbed Clinica de Medicina Traditional y Natural in Matanzas is quiet today – Cubans prefer solar and thalassotherapy in the summer, in the run-up to *carnaval*.[3] But its very existence in the heart of the sleepy provincial state hospital Faustino Perez in Matanzas[4] evinces a quiet but radical revolution in health service organization. We were there to meet Diaz's students, the directors Vivian Sanchez and Johann Perdomo, who also run a residency program for doctors and health workers in traditional and natural medicine based at the local university.

Unlike their counterparts in China who are wont to appeal to the authority of their unbroken tradition, Diaz and Perdomo readily recognize that their therapeutic practice corresponds only loosely to anything recognizably Chinese. For them, Medicina Traditional y Natural means Cuban herbs, needling and moxa-cautery to treat local conditions, delivered according to enduring Chinese diagnostic principles – just another instance of the adaptation of Chinese medical traditions that has occurred throughout history. It is clear that they view this as a virtue, not a weakness, and as evidence of a proud Cuban capacity for survival on scarce resources. This position is more or less consistent with the emerging consensus among historians that 'Chinese' medicine is a modern creation, defined in contrast to the loose bundle of traditions known as Western medicine that arrived in China in the late 18th and 19th centuries.

At first, when asking around at the boarding house it seemed that people knew nothing about acupuncture. Johann said 'ask about the *agujitas*, the little needles.' Back in our Havana garden amid some of Cuba's estimated 6300 plant species, the lively young cleaner from the rural Western part of the island had inherited a robust knowledge of medicinal wild herbs from her grandmother: sweet tamarind for liver complaints, fevers and asthma; and mariposa, the national flower, everywhere. (Cuba hardly ever needed to import Chinese materia medica.) As she applied a compress to one of our wrists, we asked

---

[3] Johann Perdomo was referring to playing on the beach. Thalassotherapy is salt therapy, a 19th century Polish vogue for treating asthma and pneumonia based on the observation that their salt miners were resistant to respiratory problems. The therapy involved treatment in natural salt caves.
[4] Matanzas, *lit.* 'the killings' by Cubans of their Spanish masters (1895) and the subsequent retaliatory slaughter.

her about *agujitas*, "everyone knows the little needles are good for pain – pain of the neck, lumbar pain, headache." So too said all the taxi drivers, a cook, and a hotelier. The latter added, "it works very well for our Cuban psychological problems. Normally we don't suffer so much from 'nerviosa' as other people... you know, we have sun and music. But we women get stressed because we have our jobs *and* do the housework." The *agujitas* have been used by auxiliary medical staff since 1962. Their acceptance may be related to a pre-existing South American culture of medical needling still in evidence in Guatemala, and/or the absorption of earlier Chinese healing practice, rather than socialist technology transfer, but this history awaits further research (Kadetz 2008). For the moment we can only observe that elements of acupuncture have been absorbed seamlessly into Cuba's own medicine and are distinct from Chinese acupuncture in dedicated clinics.

Not narrowly defined as complementary or alternative medicine as in the West, Chinese medicine at Matanzas is used for much more than the treatment of 'chronic' ailments. At Faustino Perez, Perdomo and Sanchez have transformed the old outpatient acupuncture department for the treatment of chronic pain into a front-line medical service with an emergency room and hospital beds for acupuncture. In 2008, 10% of patients passing through the hospital's accident and emergency service received some form of Medicina Traditional y Natural treatment. By 2007 with the extension of the emergency service initiative to all patients, 54% of all inpatients at Faustino Perez had received at least one such treatment; 12–13 tons of herbs are delivered every year. Chinese medicine has a new application in Cuban emergency medicine, notably for acute stroke, heart attack and dissecting aneurysm, in addition to more orthodox emergency approaches. Apart from pain, high blood pressure, acute asthma and gastric disorders are regularly treated. Trials such as the use of Chinese medicine in the rehabilitation of patients suffering hemiplegia following ischemic stroke, allow for a wide range of physical therapies that have constituted Chinese medicine to be offered. With the softening of USA diplomacy it will be interesting to see whether Cuban health authorities will get wise to the amount of money that is being spent on complementary and alternative medicine worldwide. Their well-established health tourism, sun and surgery packages could profitably add *Taiji quan*, Chinese massage, Cuban herbs and acupuncture for stroke sufferers.

With the mainstreaming of Medicina Traditional y Natural the volume and range of their clinical work has generated the conditions to develop a strong program of effectiveness research which will address the anxiety of commentators such as MacDonald (1999), who fear that there is a 'real danger ... that the ever present stress of economic restriction may empower an anti-technology/anti-science lobby that will lead to such modalities as herbalism being accepted in toto because it is 'Cuban' and 'cheap' (1999, 232–235). Diaz's book provides a robust analysis of the types of method that would be fit for purpose in evaluating practice; he critiques the limitations of the randomized controlled trial (RCT) for Medicina Traditional y Natural and therapeutics more widely. Although the RCT is good for testing the many simples in traditional materia medica, it is clearly inadequate, for example, for polypharmacy, and for traditions that use a range of techniques simultaneously, in various combinations, in the course of a patient's illness. Diaz goes further, providing a critique of the domination of medicine in capitalist states by the interests of large biotechnology and pharmaceutical companies with an overwhelming interest in promoting a saleable medicine, shrink-wrapped and branded.

THE EVIDENCE MOSAIC

WHO figures on medical provision make it absolutely clear that to have any influence on the real circumstances of sickness and healthcare worldwide it is essential to evaluate the appropriateness and efficacy of traditional and plural medicine. Is it just because traditional and plural medicine is the reality for the majority of the world that they have been increasingly funding it for the 30 years since Alma Ata? And if that is the case, then is it, shockingly, merely for the poor, and irrelevant for people in the first world who can afford proper medicine? Or can we establish those elements of Chinese medicine that are effective and attractive, the theories, the techniques, the substances, or the ability to respond to the patient as a biopsychosocial being?

The Cuban experience forces us to confront the question that if continuity in tradition is such an elusive thing, how do we define those aspects of the tradition to go on trial?

AUTHENTICITY

If we ignore, for the moment, the use of history to pursue a core identity for Chinese medicine, we can assign historical inquiry another role in the establishment of research directions. There are, for example, plenty of simples that can be mined from the Chinese materia medica, (single drugs for single symptoms, universally applicable) rather than complex concoctions blended together according to the classic system of Chinese medical potencies and tailored to the individual. These simples lend themselves to testing via the RCT. In our experience *Juhua* 菊花 (chrysanthemum) is now widely recommended by Chinese medical practitioners for high blood pressure. High blood pressure was never a disease category in the past, and thus this treatment is not historically authentic Chinese medicine but a modern hybrid. This raises the thorny problem of matching old drugs to modern symptoms.

When searching past records for modern cures proper historical attention must be paid to the definition of the diseases that were treated in the past. If we are looking for a cure for TB in ancient materia medica, how do we pragmatically extrapolate from the complex symptoms in the modern disease category to those in the ancient Chinese texts? There is no doubt that this kind of scientific enterprise can produce modern drugs. The development of *qinghao* 青蒿 (artemesinin) for *nue* 虐 (intermittent fever) into the mass-produced treatment of choice today for malaria is a case in point. Rigorous history has descriptive power and the capacity to focus attention on areas likely to be fruitful for empirical research. Equally, it can serve to prevent researchers developing pointless and random hypotheses. Trials of acupuncture for chronic pain relief which test specific acupuncture points in the classic tradition against a control of the random insertion of needles fail to recognize that needling in common usage did not generally, in the larger historical trajectory, adhere to the classic point system (Cummings 2009).

Many major obstacles to building a modern evidence base for the Chinese pharmacopeia are also not exclusive to the field. Practicable and affordable methods for evaluating the art of combining and adjusting many herbs to individual patients and adjusting the concoction to the course of their illness do not exist, and await more sophisticated research methodologies appropriate to polypharmacy. The problems are as germane to geriatric medicine in orthodox medical care as to Chinese drug therapy. Seen in this light, the opposition between orthodox and alternative medicine dissolves and the antagonistic rhetoric of their respective proponents and detractors emerges as one that may be as much motivated by the maintenance of social and professional boundaries as by the pursuit of scientific and intellectual rigor.

The attribution of Chinese potencies to Cuban herbs and drugs, however, does demand another kind of engagement with the changing historical identity of Chinese medicine and the continuity and value of its systems and traditions. Diaz and his colleagues insist that the future of Cuban Chinese medicine lies in understanding and teaching the theoretical foundations of Chinese medicine and philosophy alongside its techniques. They have a great thirst for higher-quality translations and secondary literature which is hard to come by in Cuba. Of course these theoretical constructs of physiology and pathogenesis are different from the material and biochemical constructs of Western medical orthodoxy. The Chinese physiopathological theories used in Cuban Chinese medicine make predictions that are testable. A cost-effective approach to this might be to carry out experiments that test the value of these theories in predicting the therapeutic benefit of Cuban herbs (see Vignette 13.1).

VIGNETTE 13.1 SCIENCE, EVIDENCE AND COMPLEMENTARY, ALTERNATIVE AND TRADITIONAL MEDICINE
ADRIAN RENTON

Over the last few years complementary, alternative and traditional medicines have come under increasing pressure to provide evidence of effectiveness. This has come from a number of sources, including Europe-wide moves to standardize regulatory structures and the activities of the 'Bad Science' bloggers, academics and journalists who have pursued a Dawkinsesque crusade against most treatments and other health interventions which are not grounded in the dominant scientific materialist ontology and some that are, such as dietary supplements.

We have an obligation empirically to test the safety and effectiveness of any preventive or treatment intervention in health. And this is the case whether that intervention is labeled orthodox, traditional, complementary or alternative, or indeed comprises a pill, a manipulation, a needle or promoting change in a health-related behavior. I also think that those offering such interventions are under an obligation not to make claims for safety or effectiveness where they have no evidence to support those claims.

However, we know that in many of the most developed societies almost 50% of people use some type of complementary, alternative or traditional medicine in any year and, according to the World Health Organization, in some Asian and African Countries 80% of the population rely on traditional medicine for their primary healthcare. So there's a lot of it about. We also know that the properties and clinical values of, for example, many plant-based preparations have been known for many years, certainly long before the advent of the RCT or even the development of modern chemistry. Moreover, Chinese medicine pioneered an understanding of exercise interventions and an awareness of environmental influences on health which are only now being accepted in the West.

Conducting randomized double-blind placebo-controlled clinical trials of each traditional treatment for each condition is currently not an option. Costs to bring a new pharmaceutical drug to market are disputed, but probably somewhere in the region of £500m. Biotechnology and pharmaceuticals have in the past been able to recover these R&D costs through exercising intellectual property rights. This route is usually not open to traditional medicine, or for that matter to initiatives aimed at disease prevention which are not biotech or pharma based.

In many cases traditional treatments used in the context of constructs of physiology and pathogenesis (which often consider the individual in his or her environment) are quite different from the material and biochemical systems that we now consider orthodox. The role of science is to develop theories which make predictions about phenomena that can be tested, and then to test them. The physiopathological theories used by traditional medicines make predictions which are testable. Therefore, we can and should develop scientific experiments to test them.

Given the range of traditional treatments and conditions for which they are used, perhaps it might be more cost-effective, as a start, to carry out experiments that test for the predictive value of the physiological, pathological and diagnostic systems used, including the stability of diagnosis between observers/practitioners, and prediction of therapeutic benefit from observed physiological effects rather than picking off condition–treatment combinations for trial, one by one. A few carefully designed experiments would be affordable; and if they generated evidence that the physiological and pathological theories used by traditional medicines made successful predictions about observable phenomena, then strong arguments could be made for greater public investment in research programs. In an era of evidence-based medicine, accumulating evidence might be expected to translate into growing public investment.

ART OF CHINESE MEDICINE

Without considering ancient theory and traditional approaches to practice, research into Chinese medicine might be no different from research into any kind of medicine. In the identification of potent substances and effective practices for universal application, the search for continuity in tradition can easily seem like an academic distraction or something that should be relegated to the museum of human history. To be sure, research free from cultural baggage leads to essential new knowledge, such as the wonder drug artemesinin in the treatment of malaria (although this research is also based on trawling traditional texts). But this is a style of knowledge that inherently ignores cutting-edge scientific issues of efficacy that are firmly grounded in social and personal context, the physiology of individual patient responses, and the plurality of therapeutic reality. It is an approach that threatens to undermine the art of medicine. In the search for a knowledge and practice that has survived the long durée – the diachronic continuities to be found within particular geographic, social and cultural terrains – we should not avoid describing that human art of medicine that is keyed to time, place and individual just because it cannot be replicated in a clinical context.

If the art of medicine lies in identifying the right mix of remedies to treat a patient as a biopsychosocial being within their own specific environment, then the art of public health must be to weave together medical traditions for a population made up of just those individuals aggregated into social groups and taken within their own unique sociopolitical, geographical and cultural circumstances. Chinese medicine has certainly contributed to Cuba's medical autonomy: the *agujitas* have embedded themselves invisibly into the community imagination of natural medicine, and state-sponsored Chinese exercise systems and acupuncture are raising their profile both in the community and in medical institutions.

Resources devoted to the teaching, research and development of traditional medicine in China can hardly be matched in Cuba, and from the standpoint of quality of teaching and resources (books, herbs, education) it is easy to be critical. Yet, the moral power of Cuba's revolutionary rhetoric, its international record in humanitarian and medical aid and exchange, and a particular combination of pride in tradition as well as a belief in the power of change, are a huge resource for Medicina Traditional y Natural. They have created a power politics and economics that are simply different from those that govern research into traditional medicine in developed countries – and one which allows them to imagine a different kind of effectiveness for traditional medicine (Feinsilver 2009).[5] The example of 'Cuban' Chinese medicine demonstrates that we can only ever hope to understand 'medicine' – and that includes making informed and meaningful judgments about effectiveness – by way of multidisciplinary research efforts that examine what it is that we wish to examine and how it came to be that way. Further, the medical research traditions that exist in Cuba, together with the extensive use of Medicina Traditional y Natural within the public health system and the use of indigenous materials within the Chinese medical theoretical framework, place it in a strong position to carry out research which tests, forensically, the predictive value of the theoretical framework as well as the effectiveness of its individual techniques.

Whereas in China top-down Party-led public health directives were a feature of the integration of modern and traditional medicines that began in the 1950s, Cuba's unique military context, its emphasis on the value of 'changing

---

[5] Cuba's conspicuous success in providing more humanitarian aid per capita than the US and China, and its training of doctors as an 'export commodity', has reinforced the moral power of its revolutionary rhetoric and ranked it among the world's top medical powers.

all that needs to be changed' (Castro, see above) provides an alternative space for investigating the modification and expansion of traditional medical techniques in the modern world, and its value in practice. Our own mission to chart the integration of Chinese medicine into the Cuban public health system was inconclusive. A full appreciation of the Cuban Chinese Medical Revolution requires a much more in-depth study into the institutions, practitioners and educators as well as the experience of the 20–30 million patients treated with Medicina Traditional y Natural in Cuba each year. For the purposes of this chapter it has been replaced by a meditation on the value of authenticity in traditional medicine and the design of innovative research projects that involve history in their making.

The future seems bright: Diaz, Sanchez and Perdomo have the institutions, the right kind of socialist pedigree and plenty of aspiration. They still need resources, better teaching and a clearer account of what aspects of traditional medicine they want to research, but to conclude with Diaz, quoting José Martí:

".. toda ciencia empieza en la imaginación, y no hay sabio sin el arte de imaginar..."[6]

José Martí

---

[6] All science begins in the imagination and there is no knowledge without the art of imagining.

REFERENCES

Acosta Martínez, B., 2000. Editorial: 'Palabras de recibimiento al III Congreso Internacional de Medicina Tradicional, Natural y Bioenergética, celebrado en la Facultad de Ciencias Médicas de Holguín del 7 al 11 de Junio del 2000.' Correo Científico Médico de Holguín 4 (1).

Barnes, L., 2009. Practitioner decisions to engage in Chinese medicine: cultural messages under the skin. Med. Anthropol. 28 (2), 141–165.

Castro, F., 2000. Fidel Castro, May 1st, 2000, Plaza de Revolucion.

Chomsky, A., 2000. The threat of a good example: health and revolution in Cuba. In: Kim, J.Y., Millen, J., Irwin, A., et al. (Eds.), Dying for Growth: Global Inequality and the Health of the Poor. Common Courage Press, Monroe, Maine.

Cummings, M., 2009. Modellvorhaben Akupunktur—a summary of the ART, ARC and GERAC trials. Acupunct. Med. 27 (1), 26–30.

Delgado, G., 1995. La medicina China y su presencia en Cuba. Cuadernos de Historia de la Salud Pública.

Diaz, M., 2005. En Defensa de la Medicina y de su Método Científico (Safeguarding Medicine and its Scientific Method). Impresines Hel Ltda, Bogotá, Colombia.

Dirección Provincial de Salud-Matanzas. 2008. Departamento de registros médicos y estadísticas de salud. Modelo 241–458–01.

Feinsilver, J.M., 1995. Healing the Masses: Cuban Health Politics at Home and Abroad. University of California Press, California.

Feinsilver, J., 2009. Cuba's medical diplomacy. In: Font, M., (Ed.), A Changing Cuba in a Changing World. Bildner Center for Western Hemisphere Studies, City University of New York, New York, pp. 273–286.

Hsu, E., 2002. 'The Medicine from China has rapid effects': Chinese medicine patients in Tanzania. Anthropol. Med. 9 (3), 291–313.

Kadetz, P., 2008. The transfer of acupuncture to indigenous Guatemala: a model for understanding change in an indigenous medical system. MA Dissertation, Oxford University, Oxford.

Lei, S. H., 雷祥麟, 2002. How did Chinese medicine become experiential? The political epistemology of Jingyan. Positions 10 (2), 333–364.

Lo, V., 2009. But is it history of medicine?: 20 years in the healing arts of China. Soc. Hist. Med. 2009 (1).

MacDonald, T. H., 1999. A Developmental Analysis of Cuba's Health Care System

Since 1959. Studies in Health and Human Services, vol. 32. Edwin Mellen Press, Lewiston, Queenston, Lampeter, pp. 232–235 (p. 233).

Ministerio de Salud Pública, 2003. Dirección nacional de registros médicos y estadísticas de salud.

Ministerio de Salud Pública, 2008. Dirección nacional de registros médicos y estadísticas de salud. Anuario Estadístico de Salud.

Roig de Leuchsenring, E., 1965. Medicos y Medicina en Cuba. Historia, Biografia, Costumbrismo. Academia de Ciencias de Cuba, La Habana.

Scheid, V., 2007. Currents of Tradition in Chinese Medicine 1626 – 2006. Eastland Press, Seattle.

Taylor, K., 2005. Medicine in Early Communist China. RoutledgeCurzon, London.

Zhan, M., 2009. Other-Worldly. Duke University Press, Durham and London.

The Cuban Chinese medical revolution

Redescribing biomedicine: toward the integration of East Asian medicine into contemporary healthcare

Kathryn Montgomery

"*But health is whatever works/and for as long…*"

John Stone, 'He Makes a House Call'

Beneficiaries of Western biomedicine attribute the strength and the authority of its practices to science. Physicians occasionally remind themselves (and, more rarely, their patients) that much of what they prescribe has been tested by time rather than in laboratories or with randomized controlled trials. This is equally true for much of what they know and believe. No-one quite understands how aspirin works; fevers of unknown origin are likely to remain just that; over time musculoskeletal disorders elude effective surgical treatment and are handed over to physical therapists. Yet when credit for the prodigious improvement in health and longevity is handed out, even knowledgeable people ignore the importance of clean water, safer births and more productive agriculture and focus entirely on advances in biological science and medical technology. Even the expert team recently assembled by the US National Institutes of Health to study baffling maladies, otherwise undescribed and resistant to treatment, sees evidence of advancing science rather than medicine's ineradicable uncertainty (Henig 2009). For almost everyone, physician and patient, biomedicine remains reassuringly solid, scientific, even infallible until – usually at some life-defining moment – it's not.

How different East Asian medicine appears to be! Its description of bodily states of *qi* transformation, of pulses and tongues, meridians, acupuncture and herbal medicaments seems clearly 'cultural.' These are practices inherited from a venerable past, and the policymakers of today have encouraged their scientific development. 'Placebo!' my biomedical colleagues are likely to say, not always ungenerously but almost never acknowledging that numerous studies have established the importance of the placebo effect in their own practice (Brody & Brody 2000; Finniss et al 2010).

Biomedicine's faith in science as the unmediated discovery of reality means that biomedicine is not self-reflective. Meanwhile, complementary and alternative medicine, faced with the power imbalance between the two regimes, is inspired to wrestle with important questions about the nature of skill, the constitution of evidence, the role of autonomy in standardized practice, and the challenges of 'integration' in a range of circumstances outside

229

East Asia. Above all, complementary and alternative medicine must seek out and defend appropriate research methodologies for questions that biomedicine for the most part neglects, even fails to recognize. For this reason, the discussions and debates contained in this book are not only a major contribution to the theory and practice of Asian medicine but also a reminder to biomedicine that there are things not dreamt of in its philosophy.

Medical practice in both traditions is uncertain. Almost a century and a half ago in *Middlemarch,* a novel by George Eliot originally intended to be entirely about medicine, Dorothea Brooke's opinionated uncle pointed out that 'every dose you take is an experiment' (Eliot [1871–72] 1997, 93). Despite the value of randomized controlled trials in establishing pharmaceutical efficacy, this is as true (if not quite as dangerous) now as then. Medical practice is negotiated between scientific generalizations and the individual patient. How do the results of a randomized controlled trial, even a pragmatic one, apply to this one patient in all her complex particularity? The answer is never completely certain. Thus, every patient is to some extent an experiment, a data point in the ongoing enterprise of clinical reasoning, and wise physicians keep track of both ordinary and remarkable cases, however informal the series, however fallible their memory. This is necessary because biomedicine is no more a science than it has ever been. It is a practice although a scientific and technological one: the care of sick people who have asked for help. Physicians continue to learn details of its uncertain variability in diagnosis, prognosis, and treatment throughout their careers. If someday the catalogs of pharmaceuticals and clinical practices, Western or Asian, are thoroughly researched and those studies made readily available to every clinician, those practices will of course be more scientific. But in the Newtonian, positivist sense we popularly assume, they will never constitute a science. Clinicians will still be revered for their interpretive judgment, the virtue of practical reasoning which in the *Nicomachean Ethics* Aristotle called *phronesis* (1139b–1142a), because even the most comprehensive studies of efficacy and effectiveness must themselves be studied for their applicability to the individual patient.

Thus, an integration of biomedicine and Asian medicine cannot take place on what are understood to be biomedicine's epistemological terms. Although herbal medicine, acupuncture, and Ayurveda may be improved by standardization, studies of the acquisition of clinical skill, and pragmatic trials, they will not become sciences. The best hope for the integration of Asian medicine into contemporary healthcare lies in a redescription of clinical medicine as it is currently practiced in the Western tradition. Experiments in the clinical validation of Asian medicine, especially those that seek alternatives to explanatory randomized controlled trials or otherwise challenge the hierarchy of evidence-based medicine, can play an important part in that redescription.

A redescription of biomedicine would take into account currently unquantified aspects of biomedical practice as well as the science-ignoring methods of clinical education that now are ignored. Alvan Feinstein, who taught us how to apply epidemiology to individual patients in his classic *Clinical Judgment* (1967), was ideally placed to point out the drawbacks of evidence-based medicine. And point them out he did! In a retrospective essay on his life's work, he observed that despite evidence-based medicine's undoubted contribution to clinical knowledge, it borrows its methods from engineering, mathematical theory, and testing psychology, rather than from clinical practice. In the process it ignores medicine's ongoing need for reliable clinical data, a sound taxonomy of disease, and attention to the nature of clinical reasoning. Instead, he argued, clinical studies should focus on all that evidence-based medicine systematically eliminates: 'patterns of symptoms, severity of illness, effects of comorbid conditions, timing of phenomena, rate of progression of illness, functional capacity, and other clinical distinctions that demarcate major prognostic and therapeutic differences among groups of patients who otherwise seem deceptively similar because they have the same diagnosis, laboratory results, and demographic status' (Feinstein 1994). Citing Apgar scores and the staging of cancer as examples, he called for a bottom-up study of medical practice that he labeled 'medicine-based evidence.' Such work is vitally important to practice because it gives numbers to phenomena that have been unquantified and therefore disregarded. For, as he notes, "All the basic issues... [are] qualitative: The new procedures . . . emerge from descriptive solutions to the basic problems in clinical data and clinical taxonomy."

Despite the excellence of the quantitative expressions, the forced expiratory volume of respiration does not indicate a patient's dyspnea, and a depressed S-T segment does not indicate angina pectoris in daily life. Besides, many of the most important clinical events are intrinsically human reactions and sensations – pain, discomfort, disability, general functional capacity, depression, anxiety, and gratification – that cannot be measured with any technologic test. His critique might well have been written by a student of Asian medicine.

Since Feinstein wrote, there have been a few developments along these lines but not as many as he hoped. None have been accompanied by any alteration in research focus or philosophy of medicine. The intensity of pain – a subjective data point if there ever was one – has been given a scale, but as 'the fifth vital sign' it is still primarily the province of nursing. Linda Emanuel and colleagues (2001) have studied the needs of dying patients and their families and furthered the focus of palliative care on their qualitative concerns. Atul Gawande (2007, 169–200) has recommended something like the Apgar score as a way to assess the experience of childbirth (although he ignores a nursing questionnaire – undoubtedly too long but surely adaptable – that exists for this purpose). Its results might alter the US reliance on fetal monitors and reverse its soaring rate of cesarian sections. Most recently, the opportunities and constraints of the new US healthcare plan have prompted the Department of Health and Human Services to call for comments on its criteria for evaluating home visits (Rachel Abramson, personal communication).

Feinstein's list of neglected biomedical concerns bears a remarkable resemblance to the problems engaging the theorists of Asian medicine. But it is all too easy to assimilate those 'bottom-up' improvements that address his concerns into the prevailing view that medicine is a science. What is also needed is a view of biomedicine that can see these developments as quintessential to its practice. What is needed is a phronesiology – a philosophy of medicine as a practice.

Some hints of this phronesiology can be found in the oddities that are part (albeit an overlooked one) of clinical education in biomedicine. There are at least three: the persistence of narrative as a way of knowing, the veneration of learned elders, and the use of counterweighted proverbs as guides to judgment.

The narrative case remains coin of the realm in biomedical discourse (Montgomery Hunter 1991). Even as the 'anecdotal' is scorned as unscientific, individual accounts of patient care are the medium of teaching and learning, memory and communication. Indeed, learning to hear the patient's story and transform it into a clinical case is the essential act of becoming a clinician. Single cases have disappeared from most medical journals, but their continuing value for biomedicine's scientific knowledge is evinced in the syndrome letters published in the *New England Journal of Medicine* and in that journal's defense of exempting them from peer review. The case is especially valuable in biomedicine's most confused and uncertain moments. The Australian physician who first identified the teratogenic effect of thalidomide apologized for a two-case report, but statistically his observation of two anomalies within a brief time was enormously significant. Near the beginning of the AIDS epidemic, when its symptoms were still astonishing, Gerald Weissmann and four colleagues (Abramson et al 1985) published a five-patient clinical study of an odd malady of the knee. He and his four co-authors, each from a different service at Bellevue Hospital, had swapped single anecdotes during a lunchtime. Such extreme moments emphasize that, despite the routinized, almost ritual order of its telling, the clinical case is not a scientific report but a narrative, an account of events through time that implies one or more causes of the changes it relates. Medical informatics and machine learning theory have confirmed the value of the case for its resilient combination of open hypothesizing and situational focus (Blois 1984; Schank & Abelson 1981). Patients cannot usefully be run through scanners in lieu of a good history and physical examination: radiologists want context to make good interpretations of the images they read (Saunders 2008). Physicians cannot be replaced by even very well programed computers: interpretation is needed.

The continued veneration of elders is another sign of a philosophy of biomedicine as a practice. Nothing seems more 'natural.' Even after the introduction of machine- and computer-assisted learning aids, especially in surgery, little has changed since Charles Bosk described the residency in *Forgive and Remember* (1979). This is not sentimentality or some sudden Western adoption of Asian respect for age and wisdom, but a recognition that clinical judgment is learned from people in practice. If medicine were a science, surely it could be learned primarily from books, and residency programs would vary so little that the choice among them would be a mere matter of convenience. Instead, students pursue prestigious residencies, and not only because the reputation of the institutions concerned will open further doors, but also because of the skill and knowledge and clinical judgment of the physicians who will guide (if indirectly through senior residents and fellows) their specialty training.

Perhaps the most persuasive evidence of biomedicine's phronesiology is the use of proverbs and maxims in clinical education (Montgomery 2006, Chs 8 and 9). These are not invariable rules: any pretense to generalizability they may have is undermined by the existence, as with proverbs outside medicine, of sayings that can be uttered with equal force on the other side of the question. Everything depends on the situation that calls them forth, and that of course is their lesson. Students learning physical diagnosis are advised to 'Focus!' but also to 'Notice everything!' Occam's Razor, the rule of parsimony, cuts against the rhyming Hickam's dictum: 'The patient can have as many diseases/As the patient damn well pleases' (Miller 1998). And although solid studies are hard to find, students also hear, 'Sixty-seven percent [or 75% or 89%] of diagnoses are made from the history.' This creative statistic, no matter the exact number, goes up against the habitual rhetoric of 'denial' in history-taking as in 'the patient denies alcohol use.'

Nor does biomedical research provide an overarching rule for deciding between contradictory maxims or resolving the clash of a proverb with habitual practice. Instead, medicine's working theory of clinical knowing, its *phronesiology*, also comes in proverbs and maxims that are also paired and contradictory. 'Medicine is an art', students are told; but 'Medicine is a science.' 'Avoid the anecdotal' but 'Pay attention to the stories.' 'Always do everything for every patient forever', but 'Above all do no harm.' How in the world is a clinician to choose? Even the zebra aphorism, biomedicine's overriding epidemiological rule – 'If you hear hoof beats, don't think zebras' – contains its own contradiction. How are zebras to be un-thought?

These counterweighted maxims teach clinical students and house officers that rules in the practice of biomedicine are not absolute. After years spent studying the sciences of human biology, they are learning in the clinic that rules must be interpreted. Circumstances matter. Nothing is entirely certain – not even test results. *Phronesis* is essential. For this reason, clinical education stretches on for years: its goal is the cultivation of sound clinical judgment, the practitioner's capacity for assessing the situation and for knowing when to break or stretch the rules. Contradictory proverbs and maxims embody its lessons.

Such lessons are surely available (with or without aphorisms) to beginning practitioners of Asian medicine as they acquire diagnostic skill and therapeutic acumen. Only the misdescription of biomedicine as a science prevents our seeing the commonalities.

The commonalities are fundamental. Medical practice in every culture is grounded in its duty, the care of patients. What is more, every practitioner in every tradition must negotiate the gap between a general knowledge of the field and the particular characteristics of the individual patient. Thus, practices of whatever kind are by their nature uncertain, and clinicians in every culture must diagnose and treat and prognosticate despite unforeseen human variability, the uncertain effects of treatment, and the difficulties always inherent in prediction. They face these potential uncertainties with each patient, and on many occasions they face them in circumstances of great or sudden need. They are committed to do the best they can: to observe their patients carefully, to cultivate their skills, and to test and improve their knowledge. But their control over illness is limited.

It was surely the realization of something like this that led John Stone (1980, 4–5) to declare in 'He Makes a House Call' that '. . . health is whatever works/ And for as long.' A poet and cardiologist, Stone describes a doctor's visit to a patient's garden, where '… you are in charge/Of figs, beans, tomatoes, life.' The physician's original task had been a highly technologized one, a cardiac catheterization that preceded the patient's valve replacement, but since that time – 'seven years, it was' – he has tended to her in his clinic, *attended* her survival, her flourishing. His reward is this realization of the nature and limits of his calling – to say nothing of the armload of vegetables she bestows on him as he leaves.

Medical practice focuses on the care of patients, and interpretation is essential to this task no matter how standardized and scientific that practice becomes. Room must be left for the expert's well-considered autonomy and the inspired hunches or insight that could make all the difference. Studies of the theory and practice of Asian medicine can point the way to a clearer assessment of vitally important matters: the nature of healing, the characteristics of good medical care, and the power of the patient – physician relationship – all of which are still poorly understood or seldom examined in biomedicine.

REFERENCES

Abramson, S.B., et al., 1985. Hyperalgesic pseudothrombophlebitis: new syndrome in male homosexuals. Am. J. Med. 78, 317–320.

Blois, M.S., 1984. Information and Medicine. University of California Press, Berkeley.

Bosk, C., 1979. Forgive and Remember: Managing Medical Failure. University of Chicago Press, Chicago.

Brody, H., Brody, D., 2000. The Placebo Response. HarperCollins, New York.

Eliot, G., [1871–72] 1997. Middlemarch. Penguin Classics, London.

Emanuel, L.L., Alpert, H.R., Emanuel, E.E., 2001. Concise screening questions for clinical assessments of terminal care: the needs near the end-of-life care screening tool. J. Palliat. Med. 4, 465–474.

Feinstein, A., 1967. Clinical Judgment. Williams and Wilkins, Baltimore.

Feinstein, A., 1994. Clinical judgment revisited: the distraction of quantitative models. Ann. Intern. Med. 120, 799–805.

Finniss, D.G., Kaptchuk, T.J., Miller, F., et al., 2010. Biological, clinical, and ethical advances of placebo effects. Lancet 375, 686–695.

Gawande, A., 2007. Better: A Surgeon's Notes on Performance. Henry Holt, New York.

Henig, R.M., 2009. What is wrong with Summer Stiers. N. Y. Times Mag. (accessed at nytimes.com; 10.08.10).

Miller, W.T., 1998. Occam versus Hickam. Semin. Roentgenol. 33, 213.

Montgomery Hunter, K., 1991. Doctors' Stories: The Narrative Structure of Medical Knowledge. Princeton University Press, Princeton.

Montgomery, K., 2006. How Doctors Think: Clinical Judgment and the Practice of Medicine. Oxford University Press, New York.

Saunders, B., 2008. CT Suite: The Work of Diagnosis in the Age of Noninvasive Cutting. Duke University Press, Durham.

Schank, R.C., Abelson, R.P., 1981. Scripts, Plans, Goals and Understanding: An Inquiry Into Human Knowledge. Erlbaum, Hillsdale, NJ.

Stone, J., 1980. In All This Rain. Louisiana State University Press, Baton Rouge.

INDEX

Note: Page numbers followed by *b* indicate boxes, *f* indicate figures, *t* indicate tables, and *np* indicate footnotes.

INDEX

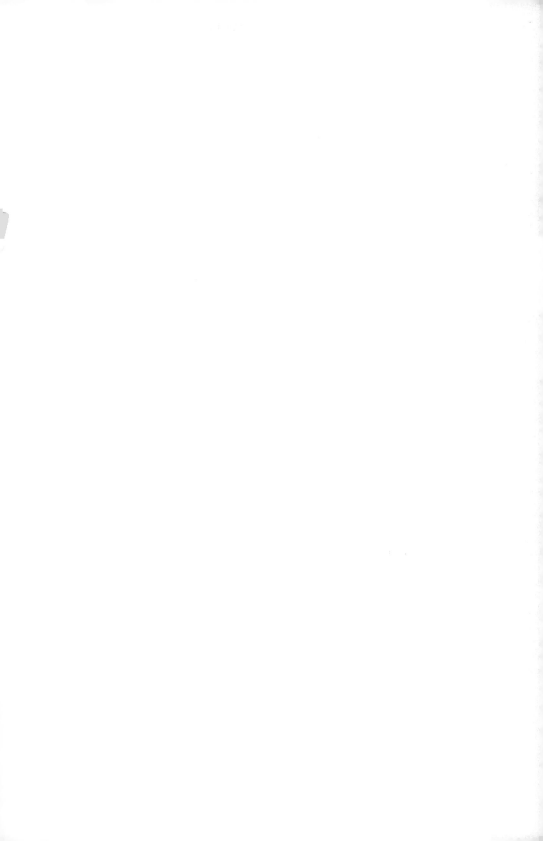